MW00626518

Dose Finding in Drug Development

Series Editor
M. Gail, K. Krickeberg, J. Samet, A. Tsiatis, W. Wong

Statistics for Biology and Health

Borchers/Buckland/Zucchini: Estimating Animal Abundance: Closed Populations.

Burzykowski/Molenberghs/Buyse: The Evaluation of Surrogate Endpoints

Everitt/Rabe-Hesketh: Analyzing Medical Data Using S-PLUS.

Ewens/Grant: Statistical Methods in Bioinformatics: An Introduction. 2nd ed.

Gentleman/Carey/Huber/Izirarry/Dudoit: Bioinformatics and Computational Biology Solutions Using R and Bioconductor

Hougaard: Analysis of Multivariate Survival Data.

Keyfitz/Caswell: Applied Mathematical Demography, 3rd ed.

Klein/Moeschberger: Survival Analysis: Techniques for Censored and Truncated Data, 2nd ed.

Kleinbaum/Klein: Survival Analysis: A Self-Learning Text. 2nd ed.

Kleinbaum/Klein: Logistic Regression: A Self-Learning Text, 2nd ed.

Lange: Mathematical and Statistical Methods for Genetic Analysis, 2nd ed.

Manton/Singer/Suzman: Forecasting the Health of Elderly Populations.

Martinussen/Scheike: Dynamic Regression Models for Survival Data

Moyé: Multiple Analyses in Clinical Trials: Fundamentals for Investigators.

Nielsen: Statistical Methods in Molecular Evolution

Parmigiani/Garrett/Irizarry/Zeger: The Analysis of Gene Expression Data: Methods and Software.

Salsburg: The Use of Restricted Significance Tests in Clinical Trials.

Simon/Korn/McShane/Radmacher/Wright/Zhao: Design and Analysis of DNA Microarray Investigations.

Sorensen/Gianola: Likelihood, Bayesian, and MCMC Methods in Quantitative Genetics.

Stallard/Manton/Cohen: Forecasting Product Liability Claims: Epidemiology and Modeling in the Manville Asbestos Case.

Therneau/Grambsch: Modeling Survival Data: Extending the Cox Model.

Ting: Dose Finding in Drug Development

Vittinghoff/Glidden/Shiboski/McCulloch: Regression Methods in Biostatistics: Linear, Logistic, Survival, and Repeated Measures Models.

Zhang/Singer: Recursive Partitioning in the Health Sciences.

Naitee Ting

Editor

Dose Finding in Drug Development

With 48 Illustrations

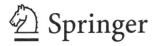 Springer

Naitee Ting
Pfizer
New London, CT 06320
naitee.ting@pfizer.com

Series Editors:

M. Gail
National Cancer Institute
Rockville, MD 20892
USA

K. Krickeberg
Le Chatelet
F-63270 Manglieu
France

J. Samet
Department of Epidemiology
School of Public Health
Johns Hopkins University
615 Wolfe Street
Baltimore, MD 21205-2103
USA

A. Tsiatis
Department of Statistics
North Carolina State University
Raleigh, NC 27695
USA

W. Wong
Sequoia Hall
Department of Statistics
Stanford University
390 Serra Mall
Stanford, CA 94305-4065
USA

Library of Congress Control Number: 2005935288

ISBN-10: 0-387-29074-5
ISBN-13: 978-0387-29074-4

Printed on acid-free paper.

© 2006 Springer Science+Business Media, Inc.
All rights reserved. This work may not be translated or copied in whole or in part without the written permission of the publisher (Springer Science+Business Media, Inc., 233 Spring Street, New York, NY 10013, USA), except for brief excerpts in connection with reviews or scholarly analysis. Use in connection with any form of information storage and retrieval, electronic adaptation, computer software, or by similar or dissimilar methodology now known or hereafter developed is forbidden.
The use in this publication of trade names, trademarks, service marks, and similar terms, even if they are not identified as such, is not to be taken as an expression of opinion as to whether or not they are subject to proprietary rights.

Printed in the United States of America.   (TB/MVY)

9 8 7 6 5 4 3 2 1

springer.com

Preface

This book emphasizes dose selection issues from a statistical point of view. It presents statistical applications in the design and analysis of dose–response studies. The importance of this subject can be found from the International Conference on Harmonization (ICH) E4 Guidance document.

Establishing the dose–response relationship is one of the most important activities in developing a new drug. A clinical development program for a new drug can be broadly divided into four phases – namely Phases I, II, III, and IV. Phase I clinical trials are designed to study the clinical pharmacology. Information obtained from these studies will help in designing Phase II studies. Dose–response relationships are usually studied in Phase II. Phase III clinical trials are large-scale, long-term studies. These studies serve to confirm findings from Phases I and II. Results obtained from Phases I, II, and III clinical trials would then be documented and submitted to regulatory agencies for drug approval. In the United States, reviewers from Food and Drug Administration (FDA) review these documents and make a decision to approve or to reject this New Drug Application (NDA). If the new drug is approved, then Phase IV studies can be started. Phase IV clinical trials are also known as postmarketing studies.

Phase II is the key phase to help find doses. At this point, dose-ranging studies and dose-finding studies are designed and carried out sequentially. These studies usually include several dose groups of the study drug, plus a placebo treatment group. Sometimes an active control treatment group may also be included. If the Phase II program is successful, then one or several doses will be considered for the Phase III clinical development. In certain life-threatening diseases, flexible-dose designs are desirable. Various proposals about design and analysis of these studies are available in the statistical and medical literature.

Statistics is an important science in drug development. Statistical methods can be applied to help with study design and data analysis for both preclinical and clinical studies. Evidences of drug efficacy and drug safety in human subjects are mainly established on the findings from randomized double-blind controlled clinical trials. Without statistics, there would be no such trials. Descriptive statistics are frequently used to help understand various characteristics of a drug. Inferential statistics helps quantify probabilities of successes, risks in drug discovery and development, as well as variability around these probabilities. Statistics is also an important decision-making tool throughout the entire drug development process. In clinical trials of all phases, studies are designed using statistical principles. Clinical data are displayed and analyzed using statistical models.

This book introduces the drug development process and the design and analysis of clinical trials. Much of the material in the book is based on applications of statistical methods in the design and analysis of dose-response studies. In general, there are two major types of dose-response concerns in drug development—concerns regarding drugs developed for nonlife-threatening diseases and those for life-threatening diseases. Most of the drug development programs in the pharmaceutical industry and the ICH E4 consider issues of nonlife-threatening diseases. On the other hand, many of the NIH/NCI sponsored studies and some of the pharmaceutical industry-sponsored studies deal with life-threatening diseases. Statistical and medical concerns in designing and analyzing these two types of studies can be very different. In this book, both types of clinical trials will be covered to a certain depth.

Although the book is prepared primarily for statisticians and biostatisticians, it also serves as a useful reference to a variety of professionals working for the pharmaceutical industry. Nonetheless, other professions – pharmacokienticists, clinical scientists, clinical pharmacologists, pharmacists, project managers, pharmaceutical scientists, clinicians, programmers, data managers, regulatory specialists, and study report writers can also benefit from reading this book. This book can also be a good reference for professionals working in a drug regulatory environment, for example, the FDA. Scientists and reviewers from both U.S. and foreign drug regulatory agencies can benefit greatly from this book. In addition, statistical and medical professionals in academia may find this book helpful in understanding the drug development process, and the practical concerns in selecting doses for a new drug.

The purpose of this book is to introduce the dose-selection process in drug development. Although it includes many preclinical experiments, most of dose-finding activities occure during the Phase II/III clinical stage. Therefore, the emphasis of this book is mostly about design and analysis of Phase II/III dose–response clinical trials. Chapter 1 offers an overview of drug development process. Chapter 2 covers dose-finding in preclinical studies, and Chapter 3 details Phase I clinical trials. Chapters 4 to 8 discuss issues relating to design, and Chapters 9 to 13 discuss issues relating to analysis of dose–response clinical trials. Chapter 14 introduces power and sample size estimation for these studies. For readers who are interested in designs involving life-threatening diseases such as cancer, Chapters 4 and 5 provide a good overview from both the nonparametric and the parametric points. In planning dose–response trials, researchers are likely to find PK/PD and trial simulation useful tools to help with study design. Hence Chapters 6 to 8 cover these and other general design issues for Phase II studies. In data analysis of dose–response results, the two major approaches are modeling approaches and multiple comparisons. Chapters 9 and 10 cover the modeling approach while Chapters 11 and 12 cover the multiple comparison methods. Chapter 13 discusses the analysis of categorical data in dose-finding clinical trials.

Naitee Ting
Pfizer Global Research and Development
New London
Connecticut
Naitee.ting@pfizer.com

Contents

Preface   **v**

1 Introduction and New Drug Development Process   **1**
     1.1   Introduction 1
     1.2   New Drug Development Process 4
     1.3   Nonclinical Development 5
          1.3.1   Pharmacology 5
          1.3.2   Toxicology/Drug Safety 6
          1.3.3   Drug Formulation Development 7
     1.4   Premarketing Clinical Development 8
          1.4.1   Phase I Clinical Trials...................................... 8
          1.4.2   Phase II/III Clinical Trials................................. 10
          1.4.3   Clinical Development for Life-Threatening Diseases   12
          1.4.4   New Drug Application 12
     1.5   Clinical Development Plan 13
     1.6   Postmarketing Clinical Development 14
     1.7   Concluding Remarks 16

2 Dose Finding Based on Preclinical Studies   **18**
     2.1   Introduction 18
     2.2   Parallel Line Assays 20
     2.3   Competitive Binding Assays 20
     2.4   Anti-infective Drugs 25
     2.5   Biological Substances 25
     2.6   Preclinical Toxicology Studies...................................... 26
     2.7   Extrapolating Dose from Animal to Human 28

3 Dose-Finding Studies in Phase I and Estimation
of Maximally Tolerated Dose   **30**
     3.1   Introduction 30
     3.2   Basic Concepts 30
     3.3   General Considerations for FIH Studies 32

	3.3.1	Study Designs	33
	3.3.2	Population	35
3.4	Dose Selection		37
	3.4.1	Estimating the Starting Dose in Phase I	37
	3.4.2	Dose Escalation	40
3.5	Assessments		42
	3.5.1	Safety and Tolerability	42
	3.5.2	Pharmacokinetics	43
	3.5.3	Pharmacodynamics	43
3.6	Dose Selection for Phase II		46

4 Dose-Finding in Oncology—Nonparametric Methods   **49**
4.1	Introduction		49
4.2	Traditional or 3 + 3 Design		50
4.3	Basic Properties of Group Up-and-Down Designs		51
4.4	Designs that Use Random Sample Size: Escalation and A + B Designs		52
	4.4.1	Escalation and A + B Designs	52
	4.4.2	The 3 + 3 Design as an A + B Design	53
4.5	Designs that Use Fixed Sample Size		53
	4.5.1	Group Up-and-Down Designs	54
	4.5.2	Fully Sequential Designs for Phase I Clinical Trials	54
	4.5.3	Estimation of the MTD After the Trial	54
4.6	More Complex Dose-Finding Trials		55
	4.6.1	Trials with Ordered Groups	55
	4.6.2	Trials with Multiple Agents	56
4.7	Conclusion		56

5 Dose Finding in Oncology—Parametric Methods   **59**
5.1	Introduction		59
5.2	Escalation with Overdose Control Design		61
	5.2.1	EWOC Design	61
	5.2.2	Example	62
5.3	Adjusting for Covariates		63
	5.3.1	Model	63
	5.3.2	Example	66
5.4	Choice of Prior Distributions		68
	5.4.1	Independent Priors	69
	5.4.2	Correlated Priors	69
	5.4.3	Simulations	70
5.5	Concluding Remarks		70

6 Dose Response: Pharmacokinetic–Pharmacodynamic Approach   **73**
| 6.1 | Exposure Response | | 73 |

	6.1.1	How Dose Response and Exposure Response Differ	73
	6.1.2	Why Exposure Response is More Informative.......	73
	6.1.3	FDA Exposure Response Guidance....................	73
6.2	Time Course of Response...............................		74
	6.2.1	Action, Effect, and Response...........................	74
	6.2.2	Models for Describing the Time Course of Response	74
6.3	Pharmacokinetics...		75
	6.3.1	Review of Basic Elements of Pharmacokinetics.....	75
	6.3.2	Why the Clearance/Volume Parameterization is Preferred...	76
6.4	Pharmacodynamics..		77
	6.4.1	Review of Basic Elements of Pharmacodynamics...	77
6.5	Delayed Effects and Response........................		77
	6.5.1	Two Main Mechanism Classes for Delayed Effects.	78
6.6	Cumulative Effects and Response....................		80
	6.6.1	The Relevance of Considering Integral of Effect as the Outcome Variable................................	80
	6.6.2	Why Area Under the Curve of Concentration is not a Reliable Predictor of Cumulative Response ...	80
	6.6.3	Schedule Dependence....................................	81
	6.6.4	Predictability of Schedule Dependence...............	82
6.7	Disease Progress..		82
	6.7.1	The Time Course of Placebo Response and Disease Natural History.................................	82
	6.7.2	Two Main Classes of Drug Effect	83
6.8	Modeling Methods..		84
	6.8.1	Analysis...	84
	6.8.2	Mixed Effect Models....................................	85
	6.8.3	Simulation..	85
	6.8.4	Clinical Trial Simulation	85
6.9	Conclusion...		86

7	**General Considerations in Dose–Response Study Designs**		**89**
7.1	Issues Relating to Clinical Development Plan....................		89
7.2	General Considerations for Designing Clinical Trials...........		90
	7.2.1	Subject Population and Endpoints......................	91
	7.2.2	Parallel Designs versus Crossover Designs...........	93
	7.2.3	Selection of Control......................................	93
	7.2.4	Multiple Comparisons	94
	7.2.5	Sample Size Considerations	95
	7.2.6	Multiple Center Studies	96
7.3	Design Considerations for Phase II Dose–Response Studies ..		96
	7.3.1	Frequency of Dosing.....................................	97
	7.3.2	Fixed-Dose versus Dose-Titration Designs...........	99
	7.3.3	Range of Doses to be Studied..........................	100

7.3.4   Number of Doses to be Tested 101
7.3.5   Dose Allocation, Dose Spacing 102
7.3.6   Optimal Designs 103
7.4   Concluding Remarks 103

**8   Clinical Trial Simulation—A Case Study Incorporating
Efficacy and Tolerability Dose Response**   **106**
8.1   Clinical Development Project Background 106
8.1.1   Clinical Trial Objectives 107
8.1.2   Uncertainties Affecting Clinical Trial Planning 107
8.2   The Clinical Trial Simulation Project 108
8.2.1   Clinical Trial Objectives Used for the CTS Project . 109
8.2.2   The Simulation Project Objective 111
8.2.3   Simulation Project Methods 1: Data Models and
Design Options 111
8.2.4   Simulation Project Methods 2: Analysis and
Evaluation Criteria 117
8.3   Simulation Results and Design Recommendations 120
8.3.1   Objective 1: Power for Confirming Efficacy 120
8.3.2   Objective 2: Accuracy of Target Dose Estimation ... 121
8.3.3   Objective 3: Estimation of a Potentially Clinically
Noninferior Dose Range 121
8.3.4   Trial Design Recommendations 124
8.4   Conclusions 125

9   Analysis of Dose–Response Studies—E_{max} Model   **127**
9.1   Introduction to the E_{max} Model 127
9.2   Sensitivity of the E_{max} Model Parameters 129
9.2.1   Sensitivity of the E_0 and E_{max} Parameters 129
9.2.2   Sensitivity of the ED_{50} Parameter 130
9.2.3   Sensitivity of the N Parameter 131
9.2.4   Study Design for the E_{max} Model 131
9.2.5   Covariates in the E_{max} Model 133
9.3   Similar Models 134
9.4   A Mixed Effects E_{max} Model 134
9.5   Examples 135
9.5.1   Oral Artesunate Dose–Response Analysis Example 135
9.5.2   Estimation Methodology 137
9.5.3   Initial Parameter Values for the Oral Artesunate
Dose–Response Analysis Example 138
9.5.4   Diastolic Blood Pressure Dose–Response Example . 139
9.6   Conclusions 141

10   Analysis of Dose–Response Studies—Modeling Approaches   **146**
10.1   Introduction 146

10.2   Some Commonly Used Dose–Response Models   149
        10.2.1 E_{max} Model   150
        10.2.2   Linear in Log-Dose Model   151
        10.2.3   Linear Model   151
        10.2.4   Exponential (Power) Model   151
        10.2.5   Quadratic Model   152
        10.2.6   Logistic Model   152
10.3   Estimation of Target Doses   153
        10.3.1   Estimating the MED in Dose-Finding Example   155
10.4   Model Uncertainty and Model Selection   156
10.5   Combining Modeling Techniques and Multiple Testing   160
        10.5.1   Methodology   160
        10.5.2   Proof-of-Activity Analysis in the
                  Dose-Finding Example   162
        10.5.3   Simulations   163
10.6   Conclusions   169

11 Multiple Comparison Procedures in Dose Response Studies   172
11.1   Introduction   172
11.2   Identifying the Minimum Effective Dose (MinED)   172
        11.2.1   Problem Formulation   172
        11.2.2   Review of Multiple Test Procedures   174
        11.2.3   Simultaneous Confidence Intervals   176
11.3   Identifying the Maximum Safe Dose (MaxSD)   177
11.4   Examples   177
11.5   Extensions   180
11.6   Discussion   181

**12 Partitioning Tests in Dose–Response Studies with
     Binary Outcomes   184**
12.1   Motivation   184
12.2   Comparing Two Success Probabilities in a Single Hypothesis   185
12.3   Comparison of Success Probabilities in
        Dose–Response Studies   188
        12.3.1   Predetermined Step-Down Method   188
        12.3.2   Sample-Determined Step-Down Method   190
        12.3.3   Hochberg's Step-up Procedure   194
12.4   An Example Using Partitioning Based Stepwise Methods   195
12.5   Conclusion and Discussion   197

**13 Analysis of Dose–Response Relationship Based
     on Categorical Outcomes   200**
13.1   Introduction   200
13.2   When the Response is Ordinal   201
        13.2.1   Modeling Dose–Response   201

	13.2.2	Testing for a Monotone Dose–Response Relationship	203
13.3	When the Response is Binary		207
13.4	Multiple Comparisons		210
	13.4.1	Bonferroni Adjustment	211
	13.4.2	Bonferroni–Holm Procedure	211
	13.4.3	Hochberg Procedure	212
	13.4.4	Gate-Keeping Procedure	212
	13.4.5	A Special Application of Dunnett's Procedure for Binary Response	213
13.5	Discussion		213

14   Power and Sample Size for Dose Response Studies   220

14.1	Introduction		220
14.2	General Approach to Power Calculation		221
14.3	Multiple-Arm Dose Response Trial		223
	14.3.1	Normal Response	224
	14.3.2	Binary Response	227
	14.3.3	Time-to-Event Endpoint	230
14.4	Phase I Oncology Dose Escalation Trial		233
	14.4.1	The A + B Escalation without Dose De-Escalation.	234
	14.4.2	The A + B Escalation with Dose De-Escalation	236
14.5	Concluding Remarks		238

Index   243

1
Introduction and New Drug Development Process

NAITEE TING

1.1 Introduction

The fundamental objective of drug development is to find a dose, or dose range, of a drug candidate that is both efficacious (for improving or curing the intended disease condition) and safe (with acceptable risk of adverse effects). If such a dose range cannot be identified, the candidate would not be a medically useful or commercially viable pharmaceutical product, nor should it be approved by regulatory agencies.

Each pharmacological agent (drug candidate) will typically have many effects, both desired (such as blood pressure reduction) and undesired (adverse effects, such as dizziness or nausea). Generally, the magnitude of a pharmacological effect increase monotonically with increased dose, eventually reaching a plateau level where further increases have little additional effect. Of course, for serious adverse effects, we will not be able to ethically observe this full dose range, at least in humans. Figure 1.1 illustrates a monotonic dose–response relationship, which could be for either a beneficial or adverse safety effect. Note that some types of pharmacological response exhibit a "U-shaped" (or "inverted U-shaped") dose–response pattern, but these are relatively rare, at least over the dose range likely to be of therapeutic value.

Figure 1.1 distinguishes between individual dose–response relationships—the three steeper curves representing three different individuals—and the single, flatter population average dose–response relationship. When discussing "dose–response" in drug development, it is generally implied the population average type of dose–response.

For a therapeutically useful drug, the "safe and efficacious" dose range will be on the low end of the safety dose–response curve and towards the higher end for beneficial effect. The concept of "efficacious dose range" and "safe dose range" is illustrated in Figure 1.2 and will be clarified in the following paragraphs.

Based on these dose–response curves, the maximum effective dose (MaxED) and the maximally tolerated dose (MTD) can be defined: MaxED is the dose above which there is no clinically significant increase in pharmacological effect or

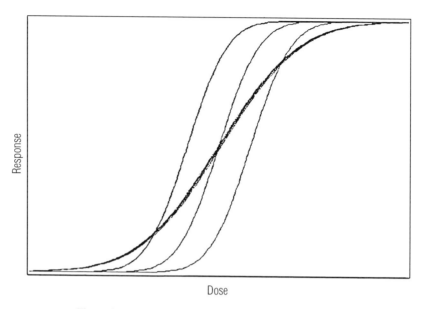

Figure 1.1. Individual and average dose–response curves.

efficacy, and MTD is the maximal dose acceptably tolerated by a particular patient population. Another dose parameter of interest is the minimum effective dose (MinED). Ruberg (1995) defines the MinED as "the lowest dose producing a clinically important response that can be declared statistically, significantly different from the placebo response".

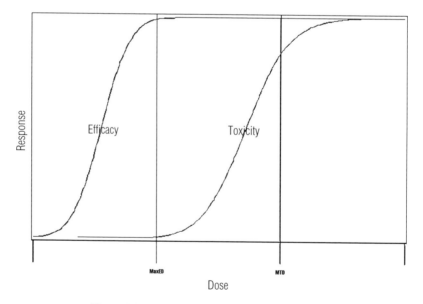

Figure 1.2. Dose–response for efficacy and toxicity.

In certain drugs, the efficacy and the toxicity curves are widely separated. When this is the case, there is a wide range of doses for patients to take; i.e., as long as a patient receives a dose between MaxED and MTD, the patient can benefit from the efficacy, and at the same time, mitigate toxicities from the drug. However, for other drugs, the two curves may be very close to each other. Under this situation, physicians have to dose patients very carefully so that while benefiting from the efficacy, patients do not have to be exposed to potential toxicity from the drug. The area between the efficacy and the toxicity curves is known as the "therapeutic window". One way to measure the therapeutic window is to use a "therapeutic index (TI)". TI is considered as the ratio of MTD over an effective dose (e.g., MaxED). Clearly, a drug with a wide therapeutic window (or a high TI) tends to be preferred by both physicians and patients. If a drug has a narrow therapeutic window, then the drug will need to be developed carefully, and physicians will prescribe the drug with caution.

It is also of interest to distinguish between the maximum effect achievable (height of the plateau) and potency (location of the response curve on dose scale). Figure 1.3 illustrates these concepts. Drugs operating by a similar mechanism of action often have (approximately) similar dose–response shapes, but will differ in potency (the amount of drug needed to achieve the same effect), e.g., Drugs A and B in Figure 1.3. Here Drug A is more potent than B because it takes less dose of A to reach the same level of response as that of B. A drug operating by a different mechanism might be able to achieve higher (or lower) efficacy—e.g., Drug C.

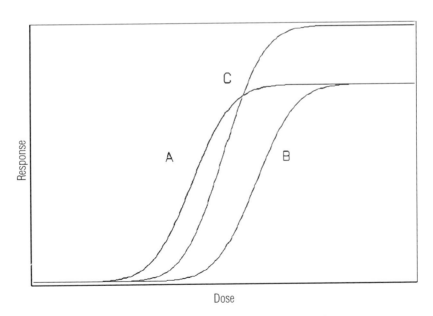

Figure 1.3. High potency drug and high efficacy drug.

The process of drug development—involving literally thousands of experiments in animals, healthy human subjects, and patients with the target disease—focuses on achieving progressively refined knowledge of the dose–response relationships for important safety and efficacy effects. Prior to human trials, extensive in vitro (outside of a living organism) and in vivo (within a living organism) experiments are conducted with the drug candidate to identify how the various effects depend upon dose (or other measures of exposure such as its concentration in the body).

Dose–response relationship for a new drug is studied both in human and in animal experiments. Human studies are referred as clinical trials, and animal studies are generally part of nonclinical studies. In either case, experiment design and data analysis are critical components for a study. Statistical methods can be applied to help with design and analysis for both nonclinical and clinical studies. Evidences of drug efficacy and drug safety in human subjects are mainly established on the findings from randomized double-blind controlled clinical trials. Descriptive statistics are frequently used to help understand and gauge various characteristics of a drug. Inferential statistics helps quantify probabilities of successes and risks in drug discovery and development, as well as variability around those probabilities. Statistics is also an important decision-making tool throughout the entire drug development process. In clinical trials of all phases, studies are designed using statistical principles. Clinical data are displayed and analyzed using various statistical models.

1.2   New Drug Development Process

Most of the drugs available in pharmacy started out as a chemical compound or a biologic discovered in laboratories. When first discovered, this new compound or biologic is denoted as a drug candidate. Drug development is a process that starts when the drug candidate is first discovered, and continues until it is available to be prescribed by physicians to treat patients (Ting, 2003). A compound is usually a new chemical entity synthesized by scientists from drug companies (also referred as sponsors), universities, or research institutes. A biologic can be a protein, a part of a protein, DNA or a different form either extracted from tissues of another live body or cultured by some type of bacteria. In any case, this new compound or biologic will have to go through the drug development process before it can be used by the general public. For purposes of this book, the focus will mostly be on the chemical compound development.

The drug development process can be broadly classified into two major components: nonclinical development and clinical development. Nonclinical development includes all drug testing performed outside of the human body. The clinical development is based on experiments conducted in the human body. Nonclinical development can further be broadly divided into pharmacology, toxicology, and formulation. In these processes, experiments are performed in laboratories or pilot plants. Observations from cells, tissues, animal bodies, or drug components are collected to derive inferences for potential new drugs. Chemical processes are involved in formulating the new compound into drugs to be delivered into human body. Clinical development can be further divided into Phases I, II, III, and IV. Clinical studies are designed to collect data from normal volunteers and subjects with the target disease, in order to help understand how the human body acts on the drug candidate, and how the drug candidate helps patients with the disease.

A new chemical compound or a biologic can be designated as a drug candidate because it demonstrates some desirable pharmacological activities in the laboratory. At the early stage of drug development, the focus is mainly on cells, tissues, organs, or animal bodies. Experiments on human beings are performed after the candidate passes these early tests and looks promising. Hence, nonclinical development may also be referred to as preclinical development since these experiments are performed before human trials.

Throughout the whole drug development process, two scientific questions are constantly being addressed: Does the drug candidate work? Is it safe? Starting from the laboratory where the compound is first discovered, the candidate has to go through lots of tests to see if it demonstrates both efficacy (the drug works) and safety. Only the candidates passing all those tests can be progressed to the next step of development. In the United States, after a drug candidate passes all of the nonclinical tests, an investigational new drug (IND) document is filed to the Food and Drug Administration (FDA). After the IND is approved, clinical trials (tests on humans) can then be performed. If this drug candidate is shown to be safe and efficacious through Phases I, II, and III of the clinical trials, the sponsor will file a new drug application (NDA) to the FDA in the United States. The drug can only be available for general public consumption in the United States, if the NDA is approved. Often, the approved drug is continually studied for safety and efficacy, for example, in different subpopulations. These post-marketing studies are generally referred as Phase IV of the clinical trials.

1.3 Nonclinical Development

1.3.1 Pharmacology

Pharmacology is the study of the selective biological activity of chemical substances on living matter. A substance has biological activities when, in appropriate doses, it causes a cellular response. It is selective when the response occurs in some cells and not in others. Therefore, a chemical compound or a biologic has to demonstrate these activities before it can be further developed. In the early stage of drug testing, it is important to differentiate an "active" candidate from an "inactive" candidate. There are screening procedures to select these candidates. Two properties of particular interest are sensitivity and specificity. Given that a compound is active, sensitivity is the conditional probability that the screen will classify it as positive. Specificity is the conditional probability that the screen will call a compound negative given that it is truly inactive.

Usually sensitivity and specificity can be a trade-off; however, in the ideal case, we hope both of these values be high and close to one.

Quantity of these pharmacological activities may be viewed as the drug potency or strength. The estimation of drug potency by the reactions of living organisms or their components is known as bioassay. According to Finney (1978), bioassay is defined as an experiment for estimating the potency of a drug, material, preparation, or process by means of the reaction that follows its application to living matters.

As discussed previously, one of the most important relationships needs to be studied for pharmacological activities is the dose–response relationship. In these experiments, several doses of the drug candidates are selected, and the responses are measured for each corresponding dose. After response data are collected, regression or nonparametric methods may be applied to analyze the results. As shown in Figure 1.2, the focus of nonclinical pharmacology is to help estimate the response curve at left. By increasing the dose or concentration of the drug candidate, if the pharmacological response does not change and stays at the low level of activity, then it can be concluded that this candidate does not have the activity under study and there is no need to develop this candidate. If the drug candidate is active, then the information about how much response can be expected for a given dosage (or concentration) can be used to help guide the design of dose selection clinical trials in human studies. Concerns relating to dose finding in nonclinical pharmacology are covered in Chapter 2.

1.3.2   Toxicology/Drug Safety

Drug safety is one of the most important concerns throughout all stages of drug development. In the preclinical stage, drug safety needs to be studied for a few different species of animals (e.g., mice, rabbits, rodents). Studies are designed to observe adverse drug effects or toxic events experienced by animals treated with different doses of the drug candidate. Animals are also exposed to the drug candidate for various lengths of time to see if there are adverse effects caused by cumulative dosing over time. These results are summarized and analyzed by using statistical methods. When the results of animal studies indicate potentially serious side effects, drug development is either terminated or suspended pending further investigations of the problem.

Depending on the duration of exposure to the drug candidate, animal toxicity studies are classified as acute studies, subchronic studies, chronic studies, and reproductive studies (Selwyn, 1988). Usually the first few studies are acute studies; i.e., the animal is given one or a few doses of the drug candidate. If only one dose is given, it can also be called a single-dose study. Only those drug candidates demonstrated to be safe in the single-dose studies can be progressed into multiple-dose studies. Single-dose acute studies in animals are primarily used to set the dose to be tested in chronic studies. Acute studies are typically about 2 weeks in duration. Repeat dose studies of 30 to 90 days duration are called subchronic studies. Chronic studies are usually designed with more than 90 days of duration. These studies are conducted in rodents and in at least one nonrodent species. Some chronic studies may also be viewed as carcinogenicity studies because the rodent studies consider tumor incidence as an important endpoint. Reproductive studies are carried out to assess the drug's effect on fertility and conception; they can also be used to study drug effect on the fetus and developing offspring.

Data collected from toxicology studies will help estimate the curve on the right-hand side of Figure 1.2. The information are not only used to identify a NOAEL (No Observed Adverse Event Level) for the drug candidate; it can also help provide guidance as to what type of adverse events to be expected in human studies. Again, results obtained from animal toxicity studies are very useful in helping design dose selection clinical trials in humans. More details about drug toxicity and dose–response are also described in Chapter 2.

1.3.3   Drug Formulation Development

As discussed earlier, a potential new drug can be either a chemical compound or a biologic. If the drug candidate is a biologic, then the formulation is typically a solution, which contains a high concentration of such a biologic, and the solution is injected into the subject. On the other hand, if the potential drug is a chemical compound, then the formulation can be tablets, capsules, solution, patches, suspension, or other forms. There are many formulation problems that require statistical analyses. The formulation problems that stem from chemical compounds are more likely to involve widely used statistical techniques. The paradigm of a chemical compound is used here to illustrate some of these formulation-related problems and how they can be related to dose selection.

A drug is the mixture of the synthesized chemical compound (active ingredients) and other inactive ingredients designed to improve the absorption of the active ingredients. How the mixture is made depends on results of a series of experiments. Usually these experiments are performed under some physical constraints, e.g., the amount of supply of raw materials, capacity of container, size and shape of the tablets. In the early stage of drug development, drug formulation needs to be flexible so that various dose strengths can be tested in animals and in humans. Often in the nonclinical development stage or in early phase of clinical trials, the drug candidate is supplied in powder form or as solutions to allow flexible dosing. By the time the drug candidate progresses into late Phase I or early Phase II, fixed dosage form such as tablets, capsules, or other formulations are more desirable.

The dose strength depends on both nonclinical and clinical information. The drug formulation group works closely with laboratory scientists, toxicologists and clinical pharmacologists to determine the possible dose strengths for each drug candidate. In many cases, the originally proposed dose strengths will need to be changed depending on results obtained from Phase II studies. These formulations are developed for clinical trial usage and are often different from the commercial formulation. After the new drug is approved for market, commercial formulation should be readily available for distribution.

1.4   Premarketing Clinical Development

If a chemical compound or a biologic gets through the selection process from animal testing and is shown to be safe and efficacious to be tested in human, it progresses into clinical development. In drug development for human use, the major distinction between "clinical trials" and "nonclinical testing" is the experimental unit. In clinical trials, the experimental units are human beings, and the experimental units in "nonclinical testing" are nonhuman subjects. As mentioned earlier, the results of these nonclinical studies will be used in the IND submission prior to the first clinical trial. If there is no concern from the FDA after 30 days of the IND submission, the sponsor can then start clinical testing for this drug candidate. At this stage, the chemical compound or the biologic may be referred to as the "test drug" or the "study drug".

An IND is a document that contains all the information known about the new drug up to the time the IND is prepared. A typical IND includes the name and description of the drug (such as chemical structure, other ingredients); how the drug is processed; information about any preclinical experiences relating to the safety of the drug; marketing information; past experiences or future plans for investigating the drug both in the United States and in foreign countries. In addition, it also contains a description of the clinical development plan (CDP, refer to Section 1.5). Such a description should contain all of the informational materials to be supplied to clinical investigators, signed agreements from investigators, and the initial protocols for clinical investigation.

Clinical development is broadly divided into four phases, namely Phases I, II, III, and IV. Phase I trials are designed to study the short-term effects; e.g., pharmacokinetics (PK, what does a human body do to the drug), pharmacodynamics (PD, what does a drug do to the human body), and dose range (what range of doses should be tested in human) for the new drug. Phase II trials are designed to assess the efficacy of the new drug in well-defined subject populations. Dose–response relationships are also studied during Phase II. Phase III trials are usually long-term, large-scale studies to confirm findings established from earlier trials. These studies are also used to detect adverse effects caused by cumulative dosing. If a new drug is found to be safe and efficacious from the first three phases of clinical testing, an NDA is filed for the regulatory agency (FDA, in the United States) to review. Once the drug is approved by the FDA, Phase IV (postmarketing) studies are planned and carried out. Many of the Phase IV study designs are dictated by the FDA to examine safety questions; some designs are employed to establish new uses.

1.4.1   Phase I Clinical Trials

In a Phase I PK study, the purpose is usually to understand PK properties and to estimate PK parameters (e.g., AUC, Cmax, Tmax, to be described in next paragraph) of the test drug. In many cases, Phase I trials are designed to study the bioavailability of a drug, or the bioequivalence among different formulations of the same drug. "Bioavailability" means "the rate and extent to which the active drug ingredient or therapeutic moiety is absorbed and becomes available at the site of drug action" (Chow and Liu, 1999). Experimental units in such Phase I studies are mostly normal volunteers. Subjects recruited for these studies are generally in good health.

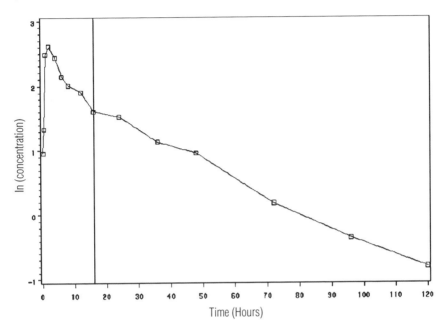

Figure 1.4. Drug concentration–time curve.

A bioavailability or a bioequivalence study is carried out by measuring drug concentration levels in blood or serum over time from participating subjects. These measurements are summarized into one value per subject per treatment period. These summarized data are then used for statistical analysis. Figure 1.4 presents a drug concentration–time curve. Data on this curve are collected at discrete time points. Typical variables used for analysis of PK activities include area under the curve (AUC), maximum concentration (C_{max}), minimum concentration (C_{min}), time to maxium concentration (T_{max}), and others. These variables are computed from drug concentration levels as shown in Figure 1.4. Suppose AUC is used for analysis, then these discretely observed points are connected (for each subject under each treatment period) and the AUC is estimated using a trapezoidal rule. For example, AUC up to 24 hours for this curve is computed by adding up the areas of the triangle between 0 hour and 0.25 hour, the trapezoid between 0.25 hour and 0.5 hour, and so on, and the trapezoid between 16 hour and 24 hour. Usually the AUC and C_{max} are first transformed using natural log, then they are included in the data analysis. Chapter 6 discusses how PK data and PK/PD models can be used to help dose selection in Phase II.

Statistical designs used in Phase I bioavailability studies are often crossover designs; i.e., a subject is randomized to be treated with formulation A first, and then treated with formulation B after a "wash-out" period; or randomized to formulation B first, and then treated with A after wash-out. In some complicated Phase I studies, two or more treatments may be designed to cross several periods for each subject. Advantages and disadvantages of crossover designs are discussed in Chow and Liu (1999). Response variables including AUC and C_{max} are usually analyzed using ANOVA models. Random and mixed effects linear/nonlinear models are also commonly used in the analysis for Phase I clinical studies. In certain designs, covariate terms considered in these models can be very complicated. How Phase I studies can help in dose finding are discussed in Chapter 3.

1.4.2   Phase II/III Clinical Trials

Phase II/III trials are designed to study the efficacy and safety of a test drug. Unlike Phase I studies, subjects recruited in Phase II/III studies are patients with the disease for which the drug is developed. Response variables considered in Phase II/III studies are mainly efficacy and safety variables. For example, in a trial for the evaluation of hypertension (high blood pressure), the efficacy variables are blood pressure measurements. For an anti-infective trial, the response variables can be the proportion of subjects cured or time to cure for each subject. Phase II/III studies are mostly designed with parallel treatment groups (in contrast to crossover). Hence, if a patient is randomized to receive treatment A, then this patient is to be treated with Drug A through out the whole study.

Phase II trials are often designed to compare one or a few doses of a test drug against placebo. These studies are usually short-term (several weeks) and designed with a small or moderate sample size. Often, Phase II trials are exploratory in nature. Patients recruited for Phase II trials are somewhat restrictive; i.e., they tend to be with certain disease severity (not too severe and not too mild), without other underlying diseases, and not on background treatments. One of the most important types of Phase II study is the dose–response study. As expressed on the left curve of Figure 1.1, drug efficacy may increase as dose increases. In a dose–response study, the following fundamental questions need to be addressed (Ruberg, 1995):

- Is there any evidence of a drug effect?
- What doses exhibit a response different from the control response?
- What is the nature of the dose–response relationship?
- What is the optimal dose?

Typical dose–response studies are designed with fixed doses, parallel treatment groups. For example, in a four-treatment group trial designed to study dose–response relationships, three test doses (low, medium, high) are compared against placebo. In this case, results may be analyzed using multiple comparison techniques or modeling approaches. In general, Phase II studies are carried out for an estimation purpose. Dose–response study designs used in Phase II are discussed in Chapters 6, 7, and 8. A special chapter (Chapter 14) is devoted for discussion on power and sample size issues.

Phase III trials are long-term (can last up to a few years), large-scale (several hundreds of patients), with less restrictive patient populations, and often compared against a known active drug (in some cases, compared with placebo) for the disease to be studied. Phase III trials tend to be confirmatory trials designed to verify findings established from earlier studies.

Statistical methods used in Phase II/III clinical studies can be different from those used for Phase I or nonclinical studies. Statistical analyses are selected based on the distribution of the variables and the objectives of the study. Many Phase I analyses tend to be descriptive, with estimation purposes. In Phase II/III, categorical data analyses are frequently used in analyzing count data (e.g., number of subjects responded, number of subjects with a certain side effect, or number of subjects improved from "severe symptom" to "moderate symptom"). Survival analyses are commonly used in analyzing time to an event (time to discontinuation of the study medication, time to the first occurrence of a side effect, time to cure). Regression analyses, t tests, analyses of variance (ANOVA), analyses of covariance (ANCOVA), and multivariate analyses (MANOVA) are useful in analyzing continuous data (blood pressure, grip strength, forced expiration volume, number of painful joints, AUC, and others). In many cases, nonparametric analytical methods are selected because the data do not fit any known parametric distribution well. In some other cases, the raw data are transformed (log-transformed, ranked, centralized, combined) before a statistical analysis is performed. A combination of various statistical tools may sometimes be used in a drug development program. Hypothesis tests are often used to compare results obtained from different treatment groups. Point estimates and interval estimates are also frequently used to estimate subject responses to a study medication or to demonstrate equivalence between two treatment groups. Statistical methods for analyzing dose–response studies are introduced in Chapters 9–13.

Although the recommendation of doses is primarily made during Phase II, in most of the cases, dose selection is further refined in Phase III. One reason for this is that Phase III exposure is long-term and with a large patient population. From an efficacy point of view, the drug efficacy from recommended doses may or may not sustain after longer duration of treatment. More importantly, from a safety point of view, a safe dose selected from Phase II results may lead to some other safety concerns after this dose is exposed for a longer time. One possibility is that drug accumulation over time may cause additional adverse events. Therefore, it is a good practice to consider incorporating more doses than just the target dose(s) in Phase III. It helps to have a dose higher than the target dose(s) so that in case the target dose(s) is not as efficacious as anticipated, we can consider this higher dose to be the effective dose. It is also useful to have a dose lower than the target dose(s) so that in case the target dose is not safe and the lower dose can be considered as a viable alternative.

After a clinical study is completed, all of the data collected from this study are stored in a database and statistical analyses are performed on data sets extracted from the database. A study report is prepared for each completed clinical trial. It is a joint effort to prepare such a study report. Statisticians, data managers, and programmers work together to produce tables, figures, and statistical reports. Statisticians, clinicians, and technical writers will then put together clinical interpretations from these results. All of these are incorporated into a study report. Study reports from individual clinical trials will eventually be culled as part of an NDA.

1.4.3   Clinical Development for Life-Threatening Diseases

In drug development, concerns for drugs to treat life-threatening diseases, such as cancer or AIDS, can be very different from those for other drugs. In the early stage of developing a cancer drug, patients are recruited to trials under open-label treatment with test drug and some effective background cancer therapy. Under this circumstance, doses of the test drug may be adjusted during the treatment period. Information obtained from these studies will then be used to help suggest dose regimen for future studies. Various study designs to handle these situations are available in statistical/oncology literatures. Examples of these types of flexible designs are covered in Chapters 4 and 5.

In some cases, drugs for life-threatening diseases are approved for the target patient population before large-scale Phase III studies are completed because of public need. When this is the case, additional clinical studies may be sponsored by National Institute of Health (NIH) or National Cancer Institute (NCI) in the United States. Many of the NIH/NCI studies are still designed for dose finding or dose adjustment purposes.

1.4.4   New Drug Application

When there is sufficient evidence to demonstrate a new drug is efficacious and safe, an NDA is put together by the sponsor. An NDA is a huge package of documents describing all of the results obtained from both nonclinical experiments and clinical trials. A typical NDA contains sections on proposed drug label, pharmacological class, foreign marketing history, chemistry, manufacturing and controls, nonclinical pharmacology and toxicology summary, human pharmacokinetics and bioavailability summary, microbiology summary, clinical data summary, results of statistical analyses, benefit–risk relationship, and others. If the sponsor intends to market the new drug in other countries, then packages of documents will need to be prepared for submission to those corresponding countries, too. For example, a new drug submission (NDS) needs to be filed to Canadian regulatory agency and a marketing authorization application (MAA) needs to be filed to the European regulatory agencies.

Often, an NDA is filed while some of the Phase III studies are ongoing. Sponsors need to be very careful in selecting the "data cut-off date" because all of the clinical data in the database up to the cut-off date need to be frozen and stored so that NDA study report tables and figures can be produced from them. The data sets stored in such an "NDA database" may have to be retrieved, and reanalyzed after filing, in order to address various queries from regulatory agencies. After these data sets are created and stored, new clinical data can then be entered into the ongoing database.

An NDA package usually includes not only individual clinical study reports, but also combined study results. These results may be summarized using meta-analyses or pooled data analyses on individual patient data across studies. Such analyses are performed on efficacy data to produce summary of clinical efficacy (SCE, also known as integrated analysis of efficacy—IAE) and on safety data to produce the summary of clinical safety (SCS, also known as integrated analysis of safety—IAS). These summaries are important components of an NDA. Increasingly, electronic submissions are filed as part of the NDA. Electronic submissions usually include individual clinical data, programs to process these data, and software/hardware to help reviewers from FDA or foreign regulatory agencies in reviewing the individual data as well as the whole NDA package.

1.5   Clinical Development Plan

In the early stage of drug development, as early as in the nonclinical stage, a clinical development plan (CDP) should be drafted. This plan should include clinical studies to be conducted in Phases I, II and III. The CDP should be guided by the draft drug label. The drug label provides detailed information on how the drug should be used. Hence, a draft label at the early stage of drug development lays out the target profile for the drug candidate. Clinical studies should be designed to help obtain information that will support this given target drug label.

One of the most important aspects of labeling information is the recommended regimen for this new drug. The regimen includes dosage and dose frequency. In the early stage of drug development, scientists need to predict the dosage and frequency as to how the drug will be labeled. Based on this prediction, the clinical development program should be designed to obtain necessary information that will support the recommended regimen. For example, if the drug will be used with one fixed dose, then the CDP should propose clinical studies to help find that dose. On the other hand, if the drug will be used as titration doses, then studies need to be designed to study the dose range for titration.

Another example is dosing frequency. Patients with chronic diseases tend to take multiple medications every day. Many patients may prefer a once-a-day (QD) drug or a twice-a-day (BID) drug. In early development of a new drug, if the best marketed product for the target disease is prescribed as a twice-a-day drug, and the preliminary information of this test drug indicates that it will have to be used three or more times a day, then the CDP needs to include studies to reformulate the test drug so that it can be used as a twice-a-day drug or a once-a-day drug, before it can be progressed into later phases of development.

A CDP is an important document to be used during the clinical development of a new drug. As a drug progresses in the clinical development process, the CDP should be updated to reflect the most current information about the drug and depending on the findings up to this point in time, the sponsor can assess whether a new version of drug label should be drafted. In case a new draft of drug label is needed, the development plan should be revised so that studies can be planned to support the new drug label.

The overall clinical development process can be viewed in two directions as shown in Figure 1.5. One is the forward scientific process, as more data and information are accumulating, we know more about the drug candidate and we design later phase studies to help progress the candidate. On the other hand, the planning is based on the draft drug label. From the draft label, we have a target profile for the drug. Depending on the drug properties to be demonstrated on the label, the sponsor needs to have Phase III studies to support those claims. In order to collect information to help design those Phase III studies, data need to be available for the corresponding Phase I or Phase II studies. Therefore, the thinking process is backward by looking at the target profile first, and then prepares the CDP according to the draft label.

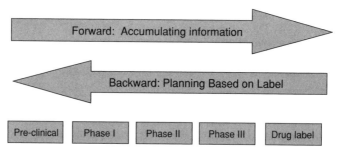

Figure 1.5. Clinical development process.

1.6   Postmarketing Clinical Development

An NDA serves as a landmark of the drug development. The development process does not stop when an NDA is submitted or approved. However, the objectives of the process are changed after the drug is approved and is available on the market. Studies performed after the drug is approved are typically called postmarketing studies, or Phase IV studies.

One of the major objectives in postmarketing development is to establish a better safety profile for the new drug. Large-scale drug safety surveillance studies are very common in Phase IV. Subjects/patients recruited in Phases I, II, and III are often somewhat restricted (patients would have to be within a certain age range, gender, disease severity or other restrictions). However, after the new drug is approved and is available for the general patient population, every patient with the underlying disease can be exposed to this drug. Problems related to drug safety that have not been detected from the premarketing studies (Phases I, II, and III) may now be observed in this large, general population.

Another objective of a Phase IV study is for the sponsor to increase the market potential for the new drug by demonstrating an improvement in patients' quality of life (QoL) and by establishing its economic value. Studies designed to achieve this objective include QoL studies and pharmaco-economic studies. Studies of this nature are often referred to as "outcomes research" studies. One of the main differences between a QoL study and an efficacy/safety study is the type of variables being studied. Although in many cases, a QoL study may include ordinary efficacy and safety endpoints, such a study will also include QoL-specific variables. These variables are typically collected from questionnaires designed for the patient to evaluate the change in life style caused by the disease and the improvement (of quality of life) brought by the medication. In general, clinical efficacy variables are measured to study the severity of symptoms, and quality of life variables are measured to study how a patient copes with life while experiencing the underlying disease. In the United States, the FDA determines whether to approve the drug based on efficacy and safety findings. However, a patient may prefer a particular drug based on how that patient feels. Among the drugs approved by FDA for the same disease, the patient tends to choose the one that is better for his/her quality of life.

Traditionally, Phase I, II, and III studies are used to establish the efficacy and safety of a drug, and Phase IV is used to study QoL. Recently, there are many changes in the field of outcomes research. For example, the new name of many of these variables is "patient reported outcome (PRO)". Generally, PRO includes more variables than just QoL. Another important change is that more and more Phase II/III studies are designed to collect and analyze PRO data. Furthermore, FDA and other regulatory agencies are more involved in reviewing and labeling PRO findings.

Pharmaco-economic studies are designed to study the direct and indirect cost of treating a disease. In these studies, costs of various FDA approved drugs are compared. Costs may include the price of the medication, expenses for monitoring the patient (physician's charge, costs of lab tests, etc.), costs for treating side effects caused by a treatment, hospital charges, and other items. Analyses are performed on these studies to demonstrate the cost-effectiveness. By showing that the new drug overall costs less than another drug from a different company, the sponsor can increase the competitive advantage by marketing this new drug.

Results obtained from "outcomes research" studies can be used by the pharmaceutical company to promote the new drug. For example, if the new drug is competing against another drug treating the same disease, the company may be able to show that the new drug improved the patient's quality of life beyond the improvement provided by the competing medication. Based on the results from the pharmaco-economic studies, the company may also be able to demonstrate that the new drug brought overall savings to both the patients and the insurance carriers. These studies help evaluate other properties or characteristics of the new drug in addition to its medical value. The results from these studies may be used to increase the market potential for the new drug.

Finally, another type of study frequently found during the postmarketing stage is the study designed to use the new drug for additional indications (symptoms or diseases). A drug developed for disease A may also be useful for disease B, but the pharmaceutical company may not have sufficient resources (budget, manpower, etc.) to develop the drug for both indications at the same time. In this case, the sponsor may decide to develop the drug for disease A to obtain approval for drug to be on the market first, and then develop it to treat disease B. There are also other situations that this strategy can be useful. Hence, Phase III, IV studies designed for "new indications" are very common.

Occasionally, in postmarketing studies, we may see that a drug is efficacious at a lower dose than the dosage recommended in the drug label. This lower dose tends to provide a better safety profile. When this is the case, drug label could be changed to include the lower dose as one of the recommended doses. On the other hand, it is seen that the recommended dose may work for many patients, but the dose is not high enough for some other patients. When this is the case, an increase in dose may be necessary. Based on Phase IV clinical trials, if there is a need to label a higher dose, the sponsor would negotiate with the regulatory agencies to modify the drug label to allow a higher dose to be prescribed.

1.7   Concluding Remarks

Based on the drug development process described above, it is obvious that selecting the right dose for a new drug is a very important process. Without dose information, it is not possible for a physician to prescribe the drug to patients. One of the regulatory guiding documents describing the importance and practical difficulties in the study of the dose–response relationship is ICH (International Conference on Harmonization) E4 (1994) Guidance. Readers are encouraged to refer to this document for some of the regulatory viewpoints.

Studying and understanding the dose–response relationship for a new drug is an evolving, nonstop process. It started at the time when the new drug was first discovered in the laboratory. Unless this newly discovered compound shows increasing activities as the concentration increases, it would not be progressed into further development. This increasing relationship is continually studied in tissues, in animals, and eventually in humans. Phase I clinical trials are designed to collect information that will support the study of dose–response relationship for Phase II. Dosing information is one of the most important considerations in Phases II and III clinical studies. Finally, before, during and after the NDA process, dose selection is being considered by the sponsor, the regulatory agencies, and the general public. Even after the drug is approved and available on the market, new drug doses are still studied carefully and the level of investigation depends on responses observed from the general patient population. When necessary, dose adjustment based on postmarketing information is still a common practice.

References

Chow, S.C., and Liu, J.P. 1999. *Design and Analysis of Bioavailability and Bioequvalence Studies*. New York: Marcel Dekker.

Finney, D.J. 1978. *Statistical Methods in Bilogical Assay*. 3rd ed., London: Charles Griffin.

ICH-E4 Harmonized Tripartite Guideline. 1994. *Dose-Response Information to Support Drug Registration*.

Ruberg, S.J. 1995. Dose response studies I. Some design considerations. *Journal of Biopharmaceutical Statistics* 5(1):1–14.

Selwyn, M.R. 1988. *Preclinical Safety Assessment, Biopharmaceutical Statistics for Drug Development* (K.E. Peace, editor), New York: Marcel Dekker.

Ting, N. 2003. *Drug Development, Encyclopedia of Biopharmaceutical Statistics*. 2nd ed. New York: Marcel Dekker, pp. 317–324.

2
Dose Finding Based on Preclinical Studies

DAVID SALSBURG

2.1   Introduction

Before it can ever become a new drug, the candidate starts as a small molecule generated through a synthetic process or as a protein or antibody purified from a cell culture or from a modified animal or egg. There is often some biological theory that supports the creation of this candidate. It might be based upon inserting a specific human gene into the DNA of the culture, or some specific configuration of the small molecule that is designed to "fit" into a three-dimensional structure on the surface of a cell known as a receptor. It might, however, be a candidate generated by a mass process that creates a large number of different molecules of similar structure, that are then tested in a screen where microtubules contain specific types of cultured cells designed to "respond" in some measurable way to a "hit".

The creation of biologic and mass throughput screening for small molecules produce problems that can be approached with statistical techniques. However, these problems are beyond the scope of this book. Instead, we start with a nominated candidate, a chemical compound or biologic that has been selected as a potential drug. The next set of studies, both in vivo (within a living organism), and in vitro (outside of the living organism), are aimed at categorizing the dose response of this compound. To fix ideas, consider the rat foot edema assay.

An irritant substance is injected into one of the hind paws of a rat. After a fixed amount of time, the paw will swell with edema, due to inflammation. If the animal is medicated with an anti-inflammatory drug, the amount of swelling will be less. Both hind paws are measured by their displacement of a heavy fluid (usually mercury), and the difference in those measurements is the degree of inflammation. In a typical day's run, 5 to 10 animals will be left untreated, a similar number will be treated with a drug known to be an effective anti-inflammatory, and similar numbers will be treated with increasing doses of the new candidate drug.

This is an example of a modified three-point assay. In a three-point assay, the candidate is measured at two different dose levels, and a known active compound is measured at a known effective dose level. In a modified three-point assay, more than two doses of the candidate will be used, but only one dose of the known positive. A graph of log-dose versus effect is constructed as in Figure 2.1. The points of the candidate effects are used to produce a straight line. A parallel line is drawn through the effect of the positive control, and the antilog of the difference in the x-direction between those two lines is taken as the relative potency. If the relative potency, for instance, is 1:4 and the standard dose of the positive control is 5 mg/day, then we could predict that the candidate will be effective in human trials at 20 mg/day. The negative control is not used in this calculation. However, it is used to make an initial test of significance between the positive and negative controls. This test is used to discard runs that may have anomalous variability.

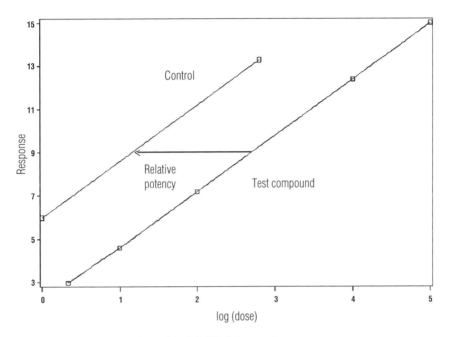

Figure 2.1. Modified three-point assay.

In an ideal world, this one study should be sufficient to establish the dose needed in human trials. Unfortunately, there is no such ideal world. Extrapolation of this initial assay assumes that (1) the dose–response lines are parallel, (2) the effect on the lab measurement is exactly the same as the effect on the clinical measure of patient response, (3) the new compound will be metabolized and be bio-available to the same degree that it was with the lab preparation, and (4) we can scale up the response on a simple mg/kg basis from lab animal to human.

It also requires the existence of a known positive as the "stalking horse". Few of these assumptions will hold true for most of the compounds, and, therefore, preclinical studies often require a number of different approaches to the problem, each with similar flaws when it comes to extrapolation. The use of different kinds of studies leads to further problems. It is axiomatic in biological research that if you ask the same question twice, you will get two different answers. The resulting ambiguity makes the choice of dose in humans difficult in most cases.

2.2   Parallel Line Assays

The phrase "three-point assay" was an attempt to establish quick and accurate tests of potency for digitalis preparations in the 1920s (see Burns, 1937). This assay used a standard of known potency and two titrations of the test material. A straight line was drawn between the two test results on a semi-log paper, another line was drawn parallel to that, through the result for the standard, and the relative potency was computed. Modern pharmacological studies use more than two doses of the test compound and usually include a negative control. However, the general approach is the same.

This type of assay can be conducted using live animals, preparations of animal tissue, or cell cultures. What are needed are a numerical response and a known positive compound. When the known positive is evaluated at more than one dose, there are two general ways that the data are analyzed. One method is to assume that the lines are parallel and to fit a restricted pair of straight lines with common slope, usually by least squares. The other method is to fit different lines to the standard and to the test compound. In that case, relative potency cannot be reported as a single number. Instead, the usual procedure is to report relative potency as a function of dose, or to report the relative potency at the animal dose equivalent to the human dose for the standard.

The previous paragraphs describe the computation of relative potency between two compounds. Potency is defined in Goodman and Gilman (1970, p. 20) as the difference in dose or log-dose between the dose associated with a minimum effect and the dose associated with a maximum effect. Although it is a useful concept in pharmacology, it provides very little information about the dose that might be useful in human trials. When there is no "stalking horse" available against which the relative potency can be estimated, then the problem is approached in a different fashion.

2.3   Competitive Binding Assays

The concept of competitive binding arises from the standard first-order chemical kinetics and this was most fully developed by Sir John Gaddum in the 1930's (Burgen and Mitchell, 1978). The idea here is that there are "receptor" sites on animal tissue. An "agonist" is a small molecule that fits into the receptor site and triggers the tissue to do something. If the tissue is a smooth muscle, it contracts. If it is glandular, it secretes some specific hormone. In animal preparations, as a whole, it might involve physiological changes such as drops in blood pressure. There is another small molecule called the "antagonist" which competes with the agonist for the receptor site. When the site is occupied by the antagonist, it blocks that site from the agonist and thus blocks the response.

In the Gaddum model, there are a fixed but large number of receptors and a larger number of agonist and antagonist molecules. For a given receptor site, the agonist and antagonist molecules compete with each other, but the binding is only fleeting. How the preparation responds as a whole depends on the percentage of sites responding to agonists. Thus, the degree of gross tissue response is a function of the relative proportions of agonist and antagonist molecules. To go further, we shall need a little notation. However, first, to fix ideas, consider a specific competitive binding assay: the guinea pig trachea response to beta-agonists.

A strip of trachea with its smooth muscle is suspended in a nutrient bath, one end anchored to the side of the bath, the other end anchored to a strain gauge. When the agonist is introduced into the flow of nutrient, the muscle contracts, and the degree of contraction is measured on the strain gauge. If the antagonist is also introduced, it will take a larger amount of agonist to produce the same degree of contraction. Although the guinea pig trachea is used here as a concrete example, this general model can be applied to any type of preparation where measurements of response can be made.

Let

A represent the event of a free agonist;
B represent the event of a free antagonist;
R represent the event of a receptor site;
AR represent the event of an agonist/receptor complex;
BR represent the event of an antagonist/receptor complex; and
(X) represent the number of events of type X.

First-order kinetics are changes in the amount of material of a given type, where the rate of change is proportional to the amount of material at a given time, described by the differential equation:

$$y'(t) = ky(t)$$

where k is the rate constant.

There is a probabilistic version of this, where the differential equation describes the expectation of a Poisson process. See McQuarrie (1967) for a complete derivation.

First-order kinetic relationships are typically symbolized as

$$X \xrightarrow{k} Y.$$

In the competitive binding model, the relationship between free agonist (or antagonist) and free receptors and a complex of agonist (or antagonist) and receptors is symbolized as

$$A + R \underset{k_{2A}}{\overset{k_{1A}}{\rightleftharpoons}} AR$$

$$B + R \underset{k_{2B}}{\overset{k_{1B}}{\rightleftharpoons}} BR$$

where k_{1A} is the rate constant governing the reaction

$$A + R \xrightarrow{k_{1A}} AR$$

where k_{2A} is the rate constant for the reaction

$$A + R \xleftarrow{k_{2A}} AR$$

Similarly, it is done for k_{1B} and k_{2B}.

We let the ratio of rate constants be

$$K_A = k_{1A}/k_{2A} \text{ and } K_B = k_{1B}/k_{2B}.$$

The first-order kinetic equations can be written as

$$d(A)(R)/dt = k_{1A}(A)(R)$$

$$d(AR)/dt = k_{2A}(AR).$$

At equilibrium, the rates of change in the total number of molecules and complexes are equal, and therefore,

$$k_{1A}(A)(R) = k_{2A}(AR) \quad \text{or} \quad K_A(A)(R) = (AR) \tag{2.1}$$

and similarly,

$$K_B(B)(R) = (BR). \tag{2.1'}$$

There are three types of complexes, AR, BR, and R (unbound receptors). The total number of receptors not bound to agonist A is

$$(R) + (BR) = (R)[1 + K_B(B)]. \tag{2.2}$$

If $a = $ the proportion of receptors bound to agonist A, then

$$a/(1 - a) = (AR)/[(R) + (BR)] = (R)K_A(A)/(R)[1 + K_B(B)] \tag{2.3}$$

or

$$K_A(A) = [a/(1 - a)][1 + K_B(B)]. \tag{2.4}$$

This derivation assumes that the same number of molecules of A and of B are needed to form a complex with a given receptor site. If, more generally, it takes n_A molecules of A and n_B molecules of B to form a complex, then

$$K_A(A)^{n_A} = [a/(1 - a)][1 + K_B(B)^{n_B}]. \tag{2.4'}$$

Formula (2.4') is not found in most of the pharmacology textbooks. Pharmacologists who are unaware of this general version sometimes try to force their data to fit the consequences of formula (2.4), even when the experimental data clearly indicate that n_A/n_B is considerably different from 1.0.

In an experimental set-up, we can saturate the solution with agonist and make our measurement on the tissue. Then, we can introduce a specific amount of antagonist and measure the difference in effect. The ratios of these two measures is proportionate to a, the proportion of receptor sites occupied by the agonist A in the presence of this amount of antagonist. The unknown kinetic constants are usually estimated in the following type of experiment.

Suppose the test compound is designed to be an antagonist, we introduce a fixed amount of the test compound. Then, for increasing levels of agonist, we measure the response of the preparation (as in the example of contraction of the trachea muscle). This leads to a sequence of sigmoidal curves of response ($= a$) versus log(A), as in Figure 2.2.

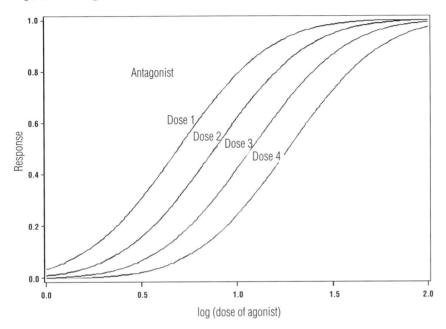

Figure 2.2. Parallel dose–response curves for increasing doses of agonist.

A few words about interpretation of graphs as seen in Figure 2.2: The parallelism of these curves assumes that the preparation has remained fresh and responds equally well across the time it takes to do the experiment. Careful pharmacologists include runs with a known antagonist from time to time to check on the ability of the preparation to continue responding. As the dose of antagonist increases, some of the binding may become noncompetitive, and the upper portion of the sigmoidal curve will fail to reach the maximum response level. It is very difficult to measure the response on a continuous basis, so the actual data usually consists of points at different levels of log (agonist). The response includes some random noise, and hence those points have to be fit to an appropriate sigmoid.

Many different methods have been proposed for fitting these data to a sigmoid, including probits, logits, and angle transformations. In practice, where the potency of the test compound is unknown, some of the curves will contain a large number of points on the lower end of the curve (where the tissue fails to respond to agonist). Inclusion of all these points can bias the estimates of rate constants that emerge.

According to a statistical folk theorem all the different models of sigmoid curves fit just as well in the center of the curve but differ greatly in the tails. It has been my experience that the best thing to do is to truncate the data points that appear to lie on either the lower or upper tail of the curve and fit a straight line to the middle. This procedure seems to lead to the most consistent estimates of the rate constants.

In 1949, Schild (1949) proposed a method of deriving a relative potency measure from this type of set up. Let

$$n = n_A/n_B.$$

Then formula (2.4′) becomes

$$K_A(A) = [a/(1 - a)][1 + K_B(B)^n] \tag{2.4″}$$

and to solve a, we have

$$a = K_A(A)/[1 + K_B(B)^n + K_A(A)]$$
$$= K_A e^{\log(A)}/[C_B + K_A e^{\log(A)}] \tag{2.5}$$

$$C_B = 1 + K_B(B)^n$$

and $C_B^{-1} = \exp\{-\log[1 + K_B(B)^n]\} = e^{-H}$

where $H = \log[1 + K_B(B)^n]$

or

$$a = K_A e^{\log(A)-H}/[1 + K_A e^{\log(A)-H}]. \tag{2.6}$$

Formula (2.6) is the theoretical description of the sigmoidal curves in Figure 2.2.

Let x be the multiple of A, needed to induce the same effect in the presence of (B) molecules of antagonist when (B) = 0. At (B) = 0, $x = 1$. Formula (2.5) implies

$$a/(1 - a) = xK_A(A)/[1 + K_B(B)^n] \tag{2.7}$$
$$= K_A(A) \quad \text{when} \quad (B) = 0. \tag{2.8}$$

When (B) is much smaller than (R), we can assume that (B) is close to zero and set (2.7) equal to (2.8), or

$$x/[1 + K_B(B)^n] = 1, \text{ or } x - 1 = K_B(B)^n$$
$$\log(x - 1) = \log(K_B) + n\log(B).$$

If we define the symbol pA_x by

$$pA_x = -\log(B), \quad \text{then}$$
$$\log(x - 1) = \log(K_B) - npA_x \tag{2.9}$$

which shows that $\log(x - 1)$ is linear in pA_x with slope $-n$.

We can now take at the center point of each sigmoid, the median doses of agonist needed to reduce the different doses of antagonist to the same effect, to derive values of x and pA_x. The plot of $\log(x - 1)$ versus pA_x should appear to be linear with slope $-n$. Schild suggested that we extrapolate that line to $x = 2$

and take the resulting value of pA_2 as a measure of the potency of the test compound. In fact, in most experimental set-ups pA_2 is not observable. It is well within the random noise at very low doses of agonist. However, it has the appeal of an easily explained measure. It is the dose of antagonist at which twice as much agonist is needed to have an effect than if the antagonist were not there. Families of compounds can be ordered by their values of pA_2, and relative potency can be computed. Where there are no other such compounds, the pA_2 can be taken as a minimally effective dose.

Pharmacologists who are unfamiliar with the more general version of Gaddum's model will sometimes try to fit a line with slope (-1) to the plot for estimating pA_2. It has been my experience that plots of pA_x versus $\log(1-x)$ tend to be quite linear, and deviations from a slope of -1 can be easily seen. In fact, it often happens that highly selective antagonists involve competitive binding where n is substantially greater than 1.0. Allowing the data to provide the estimate of $n (= n_A/n_B)$ produces much more accurate predictions of human doses than trying to force the points into a line with slope -1.

2.4 Anti-infective Drugs

The most successful extrapolation of dose directly from preclinical studies to humans occurs with anti-infective drugs. Candidates for potential use as anti-infective drugs are routinely tested against cell cultures of specific infectious agents. The concentration of drug needed to inhibit or kill the infective agent is determined by serial dilution of the candidate compound against specific cultures. This provides a spectrum of activity for the candidate drug.

It also provides the mean inhibitory concentration (MIC) for the compound against each of the specific infections. Once the candidate drug has passed safety tests in toxicology and has been introduced into human Phase I trials, the pharmacokinetic parameters of the drug in peripheral blood are estimated. If the pharmacokinetic parameters indicate that the MIC can be reached in peripheral blood, the compound is a candidate for an anti-infective drug against that particular agent, and the dose is determined by the pharmaco-kinetics as the dose that will produce the needed MIC for a sufficiently long period of time.

2.5 Biologic

Many biologic are proteins that produce highly specific responses in cell cultures or that produce antibody–antigen reactions in vitro. Radio-immune assays are available for specific antibody–antigen reactions, and so concentration of the biological candidates can be measured directly against its ability to form antibody–antigen complexes. Similarly, when proteins produce specific responses in cell cultures, the degree of response can be measured as a function of the concentration of the biologic.

Thus, the projection of human doses for most biologic is similar to the projection of human doses for anti-infective agents. Once the necessary concentration of the agent is determined, the human pharmaco-kinetics can be used to determine the dose that will produce that concentration.

2.6   Preclinical Toxicology Studies

Before going into human trials, candidate drugs and biologic undergo extensive safety evaluation in several species of animal. The legal requirements in the United States are spelled out in regulations promulgated by the Food and Drug Administration for the filing of an Investigational Drug Exemption (IND; U.S. Federal Register, 1988). The regulations call only for sufficient preclinical studies to "assure the safety and rights" of the human subjects who take part in Phase I, II, and III studies. Similar regulations govern the introduction of new drugs and biologic into human subjects in the European Union and other nations. In addition, guidelines such as ICH S2A (1996) have been issued from time to time, to describe the expected preclinical toxicology studies in greater detail. Mayne (1993) provides a general summary of the types of studies currently being used. Salsburg (1986) provides a detailed discussion of the methods of statistical analysis used in those studies.

The outcome of all toxicological studies will affect the attitude of regulatory authorities and the medical community about the new drug and may produce regulatory limitations on its use when it is marketed. However, only one type of study is actually used in setting the initial doses in human trials. This is the 60–90 day subchronic toxicity study.

Under current guidelines, subchronic studies are run on three species, at least one of which is nonrodent. In practice, this means rats, mice, and dogs are used for most drugs. For biologic that might induce severe immune reactions in other than human species, the subchronic studies are usually run on primates, often monkeys.

The fundamental law of toxicology was first stated by Paracelsus in the 16th century: "Only the dose makes a thing not a poison." Or, to put it in modern terms, everything is a poison at a sufficiently high dose, and everything is nontoxic at a sufficiently low dose. Because of this, it is widely recognized that acceptable toxicological studies must include at least one dose that is high enough to cause damage to the animal. To be acceptable for predicting human toxicity, it must also include at least one dose that has no apparent toxic effect on the animals.

The typical subchronic toxicology study will include a control group and at least three doses of the new compound. In cases where the new compound can be taken orally, it is usually introduced into the drinking water or food of the animals. In some cases, the taste or the mechanical properties of the compound cause the animals to reject it in food, and the material is force-fed by gavage. In cases where the test compound has to be injected, the control group is injected with the carrier. The highest dose used may be adjusted soon after the study begins to assure that the dose is high enough to induce a reduction in weight or some other obvious effect on the living animal.

One problem with the analysis of data from these studies is that highly social animals like mice are sometimes housed several in a single cage. If the test compound is introduced in food or water, there is no way of knowing how much individual animals may ingest, and the unit of experimentation becomes the cage.

At the end of the trial period, the animals are sacrificed and examined in terms of both gross and histopathology. In addition, blood and urine are taken from the animals over the course of the study to be analyzed.

The data and pathology from high-dose animals are examined to determine the lesions that can be associated with the test treatment. The pharmacology and other aspects of the test compound's biological activity are used to propose possible lesions that might be expected from the test material. These are identified if found in high-dose animals, along with unexpected abnormalities that might be seen. The controls are next examined to determine whether any of the abnormalities found in the high-dose group occurred there and can be attributed to the conditions of the study and not necessarily to the test treatment. From these examinations, the pathologists generate a set of putative lesions they might expect to see in the lower-dose groups. The putative lesions include both the observed lesions and any reasonable precursors that might be expected. For instance, if the high-dose animals have severe ulceration of the intestinal tract, a putative lesion would include both ulceration and the inflammation that might precede the development of ulcers.

Once a battery of putative lesions is assembled, the animals on lower doses are examined. The lowest dose that induced any of the putative lesions is considered an upper bound on the lowest dose that could induce toxicity. The highest dose that produced no animals with any of the putative lesions is labeled the "no observed effect level" (NOEL). If the high dose has not produced toxic lesions, the study is usually not accepted by regulatory authorities as an adequate one. If the lowest dose shows lesions, the study did not produce a NOEL, and it may also be necessary to redo it.

When three species are used, the lowest NOEL is usually taken for extrapolation to human trials. There are exceptions to this rule. For some compounds, one or more of the species may be unusually sensitive to the toxic effects of the treatment. For instance, rats are very sensitive to nonsteroidal anti-inflammatory drugs (NSAIDs) like aspirin and piroxicam. When rats are used in subchronic studies of these drugs, the toxic lesions in the stomach occur at doses far below those needed for efficacy in humans.

Once a NOEL is chosen, the first dose in man is taken as a submultiple of that. Usually, the first dose is 20% of the NOEL for new drugs, but there are no clear-cut regulations governing this choice. This entering dose in Phase I studies is the only use made of toxicology when it comes to setting doses in clinical studies. Once the sponsor develops experience with human dosing in Phase I studies, the limiting doses determined from those Phase I studies govern how high the doses can go in later studies.

An important exception to this occurs with cytotoxic drugs being developed for cancer chemotherapy. These drugs are designed to be toxic, albeit selectively, at the doses that will be used in humans. Doses chosen for Phase I studies are usually doses that were shown to have toxicity, but limited toxicity, in the animal studies. Unlike other drugs and biologic, where the Phase I studies use healthy volunteers, patients in Phase I studies for cytotoxic drugs are usually patients in the final stages of the cancer that will be treated.

An example of this can be seen in the development of Mithracin for the treatment of testicular cancer. Mithracin was discovered in mass screening of natural products for new antibiotics but discarded because it was as toxic to multicellular animals as it was to the bacteria. The National Cancer Institute pulled it into its standard mass screening of compounds, where it was shown to have an affinity for testicular tissue. The minimum toxic dose was used as an entering dose in human trials, and doses were slowly escalated. However, the doses that seemed effective in destroying human testicular cancers also produced severe internal bleeding in the patients. The drug was almost discarded until the clinicians began experimenting in humans with divided doses and eventually reached a regimen of dosing that is now used for this disease.

Mithracin is an extreme example of a fundamental principle in determining the toxicity of a new drug. The animal toxicology studies are useful for finding an entering dose into human studies. Thereafter, it is human experience that determines the limiting upper doses that can be used.

2.7   Extrapolating Dose from Animal to Human

There are many papers in the literature (especially in the toxicological literature) discussing whether doses can be extrapolated from animals to humans by assuming that the dose is proportional to weight or whether dose should be assumed proportional to body surface area. It has been my experience that, in most cases, it does not matter which is used. The difference is well within the prediction error of the methods.

It should be noted that no one is measuring the average body surface area of a given animal. Rather, body surface is estimated as the 2/3 power of the weight. If we consider the log transform, it can be seen that extrapolation by weight versus body surface involves the formula

$$\log(\text{dose in man}) = \log(\text{dose}) - \log(\text{weight})$$
$$\text{versus, for body surface extrapolation;}$$
$$\log(\text{dose in man}) = \log(\text{dose}) - 0.667 \log(\text{weight}).$$

If the standard deviation of the prediction runs about 1/3 the log-weight, then the difference between these two is within the random noise.

References

Burgen, A.S.V., and Mitchell, J.F. 1978. *Gaddum's Pharmacology*. 8th ed., London: Oxford University Press.

Burns, J.H. 1937. *Biological Standardization*. London: Oxford University Press.

Goodman, L.S., and Gilman, A. 1970. *The Pharmacological Basis of Therapeutics*. 4th ed., London: MacMillan.

ICH Guidance S2A. 1996. "Specific aspects of regulatory genotoxicity tests for pharmaceuticals," *International Conference on Harmonization*.

Mayne, J.T. 1993. "Preclinical drug safety evaluation," in *Drug Safety Assessment in Clinical Trials* (G. Sogliero-Gilbert, editor), New York: Marcel Dekker.

McQuarrie, D.A. 1967. Stochastic approach to chemical kinetics. *Journal of Applied Probability* 4:413–478.

Salsburg, D.S. 1986. *Statistics for Toxicologists*. New York: Marcel Dekker.

Schild, H.O. 1949. pA_x and competitive drug antagonism. *British Journal of Pharmacology* 4:277–280.

U.S. Federal Register 21-CFR1, Subpart B. 1988. *Investigational New Drug Application*. Sections 312.20–312.55.

3
Dose-Finding Studies in Phase I and Estimation of Maximally Tolerated Dose

MARLENE MODI

3.1 Introduction

Historically, drugs have been marketed at excessive doses (i.e., doses well onto the plateau of the efficacy dose–response relationship) with some patients experiencing adverse events (AEs) unnecessarily (Herxheimer, 1991; ICH-E4, 1994). Over the last 5 years, a greater effort has been made to ensure that the best benefit to risk assessment is obtained for each new drug (Andrews and Dombeck, 2004; Bush et al., 2005). The benefit to risk assessment of marketed drugs has been improved, in some cases, by postmarketing label changes, which aim to optimize the dosage regimen for the indicated populations (Cross et al., 2002). These postmarketing changes in the label may reflect the quality of drug development, regulatory review and postmarketing surveillance.

Information obtained in early clinical development about the average dose–response relationship in the intended patient population for a drug's desirable and undesirable effects is extraordinarily valuable, in that it lays the foundation for future dose–response studies (ICH-E4, 1994). Greater emphasis is being placed on the integration of information and ensuring effective decision-making during drug development. The pharmaceutical industrial sponsor of a compound is encouraged to discuss with health authorities as early as possible the type and number of clinical pharmacology studies that are needed to support labeling and approval. Also, the sponsor reviews with health authorities the use of preclinical and early clinical exposure–response information to guide the design of future dose–response, pharmacokinetic–pharmacodynamic (PK–PD) and clinical efficacy studies (FDA, 2003a,b). In this atmosphere of vigilance and information management, the selection of dose is considered a critical element of the benefit to risk assessment.

3.2 Basic Concepts

Initially, the development of a new chemical entity is influenced by its anticipated pharmacological actions in patients as suggested by its effects in animal models as well as its toxicology and PK profile in animals (Lesko et al., 2000; Peck et al., 1994). The severity of the disease state and the availability of effective and safe alternative treatments are also key factors in formulating a development plan. Each new chemical entity is evaluated against key parameters of a target profile. These key elements of the target profile are essentially the components of a draft label, which are updated as the compound proceeds through development.

In terms of facilitating drug development and increasing the likelihood of marketing a drug successfully, the inherent properties of an ideal drug are often contrasted with those of the new chemical entity. An ideal drug is effective in controlling or reversing the pathophysiology of the clinical condition for which the drug is intended. It does not adversely affect other disease processes or result in adverse interactions with other drugs. It can be administered over a broad range of doses with minimal toxicity. The ideal drug is uniformly metabolized or eliminated by other mechanisms in a predictable manner that is not altered by organ impairment and is not influenced by age, race or gender. Few, if any, drugs possess all of these characteristics.

Information collected during drug development accumulates with each new phase leading to an understanding of the drug's inherent properties that are consistently shown throughout all phases of development (Figure 3.1). A brief overview of these various phases of drug development is given in Chapter 1.

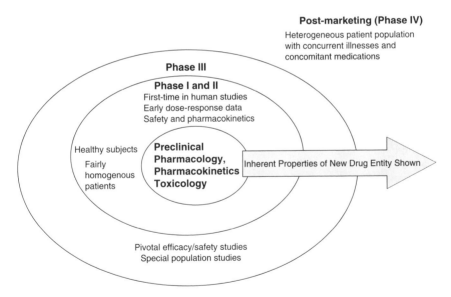

Figure 3.1. Information accumulates with each new phase of drug development and the drug's inherent properties become evident.

The information collected during drug development assists in determining the benefit-to-risk assessment for the heterogeneous population of patients that will be treated after the drug is approved for marketing. Adjustments are made to the proposed dosing regimen throughout the drug development process upon review of information related to the drug's safety profile, efficacy, and PK.

This chapter focuses on Phase I studies that are designed to provide preliminary but essential information on safety, tolerability, PK and if possible the pharmacological actions of a compound. The term Phase I has two connotations: one refers to the earliest, first-time-in-humans (FIH) studies, while the other encompasses studies of PK, metabolism, drug interactions, special populations, and other clinical pharmacology trials (ICH-E8, 1997). Dose selection is a critical activity for Phase I studies to ensure that the data collected in these clinical trials are at doses to support the recommended therapeutic dose. The purpose of dose-finding studies in Phase I is to evaluate: the compound's mechanism of action in humans, the compound's metabolic actions and PK, AEs associated with increasing doses of the compound and to gain early evidence of the compound's effectiveness (Code of Federal Regulations, 2004). A well-designed and executed Phase I program permits the design of well-controlled, scientifically valid, Phase II studies.

Traditionally, Phase I studies have been conducted in 20 to 80 young, healthy, male subjects; however, this is not a regulatory requirement (ICH-E8, 1997). Women of non-childbearing potential and older healthy subjects are now being included in early studies especially if the drug is intended for these populations. Initial evaluations in patients may be preferable for drugs with a low safety margin and in certain life-threatening disease states (see Chapters 4 and 5). Given that healthy subjects derive no benefit from receiving a new chemical entity, risk minimization is a critical ethical concern for Phase I studies (FDA, 1997; Tishler and Bartholomae, 2002).

3.3 General Considerations for FIH Studies

Ascending dose studies are usually the first clinical trials in the drug development process. The upper limit of a compound's therapeutic window is partially characterized in Phase I as these ascending dose studies usually determine the dose-limiting AEs that prevent the titration to higher doses. The primary objectives of these ascending dose studies are to estimate a maximally tolerated dose (MTD), to characterize the most frequently occurring AEs, and to gain a general understanding of the drug's PK and PD profile. The MTD is defined as the dose level below that producing unacceptable but reversible toxicity and is considered the upper limit of patient tolerance. This chapter focuses on general design concerns of Phase I clinical trials. The reader is referred to Chapters 4 and 5 for discussions of issues related to the design of dose-finding trials in life-threatening diseases.

The same pharmacological mechanisms that account for a drug's efficacy can account for many of its toxic effects, as most drug-induced (or treatment-emergent) AEs are expected extensions of a drug's known pharmacological properties (Rawlins and Thompson, 1991). These AEs are usually dose-dependent and can be predicted from animal studies. Thus, detailed knowledge of a drug's pharmacological actions assists in assessing for possible treatment-emergent AEs in the clinic. For example, both the AE of bradycardia (undesirable action) and the therapeutically desired reduction in blood pressure associated with the cardioselective beta-blocker, atenolol, are mediated through the drug's effect on beta-1 adrenergic receptors.

Treatment-emergent AEs may be unrelated to the drug's pharmacological action but may occur at higher doses or systemic exposures or upon chronic exposure to the drug. These types of AEs include withdrawal reactions, delayed reactions, failure of therapy and pharmacogenetic reactions (Edwards and Aronson, 2000). Unlike most treatment-emergent AEs, allergic drug reactions are unpredictable (Gruchalla, 2003). Some drugs (antimicrobial drugs, anticonvulsants, chemotherapeutic agents, heparin, insulin, protamine, and biologic response modifiers) are more likely to elicit clinically relevant immune responses.

Generally, ascending dose studies enroll too few subjects to observe treatment-emergent AEs that occur at a low to modest frequency. One way to visualize that only the most frequently occurring or common AEs are likely to be detected in FIH studies is to apply Hanley's Rule of Three (Hanley and Lippman-Hand, 1983). In order to ensure that one captures at least one occurrence of an AE happening at a frequency of 1:10 or greater at a 95% confidence level, the appropriate size of the safety database would be at least 30 subjects. Thus, given the small sample size of each dose group in the FIH study, it is common for these ascending dose studies to overestimate the MTD as the less frequently occurring treatment-emergent AEs and dose-limiting toxicities may not be detected (Buoen et al., 2003; Natarajan and O'Quigley, 2003).

3.3.1 Study Designs

A single dose is usually tested first, followed by multiple ascending dose studies; however, the study design is influenced by the type of compound. Study designs may be open-label, baseline-controlled or may use randomization and blinding. The most common study design used for these early studies is the parallel group, placebo-controlled, randomized, double-blind ascending dose study (Figure 3.2). Each group is typically made up of three to six subjects who receive single or multiple doses of the compound and one to two subjects who receive placebo. Safety and tolerability at the very least (in some cases PK and PD endpoints also) are evaluated before the next ascending dose group receives treatment.

Tolerability is an aspect of safety. It is a term used to indicate how well a patient is able to endure treatment such that AEs do not result in the discontinuation of treatment. A comparator drug, a marketed drug in the same class, can be included in the FIH study to evaluate the differences in tolerability between the two compounds if the comparator drug has a significant frequency of well-characterized AEs. The new chemical entity may possess a better tolerability profile than the comparator drug leading to a greater proportion of treated patients that successfully receive the full course of treatment.

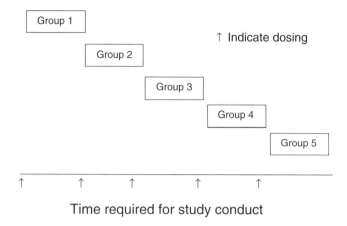

Figure 3.2. Parallel-group, placebo-controlled, randomized, double-blind ascending dose Phase I study design.

Given this early stage of drug development, not all subjects from the same dose group or cohort are dosed on the same day. This practice of spacing the dosing of subjects in a given dose group minimizes the number of subjects who are exposed to a given escalating dose of the drug and who are potentially at risk for a dose-limiting or irreversible toxicity of the drug. Should dose-limiting toxicities occur in the first few subjects of a dose group, dose escalation can be stopped without exposing all the subjects in a dose group.

Stopping rules for dose escalation need to be clearly described in the protocol. These may include reaching dose-limiting toxicities that define the MTD or seeing more frequent AEs than anticipated, that may influence the compliance of chronic administration (e.g., diarrhea or nausea). Stopping rules can also include clauses for evidence of unexpected or unique PK properties of the compound (e.g., dose- or time-dependent changes in clearance or volume of distribution, saturable absorption, presence of multiple active metabolites).

The stopping rules may be tailored for locally acting drugs or compounds with minimal toxicity. For these types of compounds, dose escalation may stop when the maximal feasible dose is reached. The maximal feasible dose is lower than the MTD, which cannot be estimated because it is not possible to administer high enough doses to reach the MTD. For some drugs where a good understanding of the pharmacological action of the drug exists in relation to the pathophysiology of the disease and efficacy of the drug, dose escalation may continue until the maximal pharmacological effect is reached in the absence of toxicity.

In general, only an average response for each dose group with respect to characterizing desirable or undesirable PD effects is obtained in the parallel-group, placebo-controlled, randomized, double-blind ascending dose study design. Although not easily appreciated, individual dose–response relationships may differ significantly from the population average relationship (see Chapter 1, Figure 1.1).

Table 3.1. Crossover, placebo-controlled, randomized, blinded study design

Group[a]	Treatment period 1	Treatment period 2	Treatment period 3
1	Placebo	Medium dose	High dose
2	Low dose	Placebo	High dose
3	Low dose	Medium dose	Placebo

[a] $N > 5$ per group

Another basic Phase I design is a crossover, placebo-controlled, randomized, blinded study (Table 3.1). In this design, a subject receives two dose levels and placebo in a randomized fashion. Like the parallel group design above, safety, tolerability, PK and PD data are evaluated before proceeding to the next treatment period. Stopping rules are clear and the study may be stopped or the doses modified based on information from the preceding treatment period. An individual subject's response is assessed at more than one dose level and before or after placebo treatment. There is a better understanding of an individual subject's contribution to the average dose response (FDA, 2003a).

The washout period between treatment periods in a crossover design is critical to ensure that there are no carryover effects from one period to another. This study design is inappropriate for drugs with long half-lives, for drugs with late toxicity, and if sensitization or tolerance develops. This study design is generally not used for FIH studies due to the general lack of information needed to rule out late toxicity, sensitization, tolerance, or to select an appropriate washout period. Sensitization is a phenomenon whereby the effects of a drug are augmented. Although it might sound counterintuitive, the same drug can evoke both tolerance and sensitization. Behavioral sensitization is a well-documented effect of repeated exposure to drugs such as amphetamine and cocaine (Pierce and Kalivas, 1997). Unlike transient drug effects, such as tolerance and withdrawal, behavioral sensitization can last as long as a year after the last drug administration in rats. The persistence of these effects implicates mechanisms distinct from those responsible for more transient drug effects.

Thus, for drugs with reversible desirable or undesirable actions, the crossover study design may provide a better understanding of the dose-concentration–response relationship than the parallel-group design as individuals receive two dose levels. In cases where it is unclear if the crossover design will be appropriate for a new chemical entity, a follow-up study to the traditional parallel-group FIH study may employ this design to better characterize individual dose- or exposure-response relationships.

3.3.2 Population

The description of the study population should identify important inclusion and exclusion criteria, demographic characteristics, baseline values of any clinically relevant variables that would be needed to understand the treatment effect related to safety, tolerability or PD. Other characteristics of the population that have implications to the extent that results can be generalized need to be clearly described (Friedman et al., 1998). Inclusion and exclusion criteria are defined according to population studied (i.e., healthy subjects or patients).

Phase I studies often include healthy subjects between 18 and 65 years old, and groups are balanced for sex and racial distribution. General exclusionary criteria are written to prevent the enrollment of subjects that are not in good health (e.g., those with evidence of underlying diseases, abnormalities, or organ impairment). Subjects are excluded if they have participated in a study with another investigational agent in the recent past or have known allergies to any of the components in the formulation of the new chemical entity or to any of the related class of compounds. Specific exclusionary criteria that are related to safety concerns may vary with the compound being studied. These specific exclusionary criteria are likely to arise due to the compound's mechanism of action (e.g., subjects with flu-like symptoms for an interferon-like drug are excluded as endogenous levels of interferon are elevated during the flu). Exclusionary criteria may also be related to preclinical toxicology findings.

There are times, however, when initial studies are best performed in patients. Often patients present with a different tolerability profile than healthy subjects (e.g., antipsychotic drugs are tolerated at significantly higher doses in patients). In some cases, the AE profile can only be studied in patients. Typically, this occurs when a drug is suspected or known to be unavoidably toxic such as those used in oncology or other life-threatening diseases. The target patient population should be considered for FIH studies when there is evidence from toxicology studies of irreversible, severe effects (e.g., cytotoxicity) or damage to an organ system, a steep toxicity dose–response curve, or the effects are not easily monitored.

Drugs for the treatment of diseases that affect the elderly are tested early in elderly subjects. Similarly, drugs intended for the treatment of diseases that typically affect women need to be tested in female subjects. In addition, the pharmacodynamic effects of the drug may be measurable only in patients (e.g., anti-hypertensive medications such as nifedipine have little or no effect on blood pressure in normotensive subjects or the glucose-lowering effect of a drug is best assessed in a diabetic patient).

The most salient issue with the administration of protein drugs is that they may induce antibody formation. Antibodies could cross react with the naturally occurring protein, conceivably neutralizing desired physiological effects in healthy subjects. This is another factor to consider when including healthy subjects versus patients.

In general, if patients are required in Phase I studies for drugs to be used in non-life-threatening diseases, patients with comorbid conditions who are receiving concomitant therapies other than for the disease under study are excluded. Phase I studies for drugs to be used in life-threatening diseases, on the other hand, may include patients who have not responded to previously administered marketed or investigational treatments. These patients are ill, may have other underlying conditions or diseases and a shortened life expectancy.

A large pool of healthy subjects willing to participate allows the rapid enrollment and completion of studies. Healthy subjects are in a normal, relatively low-risk state of health. Studies in healthy subjects offer important advantages in that they generally have a greater physiological reserve than patients do. If an AE should occur, a healthy subject is more likely to recover without suffering long-term negative consequences. Also, healthy subjects are better able to provide more frequent measures of PD endpoints and give a greater number of blood samples for PK. The drawback to enrolling healthy subjects is that pathophysiological mechanisms of the targeted disease state cannot be observed and can only rarely be accurately simulated.

3.4   Dose Selection

The most important variable in FIH studies is dose. The choice of the starting dose, dose increment for subsequent doses, and the maximal dose to be investigated are common issues that need to be addressed in the study design. Selecting a starting dose and choosing the next dose levels are challenging. An overly conservative approach may lead to an endless study, whereas a too rapid escalation can lead to unacceptable toxicity. Although not always obvious, the maximal dose considered for testing should be stated in the protocol and the rationale for the upper range of doses selected should be clearly described. It is understandable that this maximal dose may never be reached.

3.4.1   Estimating the Starting Dose in Phase I

A strategy has been proposed to determine the highest recommended starting dose of new therapeutics in adult healthy volunteers (FDA, 2002). The draft guidance presents a fairly simple method of estimating the starting dose. The maximum recommended starting dose (MRSD) in adult healthy subjects is to be derived from the no-observed adverse effect levels (NOAELs) in toxicology studies of the most appropriate species, the NOAELs converted to human equivalent doses (HED), and a safety factor is then applied. The method assumes that NOAELs and MTDs scale reasonably well across species and that the conversion to HED is reasonably accurate after normalizing dose by a body surface area (BSA) conversion factor. Another major assumption is that the determination of a NOAEL is unambiguous.

The draft guidance method for estimating a starting dose in adult healthy subjects relies solely on dose and does not employ systemic exposure data directly (Figure 3.3). While more quantitative modeling approaches are presented in other guidelines (FDA, 2003a), the draft guidance on estimating the starting dose does not recommend these approaches. However, all of the relevant preclinical data, including information on the pharmacologically active dose, the compound's full toxicology profile, and the compound's PK (absorption, distribution, metabolism, and excretion) is likely to be considered when determining the MRSD.

Toxicology studies generate basically three types of findings that can be used to determine the NOAEL: (1) overt toxicity (clinical signs, macro and microscopic

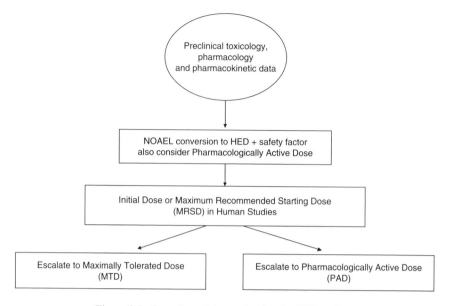

Figure 3.3. Overview of dose selection for FIH studies.

lesions), (2) surrogate markers of toxicity (serum liver enzyme levels), and (3) exaggerated pharmacodynamic effects (FDA, 2002; Sellers and du Souich, 2004). A recent review of current practices has revealed a lack of consistency in definition and application of frequently used terms such as no observed effect level (NOEL), NOAEL, adverse effect, biologically significant effect, or toxicologically significant effect (Lewis et al., 2002). Moreover, in review of current practices, no coherent criteria were found that were used to guide consistent interpretation of toxicity studies, including the recognition and differentiation between adverse effects and effects that are not considered adverse. As the interpretation of a compound's toxicology findings is the foundation of hazard and risk assessment, there is a need for consistent interpretation of toxicity (Lewis et al., 2002).

Toxicity should be avoided at the initial dose for the FIH study, but that does not necessarily mean that the starting dose will not possess any pharmacological activity. The pharmacologically active dose (PAD) should also be considered in that for a compound with limited toxicity, the PAD may be used to lower the estimate of the MRSD. However, in general, the HED is estimated from toxicology data in the most relevant species or alternatively, from the most sensitive species if the most relevant species is not known (FDA, 2002; Sellers and du Souich, 2004). Several factors could influence the choice of the most appropriate species including: (1) species differences in the compound's PK, (2) evidence indicating that a given species is predictive of human toxicity, and (3) limited cross-species pharmacological reactivity of the compound. This later point is especially important for biologic therapeutics in that many human proteins only bind to human or nonhuman primate targets, and thus species other than nonhuman primates would not be appropriate for estimation of the HED (ICH-S6, 1997).

The draft guidance advocates that the NOAEL for systemically administered compounds can be accurately extrapolated to other species and humans when doses are normalized to BSA (mg/m^2) (FDA, 2002). The work of Freireich et al. (1966) and Schein et al. (1970) using approximately 33 anti-neoplastic drugs provide the basis for this assumption. For these limited number of anti-neoplastic drugs, doses lethal to ten percent of rodents (LD$_{10}$) and MTDs in nonrodents both correlated with the human MTD when the doses were normalized to the same administration schedule and expressed in terms of BSA (i.e., mg/m^2).

Body surface area was introduced into medical oncology practice in order to derive at a safe starting dose for Phase I studies of anticancer drugs from preclinical animal toxicology data (Sawyer and Ratain, 2001). While cardiac output does correlate with BSA, the relationship between BSA and other physiologic measures relevant for drug metabolism and disposition and thus systemic exposure, such as renal and hepatic function, is weak or nonexistent (Sawyer and Ratain, 2001, Boxenbaum and Dilea, 1995, Mahmood and Balian, 1999). An analysis of the impact of allometric exponent (0.67 vs. 0.75) on the conversion of an animal dose to the HED using Eq. (3.1) is presented in Appendix A of the draft guidance (FDA, 2002).

The approach recommended in the draft guidance to convert an animal NOAEL to an HED is by using the following equation:

$$\text{HED} = \text{animal NOAEL} \times (W_{\text{animal}}/W_{\text{human}})(1 - b) \qquad (3.1)$$

where W is the weight in kg, b (equal to 0.67) is a correction factor used to convert mg/kg to mg/m^2 and the interspecies scaling factor is $(W_{\text{animal}}/W_{\text{human}})(1 - b)$.

The derivation of the interspecies scaling factor in Eq. (3.1) is presented in Appendix C of the same draft guidance. Inherent in the BSA normalization is the use of the factor, $W^{0.67}$. Other limited data besides that of Freireich et al. (1966) and Schein et al. (1970) suggest that the most accurate allometric exponent for normalizing MTDs of antineoplastic agents for interspecies extrapolation is $b = 0.75$ (FDA, 2002). Based on the analysis presented in Appendix A of the draft guidance and the premise that correcting for BSA increases clinical trial safety by resulting in a more conservative starting dose estimate, the guidance recommends that the approach of converting NOAEL doses to an HED based on BSA correction factors (i.e., $W^{0.67}$) be used for selecting starting doses of initial studies in adult healthy volunteers. Deviations from the surface area approach should be justified, and it is wise to calculate the initial dose to be used in adult healthy volunteer studies by multiple approaches (Reigner and Blesch, 2002).

Once the HED has been determined, a safety factor is applied to provide a margin of safety that allows for variability in extrapolating from animal toxicity studies to humans (FDA, 2002; Sellers and du Souich, 2004). This variability can result from: (1) uncertainties due to enhanced sensitivity to pharmacological activity in humans versus animals, (2) difficulties in detecting certain toxicities in animals, (3) differences in receptor densities or affinities, (4) unexpected toxicities and (5) interspecies differences in PK. In practice, the MRSD for the clinical trial is determined by dividing the HED by a default safety factor of 10.

In certain situations, the use of a safety factor greater than 10 is required. Criteria for using a safety factor greater than 10 include those related to toxicity such as: (1) a steep dose–response curve for important toxicities in the most relevant species or in multiple species, (2) severe toxicity or damage to an organ system in animals, (3) irreversible toxicity in animals, (4) nonmonitorable toxicity, (5) presence of significant toxicities without prodromal indicators and (6) nonpredictable and un-explained mortality. Other factors to consider include: (1) variable bioavailability between species, with poor bioavailability in the test species used to derive the HED, (2) large variability in doses or AUC levels eliciting a toxic effect, (3) questionable toxicology study design or conduct, such as few dose levels, wide dosing intervals, or large differences in responses between animals within dosing groups and (4) novel therapeutic targets. The safety factor should be increased when animal models with limited ability to evaluate the compound's toxicity are used. This may result because of very limited interspecies cross-reactivity or pronounced im-munogenicity (e.g., protein drugs likely to be pharmacologically active only in nonhuman primates), or because the compound's effect is elicited by mechanisms that are not known to be conserved between animals and humans (FDA, 2002; Sellers and du Souich, 2004).

Safety factors of less than 10 may be appropriate under some conditions (FDA, 2002; Sellers and du Souich, 2004): (1) the compound belongs to a well-characterized class, has a similar metabolic profile and bioavailability, presents similar toxicity across all the species tested including humans, and it is administered by the same route, schedule, and duration of administration, (2) the toxicity elicited is easily monitored, reversible and predictable, and a moderate to shallow dose–response relationship with toxicities are consistent across the tested species, and (3) the NOAEL is estimated from toxicity studies of longer duration than required for the proposed clinical schedule in healthy subjects. The toxicology testing in these cases should be of the highest caliber in both conduct and design.

3.4.2   Dose Escalation

It is not always necessary to escalate to doses as high as the MTD in the FIH studies. The highest single dose tested can also be defined as the pharmacologically active dose (PAD) giving the maximal effect in the absence of toxicity (Figure 3.3). However, the estimation of the PAD from preclinical pharmacology studies may not be possible if animal models of the disease are not available or the understanding of the fundamental biochemical or physiological aspects of the mechanism of action of the drug is lacking. Target site and receptors may be absent or modified in animal models precluding the estimation of the PAD in animals. Treatment in animals does not always lead to sufficiently sustained drug concentrations at the site of action in order to extrapolate the PAD to humans. PK may differ between species. Also, it is common to perform studies in animal models of disease using the intravenous or intraperitoneal route of administration which are unlikely to be the intended route of administration for patients. However, an estimation of pharmacologically active doses or targeted plasma concentrations is often helpful in guiding the dose escalation (Reigner and Blesch, 2002).

The choice of the dose escalation scheme is usually based on the type of toxicity and the steepness of the dose–response curve seen in toxicology and pharmacology experiments. Several classical methods for dose escalation have been described (Spilker, 1991): (1) starting dose (x) increased by an equal amount (x, 2x, 3x, etc.), (2) dose increased by equal percentage (e.g., by 100%), (3) modified Fibonacci (x, 2x, 3x, 5x, 7x, 9x, 12x, and 16x), and (4) a variant of the modified Fibonacci scheme where doses are increased by 100% until the first hint of toxicity followed by the modified Fibonacci scheme. Many of these methods have been traditionally used in Phase I studies in patients with cancer. A number of new study design proposals for anticancer agents address ethical concerns about treating excessive numbers of patients at subtherapeutic doses. These new study designs aim to increase the overall efficiency of the process while enhancing the precision of the recommended Phase II dose (see Chapters 4 and 5; Zhou, 2004).

Methods based on concentrations or PK guided dose escalation utilize PK parameters such as AUC or C_{max} from the preceding dose group to rationalize the dose increments for escalation (Vaidya and Vaidya, 1981; Graham and Workman, 1992; Reigner and Blesch, 2002). Doses are escalated to the MTD if appropriate, and AUC or a given PK parameter is monitored. In general, doses are escalated by doubling the dose until 40% of the AUC at the mouse LD_{10} is reached, and then conventional dose escalation begins. The underlying theme of this approach is that the AUC at the mouse LD_{10} is close to the MTD in humans although a different dose may be needed to achieve that AUC value in humans.

The PK–PD guided dose escalation can utilize target plasma concentrations established in animal models of disease and may provide a more rapid and safe completion of the FIH study as well as decrease the number of patients receiving a subtherapeutic dose. At each dose level, the PK and PD data are incorporated into an interactively updated PD model. Difficulties arise when the compound's PK differs substantially among species, dose-dependent or time-dependent changes in PK occur, or there is considerable inter- and intra-individual variability in PK or PD. In addition, it is unknown if maintaining these target plasma concentrations will ultimately lead to efficacy in the patient population. When using PK to escalate the dose, a maximally tolerated systemic exposure instead of MTD may be determined. This type of strategy can be seen as an application of the "concentration controlled clinical trial" design (Kraiczi et al., 2003).

Biomarkers can be defined as "physical signs or laboratory measurements that may be detected in association with a pathologic process and that may have putative diagnostic or prognostic utility". These can be measured objectively as indicators of biological or pathological processes or of the response to a therapeutic intervention (Rolan et al., 2003). Biomarkers can help guide dose escalation and may assist in understanding the dose–response relationship for the primary efficacy endpoint in Phases II or III (e.g., blood pressure and cholesterol reduction have been linked to heart attack or stroke-related mortality and have attained the status of surrogate endpoints; Temple, 1999). However, the shape of the dose–response relationship generated with biomarkers may differ from that of the primary efficacy endpoint, as long-term effects may not readily translate from the acute effects on the biomarker. Biomarkers may also be used to characterize the relationship between dose and undesirable effects (e.g., incidence and severity of neutropenia seen with interferon-like drugs) to facilitate the estimation of MTD.

3.5   Assessments

3.5.1   Safety and Tolerability

The use of randomization, blinding and a concurrent placebo-controlled group reduces the bias in safety assessments during the FIH study. Prespecified safety definitions (e.g., definition of dose-limiting toxicities and MTD) and stopping rules for dose escalation also ensure that safety and tolerability data are collected in an objective manner. Many have proposed that FIH studies be open-label and without concurrent placebo controls. For objective measures that are less susceptible to bias by the subject or investigator (e.g., AUC values), this could be a consideration. Unfortunately, AE reporting is often subjective.

The underlying objectives of safety and tolerability assessments in single dose FIH studies are to monitor for early signals of toxicity and to characterize the common treatment-emergent AEs. Consideration should be given to AEs that are likely after chronic use of the drug to reduce compliance in the intended patient population. Safety issues may result from the extension of the drug's pharmacological effects or be unrelated to the drug's pharmacological actions in that the toxicity is unexpected and was not seen in preclinical studies.

For multiple ascending dose studies, subchronic treatment-emergent AEs are characterized. The effect of multiple dosing on accumulation of a drug's systemic exposure is evaluated. For both single and multiple ascending dose studies, appropriate follow-up is needed to detect late toxicity (e.g., hepatotoxicity with fialuridine and antiretroviral agents; Styrt and Freiman, 1995; Kontorinis and Dieterich, 2003). Compounds that affect hematology parameters (e.g., red blood cells) may produce late toxicity like anemia, which may not appear until there has been enough time for the red blood cell population to turn over. In general, the follow-up period should not be less than four to five times the terminal half-life of the drug (provided this covers a significant portion of the AUC) or 4 weeks.

Early studies usually carefully monitor organ functions after single or multiple ascending doses (e.g., cardiovascular and pulmonary vital signs and electrocardiograms, hepatic, renal, and hematological laboratory parameters, and clinical signs and symptoms of target organ toxicity that have been identified in preclinical toxicology or pharmacology studies). One of the objectives of FIH studies is to monitor for early signals of severe toxicity, and humans are considered to be possibly more sensitive to the toxicity of the compound than the species used in toxicology studies. The critical organ functions to monitor are those identified in toxicology studies as being affected by the compound. However, a number of compounds exhibit safety concerns that were not initially detected in toxicology studies (e.g., hepatotoxicity). It is prudent to ensure that adequate safety assessments are included in the protocol to characterize the expected AEs and to identify early signals of severe or unexpected toxicity.

3.5.2 Pharmacokinetics

Most drugs have inter- and intra-subject variability in PK parameters of at least 20% to as much as several fold. Overlap in systemic exposure across various dose levels occurs when the variability in PK parameters is large (e.g., > fourfold in clearance) or if the increment in each dose escalation is low. If significant treatment–emergent events occur during a given dose escalation, it may be reasonable to repeat the same dose in the next group or proceed with a minimal dose increase.

A major objective underlying PK assessments is to detect an unexpected or unusual PK profile that could lead to severe toxicity. While important to detect, dose-dependent and time-dependent changes PK may be masked by the small sample sizes and considerable inter-subject variability in PK parameters. However, the FIH study is often the best study to show that a compound exhibits dose-independent and time-independent PK (i.e., clearance and volume of distribution is constant across doses and over time), as there are generally several dose levels tested and the PK sampling is more extensive in early studies. Further study may be required to characterize the mechanism of a compound's dose-dependent or time-dependent PK and to identify its source. PK data should be obtained rapidly from all dose groups in the single and multiple ascending dose studies if dose-dependent or time-dependent PK is suspected. If a drug exhibits dose-dependent PK such that small changes in dose have a significant effect on AUC, the drug's pharmacological effect may be increased disproportionately as well as its duration of action with increasing doses.

In multiple ascending dose studies, subjects are usually treated for several days beyond that needed to achieve steady state. PK data from the single dose FIH study is used to estimate the dosing frequency for the multiple dose study. These data are used to predict accumulation and the time required to reach steady-state plasma concentrations. In a broad qualitative sense, the appearance of metabolites are characterized in humans and compared with animal data. As drug development progresses, the PK profile of a compound is continuously refined such that predictions can be made about routes of elimination and potential drug interactions, and special populations can be identified.

3.5.3 Pharmacodynamics

It is important to determine if the drug's desired pharmacological effects occur at dose levels that humans can tolerate. Without this information, the estimated MTD cannot be put into context of a therapeutic window. For drugs with reversible pharmacological action that is readily quantifiable, PD becomes an important assessment in FIH studies. Desirable or undesirable pharmacodynamic effects may only be measurable in patients (e.g., anti-hypertensive agents). Often with antagonists, pharmacological activity can only be demonstrated with a provocative challenge. For example in exercise-induced asthma, a patient undergoes an exercise challenge to assess the pharmacological activity of a leukotriene antagonist as the targeted leukotriene pathway responsible for bronchoconstriction is operative only in the disease state (Adelroth et al., 1997).

Pharmacological effects, if these are related to exposure and are predictable from animal data, should be monitored by carefully observing subjects. If no exaggerated pharmacological effects are seen in healthy subjects and patients in early Phases I and II studies, then these exaggerated effects are unlikely to be seen in Phase III. However, it is possible that a drug could have an effect that might become apparent in patients, but was not seen in healthy subjects. The healthy subject's counter-regulatory system may be able to compensate whereas that of the patient may not. For example, counter-regulatory mechanisms induced by hypothermia include shivering, which can induce a fourfold increase in heat production, but at the expense of a 40 to 100% increase in oxygen consumption. Patients with coronary artery disease often have worse outcomes in hypothermia. However, for certain treatment–emergent events counter-regulatory mechanisms may be ineffective even in the healthy subject.

Major sources of variability in a patient's response to a given treatment are derived from PK, PD or the disease state itself provided that the patient is compliant. The drug may have a variable effect on the disease over time. For drugs having greater variability in PK than PD parameters, plasma concentration data may be better able than dose to predict the magnitude and duration of PD effects (FDA, 2003a). On the other hand, if PD variability is greater than PK variability, plasma concentration data may not predict the PD effect well. Sources of PK variability could include demographic factors (age, gender, and race), other diseases (renal or hepatic), diet, concomitant medications, and disease characteristics. Thus, assessing variability and identifying the sources of variability allows for a better understanding of the individual dose–response relationship for PD or efficacy endpoints.

Understanding a drug's pharmacological response is challenging due to the multifaceted nature of this endeavor. As a practical matter, it is easier to demonstrate a dose–response relationship for a PD effect that can be measured as a continuous or categorical variable, if the effect is obtained relatively rapidly after dosing and dissipates rapidly after therapy is stopped (e.g., blood pressure, analgesia, or bronchodilation) (FDA, 2003a). For drugs acting on the central nervous system, measuring the intensity of the pharmacological response is not always possible and several of the frequently used psychomotor performance tests suffer from limitations related to learning and practice effects (Di Bari et al., 2002). For this reason, it may not be possible to apply these tests repeatedly within the same subject.

For drugs used in the treatment of depression, anxiety and pain, rating scales are often used. The responses to rating scales may be subjective and variables such as motivation or fatigue can influence the results (Demyttenaere et al., 2005). The assessment of visual acuity in age-related macular degeneration requires the use of sham or placebo-control to minimize bias as the patient may try harder to see and lean forward during visual acuity assessments if he believes he is benefiting from treatment (Gragoudas et al., 2004). Knowledge of the disease state in relation to the selection of PD endpoints and examples of successful efforts with other drugs for the same indication or having the same mechanism of action provides a greater certainty that these data will be collected and analyzed appropriately and be ultimately usable.

PD endpoints which can be readily measured and exhibit the ideal characteristics (continuity, repeatability or the ability to obtain multiple measurements over time, reproducibility, sensitivity, and objectivity) often have an unclear relationship to the primary efficacy endpoint (Lesko et al., 2000). Sometimes the efficacy endpoint is delayed, persistent, or irreversible (e.g., stroke prevention, arthritis treatments with late onset response, survival in cancer, treatment of depression). Thus, it is not inconceivable that the shape of the dose or exposure or concentration–response relationship for the PD endpoint differs from that of the efficacy dose or concentration–response relationship (Figure 3.4).

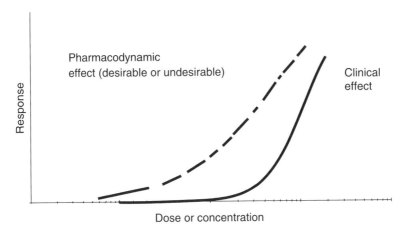

Figure 3.4. PD effect vs. clinical efficacy dose– or exposure–response relationships.

Clinical PK/PD data arise from complex and dynamic systems. Data from early studies are limited to single and short-term multiple dosing from a small number of individuals, and these data are unlikely to represent the full breadth of the intended patient population. Nonetheless, these data are invaluable in establishing exposure–response relationships that are further characterized in Phases II and III to provide a basis for dosage adjustment in subpopulations of interest and a rationale for the intended clinical dose (see Chapter 6). Various approaches have been used to model PK–PD or PD versus dose data (e.g., effect compartment, lag-time, PK–PD link, physiological feedback, indirect response models). These models in their most general form can be seen as relating PD effects to dose or exposure (see Chapter 14 for E_{max} model) to more extensive modeling efforts with successive links from dose to exposure to PD or efficacy endpoints (see Chapter 6).

3.6   Dose Selection for Phase II

In addition to examining dose or concentration response information from studies specifically designed to provide it, the entire database should be examined for possible desirable or undesirable PD effects that could be related to dose or concentration. If possible have an estimate from Phase I studies of the smallest dose that could provide any benefit. If quantifiable, select reasonable PD parameters to measure in Phase II in order to gain further information on the variability in PD and an early understanding of the influence of disease state on PD effects in Phase II. In addition, information about the relationship between PD and the proposed efficacy endpoint can be gathered in Phase II if not already known. The careful selection of PD endpoints or biomarkers are invaluable in understanding the dose or exposure response data as the development progresses from Phase I to II and reduces the likelihood of a failed Phase III study or a Phase III study where all doses rest on the plateau of the efficacy dose–response curve. Information on the duration of a PD effect along with PK data obtained in Phase I studies provides a basis for dosage interval or frequency. Identification of the common AEs and those associated with dose is extremely helpful in planning Phase II studies. Setting the upper limit of the dose range that will be explored by estimating the MTD in Phase I guides the selection of doses. While Phase I studies are generally small in size and have many limitations with respect to the breadth of information that can be gathered, a well designed Phase I program is essential for formulating hypotheses on how the drug works and forms the basis for the design of scientifically valid Phase II dose-ranging studies.

References

Adelroth, E., Inman, M.D., Summers, E., Pace, D., Modi, M., and O'Byrne, P.M. 1997. Prolonged protection against exercise-induced bronchoconstriction by the leukotriene D4-receptor antagonist cinalukast. *Journal of Allergy and Clinical Immunology* 99: 210–215.

Andrews, E., and Dombeck, M. 2004. The role of scientific evidence of risks and benefits in determining risk management policies for medications. *Pharmacoepidemiology and Drug Safety* 13:599–608.

Boxenbaum, H., and DiLea, C. 1995. First-time-in-human dose selection: Allometric thoughts and perspectives. *Journal of Clinical Pharmacology* 35:957–966.

Buoen, C., Holm, S., and Thomsen, M.S. 2003. Evaluation of the cohort size in Phase I dose escalation trials based on laboratory data. *Journal of Clinical Pharmacology* 43: 470–476.

Bush, J.K., Dai, W.S., Dieck, G.S., Hostelley, L.S., and Hassall, T. 2005. The art and science of risk management: A US research-based industry perspective. *Drug Safety* 28:1–18.

Code of Federal Regulations. 2004. *21 CFR312.21—Investigational new drug application—Phases of an investigation*.

Cross, J., Lee, H., Westelinck, A. Nelson, J., Grudzinskas, C., and Peck, C. 2002. Postmarketing drug dosage changes of 499 FDA-approved new molecular entities, 1980–1999. *Pharmacoepidemiology and Drug Safety* 11:439–446.

Demyttenaere, K., De Fruyt, J., and Stahl, S.M. (2005) The many faces of fatigue in major depressive disorder. *The International Journal of Neuropsychopharmacology* 8, 93–105.

Di Bari, M., Pahor, M., Barnard, M., Gades, N., Graney, M., Franse, L.V., Penninx, B.W., Marchionni, N., and Applegate, W.B., 2002. Evaluation and correction for a 'training effect' in the cognitive assessment of older adults. *Neuroepidemiology* 21:87–92.

Edwards, I.R., and Aronson, J.K. 2000. Adverse drug reactions: Definitions, diagnosis, and management. *Lancet* 356:1255–1259.

Food and Drug Administration. 1997. *Guidance for Industry: General Considerations for the Clinical Evaluation of Drugs*.

Food and Drug Administration. 2002. *Guidance for Industry: Estimating the Safe Starting Dose in Clinical Trials for Therapeutics in Adult Healthy Volunteers*.

Food and Drug Administration. 2003a. *Guidance for Industry: Exposure-Response Relationships – Study Designs, Data Analysis, and Regulatory Applications*.

Food and Drug Administration. 2003b. *Concept Paper: End-of-phase-2A Meetings with Sponsors Regarding Exposure-Response of IND and NDA Products*.

Freireich, E.J., Gehan, E.A., Rall, D.P., Schmidt, L.H., and Skipper, H.E. 1966. Quantitative comparison of toxicity of anticancer agents in mouse, rat, hamster, dog, monkey and man. *Cancer Chemotherapy Reports* 50:219–244.

Friedman, L.M., Furberg, C.D., and DeMets, D.L. 1998. "Study population," in *Fundametals of Clinical Trials*. 3rd ed., New York: Springer-Verlag, pp. 30–40.

Gragoudas, E.S., Adamis, A.P., Cunningham, E.T.Jr., Feinsod, M., and Guyer, D.R. 2004. Pegaptanib for neovascular age-related macular degeneration. *The New England Journal of Medicine* 351:2805–2816.

Graham, M.A., and Workman, P. 1992. The impact of pharmacokinetically guided dose escalation strategies in Phase I clinical trials: Critical evaluation and recommendations for future studies. *Annals of Oncology* 3:339–347.

Gruchalla, R.S. 2003. Drug allergy. *Journal of Allergy and Clinical Immunology* 111(2 Suppl):S548–S559.

Hanley, J.A., and Lippman-Hand, A. 1983. If nothing goes wrong, is everything all right? Interpreting zero numerators. *JAMA* 249:1743–1745.

Herxheimer, A. 1991. How much drug in the tablet? *Lancet* 337:346–348.

ICH-E4 Harmonized Tripartite Guideline. 1994. *Dose-Response Information to Support Drug Registration*.

ICH-E8 Harmonized Tripartite Guideline. 1997. *General Considerations for Clinical Trials*.

ICH-S6 Harmonized Tripartite Guideline. 1997. *Preclinical Safety Evaluation of Biotechnology-Derived Pharmaceuticals*.

Kontorinis, N., and Dieterich, D. 2003. Hepatotoxicity of antiretroviral therapy. *AIDS Reviews* 5, 36–43.

Kraiczi, H., Jang, T, Ludden, T., and Peck, C.C. 2003. Randomized concentration-controlled trials: Motivations, use and limitations. *Clinical Pharmacology and Therapeutics* 74:203–214.

Lesko, L.J., Rowland, M., Peck, C.C., and Blaschke, T.F. 2000. Optimizing the science of drug development: Opportunities for better candidate selection and accelerated evaluation in humans. *Journal of Clinical Pharmacology* 40:803–814.

Lewis, R.W., Billington, R., Debryune, E., Gamer, A., Lang, B., and Carpanini, F. 2002. Recognition of adverse and nonadverse effects in toxicity studies. *Toxicologic Pathology* 30:66–74.

Mahmood, I., and Balian, J.D. 1999. The pharmacokinetic principles behind scaling from preclinical results to Phase I protocols. *Clinical Pharmacokinetics* 36, 1–11.

Natarajan, L., and O'Quigley, J. 2003. Interval estimates of the probability of toxicity at the maximum tolerated dose for small samples. *Statistics in Medicine* 22:1829–1836.

Peck, C.C., Barr, W.H., Benet, L.Z., Collins, J., Desjardins, R.E., Furst, D.E., Harter, J.G., Levy, G., Ludden, T., Rodman, J.H., et al. 1994. Opportunities for integration of pharmacokinetics, pharmacodynamics, and toxicokinetics in rational drug development. *Journal of Clinical Pharmacology* 34:111–119.

Pierce, R.C., and Kalivas, P.W. 1997. A circuitry model of the expression of behavioural sensitization to amphetamine-like psychostimulants. *Brain Research. Brain Research Reviews* 25:192–216.

Rawlins, M.D., and Thompson, J.W. 1991. "Mechanisms of adverse drug reactions," in *Textbook of adverse drug reactions* (D.M. Davies, editor), Oxford: Oxford University Press, pp. 18–45.

Reigner, B.G., and Blesch, K.S. 2002. Estimating the starting dose for entry into humans: Principles and practice. *European Journal of Clinical Pharmacology* 57:835–845.

Rolan, P., Atkinson, A.J.Jr., and Lesko, L.J. 2003. Use of biomarkers from drug discovery through clinical practice: Report of the Ninth European Federation of Pharmaceutical Sciences Conference on Optimizing Drug Development. *Clinical Pharmacology and Therapeutics* 73:284–291.

Sawyer, M., and Ratain, M.J. 2001. Body surface area as a determinant of pharmacokinetics and drug dosing. *Investigational New Drugs* 19:171–177.

Schein, P.S., Davis, R.D., Carter, S., Newman, J., Schein, D.R., and Rall D.P. 1970. The evaluation of anticancer drugs in dogs and monkeys for the prediction of qualitative toxicities in man. *Clinical Pharmacology and Therapeutics* 11:3–40.

Sellers, E.M., and du Souich, P. 2004. "Phase I Studies (Human Pharmacology)," in *The IUPHAR compendium of basic principles for pharmacological research in humans* (P. du Souich, M. Orme and S. Erill, editors), Irvine, CA: International Union of Basic and Clinical Pharmacology, pp. 40–49.

Spilker, B. 1991. *Guide to Clinical Trials*. New York: Raven Press.

Styrt, B., and Freiman, J.P. 1995. Hepatotoxicity of antiviral agents. *Gastroenterology Clinics of North America* 24:839–852.

Temple, R. 1999. Are surrogate markers adequate to assess cardiovascular disease drugs? *JAMA* 282:790–795.

Tishler, C.L., and Bartholomae, S. 2002. The recruitment of normal healthy volunteers: A review of the literature and the use of financial incentives. *Journal of Clinical Pharmacology* 42:365–375.

Vaidya, A.B., and Vaidya, R.A. 1981. Initial human trials with an investigational new drug (Phase I and II) : Planning an management. *Journal of Postgraduate Medicine* 27: 197–213.

Zhou, Y. 2004. Choice of designs and doses for early phase trials. *Fundamental and Clinical Pharmacology* 18:373–378.

4
Dose-Finding in Oncology—Nonparametric Methods

ANASTASIA IVANOVA

4.1 Introduction

Phase I trials in oncology are conducted to obtain information on dose–toxicity relationship. Preclinical studies in animals define a dose with approximately 10% mortality (the murine LD_{10}). One-tenth or two-tenths of the murine equivalent of LD_{10}, expressed in milligrams per meters squared, is usually used as a starting dose in a Phase I trial. It is standard to choose a set of doses according to the modified Fibonacci sequence in which higher escalation steps have decreasing relative increments (100, 65, 50, 40, and 30% thereafter). Toxicity in oncology trials is graded using the National Cancer Institute Common Terminology Criteria for Adverse Events version 3.0 (available online from the Cancer Therapy Evaluation Program website http://ctep.cancer.gov). Toxicity is measured on a scale from 0 to 5. The dose limiting toxicity (DLT) is usually defined as treatment related non-hematological toxicity of Grade 3 or higher, or treatment related hematological toxicity of Grade 4 or higher. The toxicity outcome is typically binary (DLT/no DLT). The underlying assumption is that the probability of toxicity is a nondecreasing function of dose. The maximally tolerated dose (MTD) is statistically defined as the dose at which the probability of toxicity is equal to the maximally tolerated level, Γ. Alternatively, the MTD can be defined as the dose just below the lowest dose level with unacceptable toxicity rate Γ_U, $\Gamma < \Gamma_U$ (Rosenberger and Haines 2002). For example, the MTD can be defined as the dose level just below the lowest dose level where two or more out of six patients had toxicity. In the first definition, the MTD can be uniquely determined for any monotone dose–toxicity relationship; in the second, the MTD depends on the set of doses chosen for the study. In Phase I oncology studies, Γ ranges from 0.1 to 0.35. In oncology, unlike many other areas of medicine, dose-finding trials do not treat healthy volunteers, but rather patients who are ill and for whom other treatments did not work. An important ethical issue to consider in designing such trials (Ratain et al. 1993) is the need to minimize the number of patients treated at toxic doses. Therefore, patients in oncology dose-finding trials are assigned sequentially starting with the lowest dose.

Von Békésy (1947) and Dixon and Mood (1954) described an up-and-down design where the dose level increases following a nontoxic response and decreases if toxicity is observed. This procedure clusters the treatment distribution around the dose for which the probability of toxicity is equal to $\Gamma = 0.5$. To target any quantile Γ, Derman (1957) modified the decision rule of the design using a biased coin. Durham and Flournoy (1994; 1995) considered two biased coin designs in the spirit of Derman. Wetherill (1963) and Tsutakawa (1967a, b) proposed to assign patients in groups rather than one at a time. Group up-and-down designs can target a wide range of toxicity rates, Γ. Storer (1989) and Korn et al. (1994) used decision rules of group designs to suggest several designs for dose finding. Among the designs studied in Storer (1989) and Korn et al. (1994) were versions of the traditional or 3 + 3 design widely used in oncology.

Biased coin designs, group up-and-down designs, the traditional or 3 + 3 design, and its extension A + B designs (Lin and Shih 2001) are often referred to as nonparametric designs. Nonparametric designs are attractive because they are easy to understand and implement since the decision rule is intuitive and does not involve complicated calculations. Designs such as the continual reassessment method (O'Quigley et al. 1990) and the escalation with overdose control (Babb et al. 1998) are often referred to as parametric designs.

In this chapter, we describe the 3 + 3 design in Section 4.2. Basic properties of group up-and-down designs are given in Section 4.3. In Section 4.4, we review designs that use random sample size, such as the escalation and A + B designs. In Section 4.5, designs with fixed sample size are discussed. In Section 4.6, we describe more complex dose-finding situations such as trials with ordered groups and trials with more than one treatment.

4.2 Traditional or 3 + 3 Design

The most widely used design in oncology is the traditional design also known as the standard or 3 + 3 design. According to the 3 + 3 design, subjects are assigned in groups of three starting with the lowest dose with the following provisions:
  If only three patients have been assigned to the current dose so far, then:

- If no toxicities are observed in a cohort of three, the next three patients are assigned to the next higher dose level;
- If one toxicity is observed in a cohort of three, the next three patients are assigned to the same dose level;
- If two or more toxicities are observed at a dose, the MTD is considered to have been exceeded.

If six patients have been assigned to the current dose, then:

- If at most one toxicity is observed in six patients at the dose, the next three patients are assigned to the next higher dose level;

- If two or more toxicities are observed in six patients at the dose, the MTD is considered to have been exceeded.

The estimated MTD is the highest dose level with observed toxicity rate less than 0.33.

The properties of the $3 + 3$ design will be discussed later. To understand this design better we first describe group up-and-down designs.

4.3 Basic Properties of Group Up-and-Down Designs

Let $D = \{d_1, \ldots, d_K\}$ be the set of dose levels selected for the study. Let $P(d)$ denote the probability of toxicity at dose d, $p_j = P(d_j)$. We assume that $P(d)$ is an increasing function of d. The *group up-and-down design* is defined as follows.

Subjects are treated in cohorts of size s starting with the lowest dose. Let $X(d_j)$ be the number of toxicities in the most recent cohort assigned to dose d_j, $X(d_j) \sim$ Bin(s, p_j). Let c_L and c_U be two integers such that $0 \le c_L < c_U \le s$. Assume that the most recent cohort of subjects was assigned to dose level d_j, $j = 1, \ldots, K$. Then

(i) if $X(d_j) \le c_L$, the next cohort of s subjects is assigned to dose d_{j+1};
(ii) if $c_L < X(d_j) < c_U$, the dose is repeated for the next cohort of s subjects;
(iii) if $X(d_j) \ge c_U$, the next cohort of s subjects is assigned to dose d_{j-1}.

Appropriate adjustments are made at the lowest and highest doses. The process is continued until N subjects are treated. We will denote this design as UD(s, c_L, c_U).

Gezmu and Flournoy (2006) showed that assignments in group up-and-down design are clustered around the dose with toxicity rate Γ_s, where Γ_s is the solution of

$$\Pr\{\text{Bin}(s, \Gamma_s) \le c_L\} = \Pr\{\text{Bin}(s, \Gamma_s) \ge c_U\}. \tag{4.1}$$

That is, if there is a dose d_k such that $\Gamma_s = p_k$, the assignments are clustered around d_k. If $p_{k-1} < \Gamma_s < p_k$, the assignments are clustered around dose $k - 1$ or k (Ivanova, 2004).

The parameters s, c_L and c_U in a group up-and-down design are chosen so that Γ is approximately equal to Γ_s, the solution of Eq. (4.1). To find Γ_s, one needs to write (4.1) using formulae for Binomial probabilities. For example, for UD$(s, c_L = 0, c_U = 1)$, Eq. (4.1) has the form $(1 - \Gamma_s)^s = 1 - (1 - \Gamma_s)^s$ with the solution $\Gamma_s = 1 - (0.5)^{1/s}$. For most of the group up-and-down designs, closed form solutions of Eq. (4.1) do not exist but approximations can be easily obtained. Examples of group up-and-down designs can be found in Section 4.5.

4.4   Designs that Use Random Sample Size: Escalation and A + B Designs

4.4.1   Escalation and A + B Designs

In this section, we describe two types of designs that are used in dose-finding studies in oncology and other areas. Both designs do not need specification of the total sample size, since, ideally, experimentation is continued until the MTD is exceeded by one dose level. *The escalation design* is defined as follows.

Subjects are assigned in groups of size m starting with the lowest dose. Let C_U be an integer such that $0 \leq C_U < m$. Let $X(d_j)$ be the number of toxicities in a cohort of subjects assigned to dose d_j. Assume that the most recent cohort of subjects was assigned to dose level d_j, $j = 1, \ldots, K - 1$. Then

(i) if $X(d_j) \leq C_U$, the next cohort of m subjects is assigned to dose d_{j+1};
(ii) if $X(d_j) > C_U$, the trial is stopped.

The dose one level below the dose where $>C_U$ toxicities were observed is the estimated MTD.

The A + B design (Lin and Shih 2001) described below is a generalized version of the traditional or 3 + 3 design. It includes a stopping rule as in the escalation design but saves resources at lower doses. The design below does not allow dose de-escalation. We refer the reader to Lin and Shih (2001) for a description of A + B designs with the possibility of dose de-escalation. *The A + B design is* defined as follows.

Let A and B be positive integers. Let c_L, c_U, and C_U be integers such that $0 \leq c_L < c_U \leq A$, $c_U - c_L \geq 2$, and $c_L \leq C_U < A + B$. Let $X_A(d_j)$ be the number of toxicities in a cohort of size A assigned to dose d_j, and $X_{A+B}(d_j)$ be the number of toxicities in a cohort of size A + B. Subjects are treated in cohorts of size A starting with the lowest dose. Assume that the most recent cohort was a cohort of A subjects that has been treated at dose d_j, $j = 1, \ldots, K - 1$. Then

(i) if $X_A(d_j) \leq c_L$, the next cohort of A subjects is assigned to dose d_{j+1};
(ii) if $c_L < X_A(d_j) < c_U$, the cohort of B subjects is assigned to dose d_j; then, if in the combined cohort assigned to d_j, $X_{A+B}(d_j) \leq C_U$, the next cohort of size A receives dose d_{j+1}, otherwise the trial is stopped.
(iii) if $X_A(d_j) \geq c_U$, the trial is stopped.

The dose one level below the dose where unacceptable number of toxicities were observed ($\geq c_U$ toxicities in a cohort of size A or $>C_U$ toxicities in a cohort of size A + B) is the estimated MTD.

The escalation and A + B designs are constructed using general rules of group up-and-down designs. The escalation design is a group up-and-down design of the form UD(m, C_U, $C_U + 1$), with large group size. The trial is stopped as soon as the design calls for dose de-escalation. The A + B design is a combination of two group up-and-down designs UD(A, c_L, c_U) with $c_U - c_L \geq 2$ and UD(A + B, C_U, $C_U + 1$). The experimenter switches to the second design every time the first design calls for repeating the dose. The trial is stopped as soon as either design calls for dose de-escalation. In both designs, the frequency of stopping escalation at a certain dose level depends on toxicity rate at this dose as well as on toxicity at all lower dose levels. Ivanova (2006) outlined the general principles of how to select parameters in the escalation and A + B designs. Parameter C_U in the escalation design can be chosen so that $(C_U + 1)/m = \Gamma_U$, if Γ_U is specified, or $C_U/m = \Gamma$, if Γ is specified. For example, if $\Gamma_U = 0.33$, escalation design with $m = 6$ and $C_U = 1$ can be used.

Several A + B designs are presented in Table 4.1. The approximate range for Γ and the approximate value of Γ_U were computed as described in Ivanova (2006).

Table 4.1. Examples of A + B designs

Design parameters	Γ	Γ_U
A = B = 3, $c_L = 0$, $c_U = 2$, $C_U = 1$	$0.17 < \Gamma < 0.26$	$\Gamma_U = 0.33$
A = B = 4, $c_L = 0$, $c_U = 3$, $C_U = 2$	$0.25 < \Gamma < 0.31$	$\Gamma_U = 0.38$
A = B = 4, $c_L = 1$, $c_U = 3$, $C_U = 3$	$0.37 < \Gamma < 0.44$	$\Gamma_U = 0.50$
A = B = 5, $c_L = 0$, $c_U = 2$, $C_U = 1$	$0.10 < \Gamma < 0.15$	$\Gamma_U = 0.20$
A = B = 5, $c_L = 0$, $c_U = 3$, $C_U = 2$	$0.20 < \Gamma < 0.25$	$\Gamma_U = 0.30$
A = B = 5, $c_L = 1$, $c_U = 3$, $C_U = 3$	$0.30 < \Gamma < 0.35$	$\Gamma_U = 0.40$

4.4.2 The 3 + 3 Design as an A + B Design

The 3 + 3 design described in Section 4.2 can be found in Table 4.1 (Design 1). The dose most frequently selected by the 3 + 3 design has a toxicity rate above 0.17 and below 0.26 approximately. Simulation studies (Reiner et al. 1999; Lin et al. 2001) showed that the 3 + 3 design selects the dose with toxicity rate near 0.2. The approximate upper bound $\Gamma_U = 0.33$ of the probability of toxicity at the dose selected by the design is often quoted when the 3 + 3 design is described.

4.5   Designs that Use Fixed Sample Size

A trial with relatively large fixed sample size allows assigning a number of patients in the neighborhood of the MTD. The disadvantage of using a fixed sample size is that the starting dose can be too low and the sample size might not be large enough to observe a single toxic outcome in the trial or the number of toxicities in the trial might not be large enough to estimate the MTD well. The sample size usually varies from 18 to 36.

4.5.1   Group Up-and-Down Designs

In Section 4.3, we described the group up-and-down design and mentioned that the assignments for the design are clustered around the dose with probability of toxicity Γ, where Γ is the solution of Eq. (4.1). Recommended designs for different quantiles are given in Table 4.2. If the target toxicity rate is low, the group size needs to be rather large. For example, for $\Gamma = 0.1$ the group up-and-down with the smallest group size is UD($s = 6, 0, 1$). Often approximations of Γ need to be used. For example, the recommended designs for $\Gamma = 0.20$ are UD(3, 0, 1) with $\Gamma_s \approx 0.21$ or UD(5, 0, 2) with $\Gamma_s \approx 0.22$.

Table 4.2. Examples of group up-and-down designs

Targeted quantile	Group up-and-down design
$\Gamma = 0.10$	UD(6, 0, 1) with $\Gamma_s \approx 0.11$
$\Gamma = 0.20$	UD(3, 0, 1) with $\Gamma_s \approx 0.21$
	UD(5, 0, 2) with $\Gamma_s \approx 0.22$
	UD(6, 0, 2) with $\Gamma_s \approx 0.18$
$\Gamma = 0.25$	UD(4, 0, 2) with $\Gamma_s \approx 0.27$
	UD(6, 0, 3) with $\Gamma_s \approx 0.25$
$\Gamma = 0.30$	UD(2, 0, 1) with $\Gamma_s \approx 0.29$
	UD(4, 0, 2) with $\Gamma_s \approx 0.27$
	UD(5, 1, 2) with $\Gamma_s \approx 0.31$
	UD(6, 1, 3) with $\Gamma_s \approx 0.34$
$\Gamma = 0.50$	UD(1, 0, 1)* UD(4, 1, 3)*
	UD(2, 0, 2)* UD(5, 1, 4)*
	UD(3, 0, 3)* UD(6, 2, 4)*

*Targeted quantile Γ_s is exactly 0.50 for these designs.

4.5.2   Fully Sequential Designs for Phase I Clinical Trials

In a clinical setting, assigning subjects one at a time may be necessary due to time and logistical constraints. The biased coin designs (Durham et al. 1994; 1995) use the most recent outcome and a biased coin to determine the assignment of the next patient. These designs lose efficiency since they use the information from the most recent patient only. The moving average design (Ivanova et al. 2003) uses information from several subjects that have been assigned at the current dose and hence is more efficient than the biased coin designs. The moving average design has a decision rule of a group up-and-down design but uses data from the s most recent subjects instead of a new group of subjects.

4.5.3   Estimation of the MTD After the Trial

Designs that use fixed sample size require specifying an estimation procedure to use after the trial is completed. It had been shown by simulations that the isotonic regression based estimator works better than other estimators (Stylianou and Flournoy 2002; Ivanova et al. 2003). The isotonic regression estimator is essentially the maximum likelihood estimator for the isotonic model of the data. Let $N(d_j, n)$ be the number of patients assigned to dose d_j and $X(d_j, n)$ the number of toxicities at d_j after n patients have been dosed. Let $\hat{p}_j = X(d_j, n)/N_j(n)$ for all $j \in \{1, \ldots, K\}$ for which $X(d_j, n) > 0$, and $(\hat{p}_1, \ldots, \hat{p}_K)$ be the vector of these proportions. The vector of isotonic estimates $(\tilde{p}_1, \ldots, \tilde{p}_K)$ can be obtained from $(\hat{p}_1, \ldots, \hat{p}_K)$ by using the pool adjacent violators algorithm (Barlow et al. 1972). Stylianou and Flournoy (2002) described this process in detail. The dose with the value $\tilde{p}_i$ closest to Γ is the estimated MTD. If there are two of such values, the lowest of the doses is chosen except for the case where both doses have toxicity lower than Γ, in which case the higher of the two is chosen. Some authors suggested linear (Stylianou and Flournoy 2002) or logit interpolation (Ivanova et al. 2003). Methods that use interpolation allow for the estimated MTD to be between dose levels chosen for the trial.

4.6   More Complex Dose-Finding Trials

4.6.1   Trials with Ordered Groups

Sometimes patients can be stratified into two populations with possibly different susceptibility to toxicity. For example, UGT1A1 genotype might predict the occurrence of severe neutropenia during irinotecan therapy (Innocenti et al. 2004). In a study conducted by Innocenti et al. (2004), three out of six patients with the TA indel 7/7 genotype developed grade 4 neutropenia compared to 3 among 53 other patients. The two populations are referred to as *ordered* since it can be said that the probability of toxicity for the population with genotype 7/7 is the same or greater than the probability of toxicity at the same dose for the second population. Equally, the MTD (mg/m^2) for irinotecan is lower for patients with 7/7 genotype compared to other patients. Since MTDs are different, two trials need to be conducted, one for each subgroup. If one of the populations is far less prevalent, it might not be feasible to conduct both trials. One solution is to combine the two trials in one with the goal of finding two MTDs, one for each group. A parametric approach to this problem was proposed by O'Quigley et al. (1999) and O'Quigley and Paoletti (2003). Ivanova and Wang (2006) described a nonparametric design for the problem with two ordered groups and up to K dose levels tested. Assume without loss of generality that the first group is more susceptible to toxicity than the second, $G_1 \geq G_2$. Let $P^{(1 \geq 2)} = \{p_{ij}^{(1 \geq 2)}\}$ be the bivariate isotonic regression estimator (Robertson et al., 1988) of the toxicity rate for the two groups, $i = 1, 2, j = 1, \ldots, K$, obtained under the assumption $G_1 \geq G_2$ and the assumption that the probability of toxicity in each group is nondecreasing with dose. Subjects are assigned one at a time starting with dose d_1. Suppose that the most recent subject was assigned to dose d_j. Let $\tilde{p} = p_{ij}^{(1 \geq 2)}$ be the bivariate isotonic estimate of the probability of toxicity at the current dose with $i = 1$ or 2 according to the patient's group. The next subject from the same group is assigned to:

(i) dose d_{j+1}, if $\tilde{p} < \Gamma - \Delta$;

(ii) dose d_{j-1}, if $\tilde{p} > \Gamma + \Delta$;

(iii) dose d_j, if $\Gamma - \Delta \leq \tilde{p} \leq \Gamma + \Delta$.

Appropriate adjustments are made at the highest and lowest doses. Design parameter Δ was set to $\Delta = 0.05$.

4.6.2   Trials with Multiple Agents

It is common in oncology to treat patients with drug combinations. Often, the dose of one agent is fixed and the goal is to find the MTD of the other agent administered in combination. Sometimes, two or three doses of one of the agents are selected with the goal of finding the MTD of the second agent for each dose of the first agent. For example, Rowinsky et al. (1996) described a trial where five doses of topotecan and two doses of cisplatin were selected for the study. Since topotecan and cisplatin cause similar toxicities such as severe neutropenia and thrombocytopenia it was not possible to distinguish which drug caused toxicity. Ivanova and Wang (2004) suggested conducting a single trial that uses the assumption of toxicity monotonicity in both directions, that is, for each agent; toxicity is nondecreasing with dose when the dose of the other agent is fixed. Their nonparametric design for the problem uses the bivariate isotonic estimate of the probability of toxicity and is similar in spirit to the nonparametric design for ordered groups described in the previous section.

Thall et al. (2003) recently described a different setup for trials with multiple agents. The goal was to find one or more maximally tolerated combinations. Doses of both agents were increased simultaneously until the first toxicity was observed. Then nearby dose combinations were explored. They used a Bayesian (parametric) design with a five-parameter model.

4.7   Conclusion

Nonparametric designs are easy to understand by a practitioner and easier to use compared to parametric designs. These designs are flexible. Some, as the escalation and A + B designs, have an embedded stopping rule, others require specification of the sample size. All the designs mentioned in this chapter can be constructed for a wide range of values Γ. Simulation studies are a good tool to choose the best design and adequate sample size for the planned study.

Acknowledgements

The author would like to thank Vladimir Dragalin for helpful comments.

References

Babb, J., Rogatko, A., and Zacks, S. 1998. Cancer Phase I clinical trials: Efficient dose escalation with overdose control. *Statistics in Medicine* 17:1103–1120.

Barlow, R.E., Bartholomew, D.J., Bremner, J.M., and Brunk, H.D. 1972. *Statistical Inference under Order Restrictions.* New York: Wiley.

Derman, C. 1957. Nonparametric up and down experimentation. *Annals of Mathematical Statistics* 28:795–798.

Dixon, W.J., and Mood, A.M. 1954. A method for obtaining and analyzing sensitivity data. *Journal of the American Statistical Association* 43:109–126.

Durham, S.D., and Flournoy, N. 1994. "Random walks for quantile estimation," in *Statistical Decision Theory and Related Topics V* (S.S. Gupta and J.O. Berger, editors), New York: Springer-Verlag, pp. 467–476.

Durham, S.D., and Flournoy, N. 1995. "Up-and-down designs I. Stationary treatment distributions," in *Adaptive Designs* (N. Flournoy and W.F. Rosenberger, editors), Hayward, California: Institute of Mathematical Statistics pp. 139–157.

Gezmu, M., and Flournoy, N. 2006. Group up-and-down designs for dose-finding. *Journal of Statistical Planning and Inference*, in press.

Innocentt et al. 2004

Ivanova, A. 2004. Zoom-in designs for dose-finding in oncology. *UNC Technical report 04–03.*

Ivanova, A. 2006. Escalation, up-and-down and A + B designs for dose-finding trials. *Statistics in Medicine*, in press.

Ivanova, A., Montazer-Haghighi, A., Mohanty, S.G., and Durham, S.D. 2003. Improved up-and-down designs for Phase I trials. *Statistics in Medicine* 22:69–82.

Ivanova, A., and Wang, K. 2004. A nonparametric approach to the design and analysis of two-dimensional dose-finding trials. *Statistics in Medicine* 23:1861–1870.

Ivanova, A., and Wang, K. 2006. Bivariate isotonic design for dose-finding with ordered groups. *Statistics in Medicine*, in press.

Korn, E.L., Midthune, D., Chen, T.T., Rubinstein, L.V., Christian, M.C., and Simon, R.M. 1994. A comparison of two Phase I trial designs. *Statistics in Medicine* 13: 1799–1806.

Lin, Y., and Shih, W.J. 2001. Statistical properties of the traditional algorithm-based designs for Phase I cancer clinical trials. *Biostatistics* 2:203–215.

O'Quigley, J., Pepe, M., and Fisher L. 1990. Continual reassessment method: A practical design for Phase I clinical trials in cancer. *Biometrics* 46:33–48.

O'Quigley, J., Shen, J., and Gamst, A. 1999. Two-sample continual reassessment method. *Journal of Biopharmaceutical Statistics* 9:17–44.

O'Quigley, J., and Paoletti, X. 2003. Continual reassessment method for ordered groups. *Biometrics* 59:430–440.

Ratain, M.J., Mick, R., Schilsky, R.L., and Siegler, M. 1993. Statistical and ethical issues in the design and conduct of Phase I and II clinical trials of new anticancer agents. *Journal of National Cancer Institute* 85:1637–1643.

Reiner, E., Paoletti, X., and O'Quigley, J. 1999. Operating characteristics of the standard Phase I clinical trial design. *Computational Statistics and Data Analysis* 30:303–315.

Robertson, T., Wright, F.T., and Dykstra, RL. 1988. *Ordered Restricted Statistical Inference.* New York: Wiley.

Rosenberger W.F., and Haines, L.M. 2002. Competing designs for Phase I clinical trials: A review. *Statistics in Medicine* 21:2757–2770.

Rowinsky, E., Kaufmann, S., Baker, S., Grochow, L., Chen, T., Peereboom, D., Bowling, M., Sartorius, S., Ettinger, D., Forastiere, A., and Donehower, R. 1996. Sequences of topotecan and cisplatin: Phase I, pharmacologic, and in vitro studies to examine sequence. *Journal of Clinical Oncology* 14:3074–3084.

Storer, B.E. 1989. Design and analysis of Phase I clinical trials. *Biometrics* 45:925–937.

Stylianou, M., and Flournoy, N. 2002. Dose finding using isotonic regression estimates in an up-and-down biased coin design. *Biometrics* 58:171–177.

Thall, P., Millikan, R., Mueller, P., and Lee, S. 2003. Dose finding with two agents in Phase I oncology trials. *Biometrics* 59:487–496.

Tsutakawa, R.K. 1967a. Random walk design in bioassay. *Journal of the American Statistical Association* 62:842–856.

Tsutakawa, R.K. 1967b. Asymptotic properties of the block up-and-down method in bio-assay. *The Annals of Mahtematical Statistics,* 38:1822–1828.

von Békésy 1947. A new audiometer. *Acta Otolaryngology* 35:411–422.

Wetherill, G.B. 1963. Sequential estimation of quantal response curves. *Journal of the Royal Statistical Society B* 25:1–48.

5
Dose Finding in Oncology—Parametric Methods

MOURAD TIGHIOUART AND ANDRÉ ROGATKO

5.1 Introduction

The primary goal of a cancer Phase I clinical trial is to determine the dose of a new drug or combination of drugs for subsequent use in Phase II trials to evaluate its efficacy. The dose sought is typically referred to as the maximally tolerated dose (MTD) and its definition depends on the treatment under investigation, the severity and reversibility of its side effects, and on clinical attributes of the target patient population. Since it is generally assumed that toxicity is a prerequisite for optimal antitumor activity (see Wooley and Schein, 1979), the MTD of a cytotoxic agent typically corresponds to the highest dose associated with a tolerable level of toxicity. More precisely, the MTD γ is defined as the dose expected to produce some degree of medically unacceptable, dose limiting toxicity (DLT) in a specified proportion θ of patients (see Gatsonis and Greenhouse, 1992). Hence, we have

$$\text{Prob}\{\text{DLT}|\text{Dose} = \gamma\} = \theta$$

Due to the sequential nature of these trials, the small number of patients involved, and the severity of dose toxicity, designs with the following desirable properties are sought:

(1) A priori information about the drug from animal studies or similar trials should be easily implemented in the entertained model.
(2) The design should be adaptive (Storer, 1989), in the sense that uncertainty about the toxicity associated with the dose level to be given to the next patient (or cohort of patients) should be reduced when data collected thus far are taken into account.
(3) The design should control the probability of overdosing patients at each stage.
(4) The design should produce a sequence of doses that approaches the MTD as rapidly as possible.
(5) The design should take into account the heterogeneity nature of cancer Phase I clinical trial patients.

A number of statistical designs have been proposed and extensively studied in the past three decades. Nonparametric approaches to this problem have been developed by Durham and Flournoy (1994) and Gasparini and Eisele (2000). Within a parametric framework, a model for the dose–toxicity relationship is typically specified and the unknown parameters are estimated sequentially. Bayesian approaches to estimating these parameters are natural candidates for designs that satisfy properties (1) and (2) above. Among such designs, we mention the pioneering work of Tsutakawa (1972, 1980), Grieve (1987), and Racine et al. (1986). More recent Bayesian models include the continual reassessment method (CRM) of O'Quigley et al. (1990), escalation with overdose control (EWOC) described by Babb et al. (1998), the decision-theoretic approach of Whitehead and Brunier (1995), and constrained Bayesian C- and D-optimal designs proposed by Haines et al. (2003). The CRM and EWOC schemes both produce consistent sequences of doses in the sense that the sequence of doses converge to the "true" MTD in probability but EWOC takes into account the ethical constraint of overdosing patients. The last two designs are optimal in the sense of maximizing the efficiency of the estimate of the MTD. A discussion on the performance of these designs can be found in Rosenberger and Haines (2002).

In this chapter, we focus in one particular parametric, adaptive, and Bayesian method—EWOC—and present two real life applications where this approach was used. EWOC is the first statistical method to directly incorporate formal safety constraints into the design of cancer Phase I trials. In Section 5.2, we show how the method controls the frequency of overdosing by selecting dose levels for use in the trial so that the predicted proportion of patients administered a dose exceeding the MTD is equal to a specified feasibility bound. This approach allows more patients to be treated with potentially therapeutic doses of a promising new agent and fewer patients to suffer the deleterious effects of a toxic dose. EWOC has been used to design over a dozen of Phase I studies approved by the Research Review Committee and the Institute Review Board of the Fox Chase Cancer Center, Philadelphia. Also, EWOC was adopted by the University of Miami for its National Cancer Institute Cancer Therapy Evaluation Program (NCI/CTEP) approved study of Cytochlor, a new radio-sensitizing agent synthesized at UM. Additionally, EWOC has been used in trials sponsored by pharmaceutical companies such as Pharmacia-Upjohn, Jensen, and Bristol-Myers-Squibb.

In Section 5.3, we show how EWOC permits the utilization of information concerning individual patient differences in susceptibility to treatment. The extension of EWOC to covariate utilization made it the first method described to design cancer clinical trials that not only guides dose escalation but also permits personalization of the dose level for each specific patient, see Babb and Rogatko (2001) and Cheng et al. (2004). The method adjusts doses according to patient-specific characteristics and allows the dose to be escalated as quickly as possible while safeguarding against overdosing. The extension of EWOC to covariate utilization was implemented in four FDA approved Phase I studies. Section 5.4 addresses the issue of the choice of prior distributions by exploring a wide range of vague and informative priors. In Section 5.5, we give some final remarks and discussion of current and future work.

Based on the research work we describe in Sections 5.1 to 5.3, the EWOC methodology satisfies the above five desirable properties, and to our knowledge, no other design has been shown to be flexible enough to accommodate those properties simultaneously.

5.2   Escalation with Overdose Control Design

The main attribute underlying EWOC is that it is designed to approach the MTD as fast as possible subject to the ethical constraint that the predicted proportion of patients who receive an overdose does not exceed a specified value. The design has many advantages over some competing schemes such as up-and-down designs and continual reassessment method; see Babb et al. (1998). In this section, we describe the methodology in details and give a real-life example illustrating this technique.

5.2.1   EWOC Design

Let X_{min} and X_{max} denote the minimum and maximum dose levels available for use in the trial. One chooses these levels in the belief that X_{min} is safe when administered to humans and $\gamma \in [X_{min}, X_{max}]$ with prior (and hence posterior) probability 1. Denote by Y the indicator of toxicity. The dose–toxicity relationship is modeled parametrically as

$$P(Y = 1|\text{Dose} = x) = F(\beta_0 + \beta_1 x) \qquad (5.1)$$

where F is a specified cumulative distribution function. We assume that $\beta_1 > 0$ so that the probability of a DLT is a monotonic increasing function of dose. The model is reparameterized in terms of γ and ρ_0, the MTD and the probability of DLT at the starting dose, respectively. These parameters can be easily interpreted by the clinicians. This might be advantageous since γ is the parameter of interest and one often conducts preliminary studies at or near the starting dose so that one can select a meaningful informative prior for ρ_0. Assuming a logistic distribution for F, model (5.1) becomes

$$P(Y = 1|\text{Dose} = x) = \frac{\exp\left\{\ln\left[\dfrac{\rho_0}{(1 - \rho_0)}\right] + \ln\left[\dfrac{\theta(1 - \rho_0)}{\rho_0(1 - \theta)}\right]\dfrac{x}{\gamma}\right\}}{1 + \exp\left\{\ln\left[\dfrac{\rho_0}{(1 - \rho_0)}\right] + \ln\left[\dfrac{\theta(1 - \rho_0)}{\rho_0(1 - \theta)}\right]\dfrac{x}{\gamma}\right\}} \qquad (5.2)$$

Denote by y_i the response of the i th patient where $y_i = 1$ if the patient exhibits DLT and $y_i = 0$, otherwise. Let x_i be the dose administered to the ith patient and

$D_k = \{(x_i, y_i), i = 1, \ldots, k\}$ be the data after observing k patients. After specifying a prior distribution $h(\rho_0, \gamma)$ for (ρ_0, γ), denote by $\Pi_k(x)$ the marginal posterior cdf of γ given D_k. EWOC can be described as follows. The first patient receives the dose $x_1 = X_{\min}$ and conditional on the event $\{y_1 = 0\}$, the kth patient receives the dose $x_k = \Pi_k^{-1}(\alpha)$ so that the posterior probability of exceeding the MTD is equal to the feasibility bound α. Such a procedure is called Bayesian feasible of level $1-\alpha$, see Eichhorn and Zacks (1973); the corresponding sequence of doses generated by this design converges to the unknown MTD while minimizing the amount by which patients are underdosed. Calculation of the marginal posterior distribution of γ was performed using numerical integration. In practice, Phase I clinical trials are typically based on a small number of prespecified dose levels z_1, $z_2, \ldots, z_r$. In this case, the kth patient receives the dose

$$z_k = \max\{z_1, \ldots, z_r : z_i - x_k \le T_1 \text{ and } \Pi_k(x_k) - \alpha \le T_2\}$$

where T_1, and T_2 are nonnegative numbers we refer them as tolerances. The resulting dose sequence is Bayesian-feasible of level $1 - \alpha$ if and only if T_1 or T_2 is zero. We note that this design scheme does not require that we know all patient responses before we can treat a newly accrued patient. Instead, we can select the dose for the new patient based on the data currently available.

At the end of the trial, the MTD is estimated by minimizing the posterior expected loss with respect to some suitable loss function l. One should consider asymmetric loss functions since underestimation and overestimation have very different consequences. Indeed, the dose x_k selected by EWOC for the kth patient corresponds to the estimate of γ having minimal risk with respect to the asymmetric loss function

$$l_\alpha(x, \gamma) = \begin{cases} \alpha(\gamma - x) & \text{if } x \le \gamma \text{ that is, if } x \text{ is an underdose} \\ (1 - \alpha)(x - \gamma) & \text{if } x > \gamma \text{ that is, if } x \text{ is an overdose} \end{cases}$$

Note that the loss function l_α implies that for any $\delta > 0$, the loss incurred by treating a patient at δ units above the MTD is $(1 - \alpha)/\alpha$ times greater than the loss associated with treating the patient at δ units below the MTD. This interpretation might provide a meaningful basis for the selection of the feasibility bound.

The above methodology can be implemented using the user-friendly software of Rogatko et al. (2005).

5.2.2 Example

EWOC was used to design a Phase I clinical trial that involved the R115777 drug at Fox Chase Cancer Center in Philadelphia, USA in 1999. R115777 is a selective nonpeptidomimetic inhibitor of farnesyltransferase (FTase), one of several enzymes responsible for post-translational modification that is required for the function of p21(ras) and other proteins. This was a repeated dose, single center trial designed to determine the MTD of R115777 in patients with advanced incurable cancer, Hudes et al. (1999).

The dose-escalation scheme was designed to determine the MTD of R115777 when drug is administered orally for 12 hours during 21 days followed by a 7-day rest. Toxicity was assessed by the National Cancer Institute of Canada (NCIC) Expanded Common Toxicity Criteria. Dose limiting toxicity was determined by Week 3 of Cycle 1, as defined by Grade III nonhematological toxicity (with the exception of alopecia or nausea/vomiting) or hematological Grade IV toxicity with a possible, probable, or likely casual relationship to administration of R115777. Dosing continued until there was evidence of tumor progression or DLT leading to permanent discontinuation. The initial dose for this study was 60 mg/m^2 for 12 hours. Drug was supplied in 50 and 100 mg capsules, therefore the patients' dose was averaged to the closest 50 mg. In a previous pilot study, five patients received doses ranging from 100 to 300 mg/m^2 and no toxicity has been noted. An accelerated dose escalation scheme was then used whereby the dose of R115777 was increased by increments of approximately 50% in successive patients treated at 21-day intervals because no dose-limiting toxicity was encountered in any of the proceeding patients. The first patient received 240 mg/m^2, and doses for subsequent patients were selected from the set $\{360, 510, 750\}$ mg/m^2.

The dose of R115777 at which the first DLT occurred during Cycle 1 of treatment was denoted by Dl. Once a DLT occurred in any treated patient, all subsequent patients were assigned a dose based on the EWOC Algorithm using Dl as the dose upon which subsequent dose levels were derived.

Figure 5.1 shows the posterior distributions of the MTD as the trial progressed. The prior probability density function of (ρ_0, γ) was taken as

$$
h(\rho_0, \gamma) = \begin{cases} \dfrac{1}{180} & \text{if } (\rho_0, \gamma) \in [0, 0.333] \times [60, 600] \\ 0 & \text{otherwise} \end{cases}
$$

Thus, ρ_0 and γ are independent a priori, uniformly distributed over their corresponding interval. The EWOC scheme assumed (1) that the dose of R115777 below which the DLT was first observed is the safe starting dose, (2) that the maximum dose achieved will not exceed four times the value of D1, (3) that $\theta = 0.333$, and (4) that $\alpha = 0.3$. This modification of the EWOC scheme allowed rapid dose escalation at nontoxic doses of the drug, which resulted in a more efficient yet safe determination of the MTD.

Figure 5.2 shows the posterior density of the MTD after 10 patients have been treated. The posterior mode is 372, which corresponds to the 40th percentile of the distribution but by design, since $\alpha = 0.3$, patient 11 was given the dose 340.

5.3   Adjusting for Covariates

5.3.1   Model

In the previous section, the MTD was assumed to be the same for every member of the patient population; no allowance is made for individual patient differences in susceptibility to treatment. Recent developments in our understanding of the genetics of drug-metabolizing enzymes and the importance of individual patient

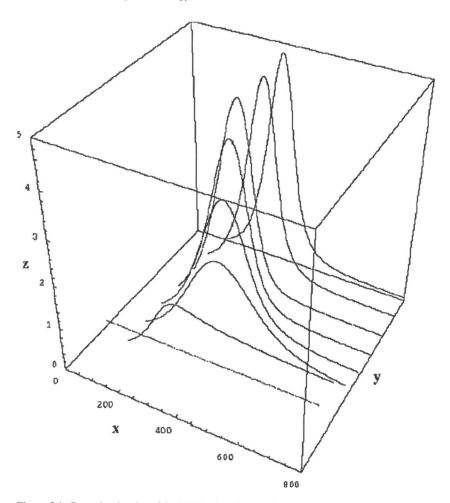

Figure 5.1. Posterior density of the MTD when the number of treated patients (from bottom to top) is 1, 5, 10, 15, 20, 25, 30, 33. The x-axis represents the MTD and the y-axis represents the number of patients.

differences in pharmacokinetic and relevant clinical parameters is leading to the development of new treatment paradigms (see for e.g., Decoster, 1989; Ratain, 1993).

In cancer clinical trials, the target patient population can often be partitioned according to some categorical assessment of susceptibility to treatment. A Phase I investigation can then be conducted to determine the appropriate dose for each patient subpopulation. As an example, the NCI currently accounts for the contribution of prior therapy by establishing separate MTDs for heavily pretreated and minimally pretreated patients. In such contexts, independent Phase I trials can be designed for each patient group according to the methods outlined above. Alternatively, a single trial might be conducted with relevant patient information

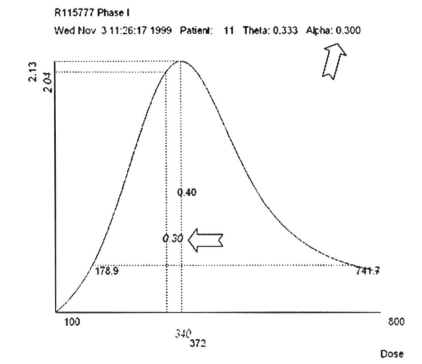

R115777 Phase I

Wed Nov 3 11:26:17 1999 Patient: 11 Theta: 0.333 Alpha: 0.300

Figure 5.2. Posterior density of the MTD after 10 patients have been treated.

directly incorporated into the trial design. Thus, the dose–toxicity relationship is modeled as a function of patient attributes represented by the vector c of covariate measurements. For simplicity of presentation, we consider the case where a single covariate observation c_i is obtained for the ith patient and the relationship between dose and response is characterized as

$$P(Y = 1 | \text{Dose} = x, \text{ Covariate} = c) = \frac{\exp\{\beta_0 + \beta_1 x + \beta_2 c\}}{1 + \exp\{\beta_0 + \beta_1 x + \beta_2 c\}}. \tag{5.3}$$

Assuming that the covariate assessment is made before the initial course of treatment, the dose recommended for Phase II testing can be tailored to individual patient needs. Specifically, the MTD for patients with covariate c is defined as the dose $\gamma(c)$ such that $P(Y = 1 \mid \text{dose} = \gamma(c), \text{ covariate} = c) = \theta$. In other words, $\gamma(c)$ is the dose that is expected to induce DLT in a proportion θ of patients with pretreatment covariate observation c. Since estimation of the MTD is the primary aim of cancer Phase I clinical trials and in order to accommodate prior information about the toxicity of the agent for selected groups of patients (if available), it is convenient to reparameterize model (5.3) in terms of $\gamma(c_0)$, $\rho_{x1}(c_1)$, and $\rho_{x2}(c_2)$ where $\gamma(c_0)$ is the maximally tolerated dose associated with a patient with covariate value c_0, and $\rho_{x1}(c_1)$, $\rho_{x2}(c_2)$ are the probabilities of DLT associated with patients with covariate values c_1 and c_2 when treated with dose levels x_1 and x_2, respectively.

5.3.2 Example

In this example, we describe the use of EWOC using the above reparameterization in a Phase I study of PNU-214565 (PNU) involving patients with advanced ade-nocarcinomas of gastrointestinal origin. Preclinical studies demonstrated that the action of PNU is moderated by the neutralizing capacity of anti-SEA antibodies. Based on this, the MTD was defined as a function of, and dose levels were ad-justed according to, each patient's plasma concentration of anti-SEA antibodies. Specifically, the MTD for patients with pretreatment anti-SEA concentration c was defined as the dose $\gamma(c)$ that results in a probability equal to $\theta = 0.1$ that a DLT will be manifest within 28 days. The small value chosen for θ reflects the severity of treatment attributable toxicities (for example, myelosuppression) observed in previous studies.

We assume that $\beta_1 > 0$ and $\beta_2 < 0$ in model (5.3) so that the probability of DLT is (1) an increasing function of dose for fixed anti-SEA, and (2) a decreasing function of anti-SEA for fixed dose since anti-SEA has a neutralizing effect on PNU. A previous clinical trial showed that patients could be safely treated at 0.5 ng/kg dose of PNU irrespective of their anti-SEA concentration. Furthermore, it was observed that patients with anti-SEA concentration equal to c (pmol/ml) could receive PNU doses up to the minimum of 3.5 and $c/30$ ng/kg without the induction of significant toxicity. Owing to the nature of the agent and as a precaution, it was also decided that no patient with anti-SEA titre greater than 5 pmol/ml should be administered a dose level greater than his/her pretreatment anti-SEA concentration.

Model (5.3) is re-expressed in terms of three parameters γ_{max}, ρ_1, and ρ_2 defined as follows. The maximally tolerated dose for patients with anti-SEA concentration c_2, $\gamma_{max} = \gamma(c_2)$, and the probabilities of DLT at dose level 0.5 ng/kg for patients with anti-SEA concentrations c_1 and c_2, $\rho_1 = \rho_{0.5}(c_1)$, and $\rho_2 = \rho_{0.5}(c_2)$. We took $c_1 = 0.01$ and $c_2 = 1800$ since these values span the range of anti-SEA concentrations expected in the trial. Since the probability of DLT at a given dose is a decreasing function of anti-SEA, we have $\rho_2 < \rho_1$. Furthermore, since the MTD was assumed to be greater than 0.5 ng/kg for all values of anti-SEA, we have $\rho_1 < \theta$. The prior distribution of $(\gamma_{max}, \rho_1, \rho_2)$ was then specified by assuming that γ_{max} and (ρ_1, ρ_2) are independent a priori, with (ρ_1, ρ_2) uniformly distributed on $\Omega = \{(x, y): 0 \le y \le x \le \theta\}$ and $\ln(\gamma_{max})$ uniformly distributed on the interval $[\ln(3.5), \ln(1000)]$.

The PNU trial was designed according to scheme described in Section 5.2. Ac-cordingly, each patient is administered the dose level corresponding to the αth fractile of the marginal posterior cumulative distribution function (CDF) of the MTD. Specifically, after $k - 1$ patients have been observed, the dose for the next patient accrued to the trial is $x_k(c) = \Pi_{k,c}^{-1}(\alpha)$, where $\Pi_{k,c}(x)$ is the marginal pos-terior CDF of the MTD $\gamma(c)$ given the data from the previous $k - 1$ patients. Prior to the onset of this trial, data from 76 patients with known pretreatment anti-SEA

concentration were treated with PNU. This data was used during the Phase I trial
in order to maximize statistical efficiency, see Babb et al. (2001) and Cheng et al.
(2004) for more details.

A total of 56 patients were treated in the Phase I trial of which three (5.4%)
experienced DLT. The data from patients with anti-SEA less than 100 pmol/ml,
treated either during or prior to the Phase I trial, are depicted in Figure 5.3. Patients
were observed to tolerate doses of PNU as high as 44% of their anti-SEA concentration without significant toxicity. None of the 96 patients treated at a dose less
than 7% of their anti-SEA concentration exhibited DLT. Of the 63 patients treated
with a dose greater than their anti-SEA/30 (the lowest permissible dose during the
Phase I trial), seven patients (11.1 per cent) manifest DLT, a rate of toxicity not
far above the targeted proportion $\theta = 0.1$.

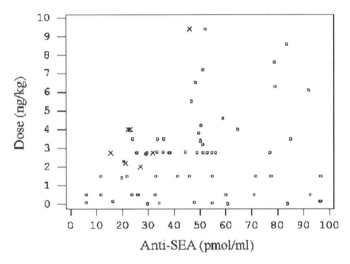

Figure 5.3. The dose level and anti-SEA of each Phase I patient with anti-SEA concentration
less than 100 pmol/ml. Patients experiencing treatment attributable dose limiting toxicity
(DLT) are indicated by a cross, those without DLT by an open circle.

Figure 5.4 shows the recommended dose level as a function of anti-SEA at both
the start and the conclusion of the trial. The latter (uppermost) curve corresponds
to the dose levels recommended for Phase II evaluation. At trial onset the recommended dose curve was nearly horizontal beyond an anti-SEA concentration
of 100 pmol/ml. In other words, nearly the same dose was recommended for all
patients with sufficiently high anti-SEA concentration. Essentially, this was a re-
flection of the fact that data from only 36 patients with anti-SEA greater than 100
were available at the start of the trial. Since all of these patients received a dose
less than 2.6% of their anti-SEA concentration (no dose exceeded 4 ng/kg) and
none experienced DLT, little was initially known about the effect of high anti-SEA
concentrations on treatment response. The amount of information gained during

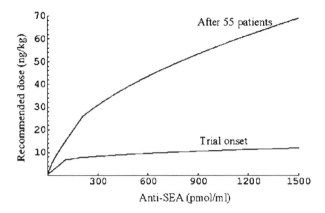

Figure 5.4. The recommended dose of PNU as a function of anti-SEA concentration at both the onset and the conclusion of the Phase I trial.

the trial is demonstrated in Figure 5.5 which shows the change in the marginal posterior distribution of $\gamma(5)$, the MTD for patients with anti-SEA equal to 5, from the start to the end of the Phase I trial.

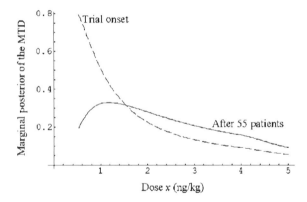

Figure 5.5. The marginal posterior distribution of the MTD for patients with anti-SEA concentration equal to 5 pmol/ml, at both the onset and the conclusion of the Phase I trial.

5.4   Choice of Prior Distributions

In this section, we address the issue of the choice of prior distributions. Specifically, we extend the class of restrictive priors used in Sections 5.2 and 5.3 by relaxing some of the constraints placed on (ρ_0, γ). We show through simulations that a candidate joint prior distribution for (ρ_0, γ) with negative a priori correlation between these two components results in a safer trial than the one that assumes independent priors for these two parameters while keeping the efficiency of the estimate of the MTD essentially unchanged.

5.4.1   Independent Priors

In Sections 5.2 and 5.3, we assumed that the support of the MTD was contained in $[X_{\min}, X_{\max}]$. That is, it was assumed that dose levels $X_{\min}$ and $X_{\max}$ could be identified a priori such that $\gamma \in [X_{\min}, X_{\max}]$ with prior (and hence posterior) probability 1. Although simulation studies showed that the logistic based model (5.2) works well in practice, the assumption that the support of γ is bounded from above is too restrictive. In the absence of toxicity, this assumption causes the dose escalation rate to slow down and in general, the target MTD will never be achieved if it lies outside the support of γ. Furthermore, because the support of the probability of DLT at the initial dose ρ_0 is $[0, \theta]$ and γ is a function of θ, the assumption of prior independence between ρ_0 and γ may not be realistic. Intuitively, the closer is ρ_0 to θ, the closer the MTD is to $X_{\min}$. We also note that when independent priors are specified for (β_0, β_1) as in Tsutakawa (1980) and Racine et al. (1986), then a negative correlation between ρ_0 and γ will result in the induced prior for these two parameters. Such observations are useful if a researcher plans to compare the EWOC methodology we described with the designs used in Tsutakawa (1980) and Racine et al. (1986). In the next section, we examine a class of prior distributions for (ρ_0, γ) defined on $[0, \theta] \times [X_{\min}, \infty)$ and study their properties through simulations.

5.4.2   Correlated Priors

For simplicity of notation, ρ_0, γ, and ν will denote both random variables and arguments of the corresponding densities.

Let ρ_0 be a random variable defined on $(0, \theta)$ and $\nu \sim N(b, \sigma_1^2)$ truncated to the interval $[b, \infty)$.

Given ρ_0 and ν, let $\gamma \sim N(\mu(\rho_0, \nu), \sigma_2^2)$ truncated to the interval (a, ν) with $a < \mu(\rho_0, \nu) < \nu$ and $a < b$. Denote by $g_{\mu(.)}(\gamma)$ the marginal distribution of γ. This density depends on the functional form of $\mu(\rho_0, \nu)$ specified below.

Model M_1: ρ_0 and γ are independent with $\rho_0 \sim U(0, \theta)$ and $\gamma \sim U(a, b)$.

Model M_2: ρ_0 and γ are independent with $\rho_0 \sim U(0, \theta)$ and γ has density $g_{\mu(.)}(\gamma)$ with $\mu(\rho_0, \nu) = (a + \nu)/2$. This prior allows the support of the MTD to extend beyond b and keeps a vague prior for ρ_0 on $(0, \theta)$.

Model M_3: ρ_0 and γ are independent with $\rho_0/\theta \sim \text{beta}(\alpha_1, \alpha_2)$ and γ has density $g_{\mu(.)}(\gamma)$ with $\mu(\rho_0, \nu) = (a + \nu)/2$. Again, the support of the MTD is extended to $[a, \infty)$ but the prior distribution for ρ_0 puts more mass near 0 for suitable choices of the hyperparameters α_1 and α_2 as in Gatsonis and Greenhouse (1992).

Model M_4: $\rho_0 \sim U(0, \theta)$ and γ has density $g_{\mu(.)}(\gamma)$ with $\mu(\rho_0, v) = (\rho_0/\theta) a + (1 - (\rho_0/\theta)) v$. Here, we introduced an a priori correlation structure between the MTD γ and ρ_0 by forcing the distribution of the MTD to concentrate towards its upper tail whenever the probability of DLT at the initial dose is close to 0.

Model M_5: $\rho_0/\theta \sim$ beta (α_1, α_2) and γ has density $g_{\mu(.)}(\gamma)$ with $\mu(\rho_0, v) = (\rho_0/\theta) a + (1 - (\rho_0/\theta)) v$. The prior structure is similar to that of model M_4 except that the prior distribution for ρ_0 puts more mass near 0 as in Model M_3.

Specification of the hyperparameters contained in the above prior distributions can be achieved with the help of clinicians and prior information about the agent. For more details about the selection of these hyperparameters and fitting the above five models in the Bayesian statistical software WinBugs (see Spiegelhalter et al., 1999; and Tighiouart et al., 2005).

5.4.3   Simulations

We compared the performance of models M_2 with M_4 and M_3 with M_5 by simulating a large number of trials from each model. An MCMC sampler based on the Metropolis-Hastings algorithm (Metropolis et al., 1953; Hastings, 1970) was devised to estimate features of the marginal posterior distribution of γ. For each of the above four models, we simulated 5000 trials, each consisting of $n = 30$ patients. Comparisons of these models were based on the proportion of patients that were assigned dose levels higher than the MTD, the proportion of patients exhibiting DLT, the average bias and the estimated MSE. We found that on the average, fewer patients were overdosed under M_4 compared to M_2 whereas the proportions of patients exhibiting dose limiting toxicity were about the same under these two models. The efficiency of the estimated MTD as measured by the root mean square error was about the same on the average. Based on the above remarks, we recommend the use of model M_4 with our proposed a priori correlation structure between ρ_0 and γ; while the efficiency of the estimated MTD is about the same under the two models; fewer patients are overdosed under model M_4. Under models M_3 and M_5, the prior distribution of the probability of dose-limiting toxicity at the initial dose is more concentrated toward zero. Since ρ_0 and γ are negatively correlated a priori under model M_5, this resulted in more patients being overdosed and exhibiting DLT under this model compared to model M_3. In other words, model M_5 uses a more aggressive scheme in search of the MTD. On the other hand, model M_5 performs much better in terms of the efficiency of the estimated MTD. Details on the above simulations can be found in Tighiouart et al. (2005).

5.5   Concluding Remarks

We described a dose-escalation scheme (EWOC) for cancer Phase I clinical trials that addresses the ethical demands that underlie cancer Phase I trials by selecting doses while controlling for the probability of overdosing patients. Simulation results presented in Babb et al. (1998) showed that (1) relative to CRM, EWOC overdosed a smaller proportion of patients, exhibited fewer dose-limiting toxicities and estimated the MTD with slightly lower average bias and marginally higher mean squared error, and (2) relative to the nonparametric dose escalation schemes, EWOC treated fewer patients at dose levels that were either subtherapeutic or severely toxic, treated a higher proportion of patients at doses near the MTD and estimated the MTD with lower average bias and mean squared error.

We also showed through a Phase I clinical trial how EWOC permits the utilization of information concerning individual patient differences in susceptibility to treatment. This extension to continuous covariate utilization made it the first method described to design cancer clinical trials that not only guides dose escalation but also permits personalization of the dose level for each specific patient. A priori information and uncertainty about the agent under consideration can easily be implemented into the methodology and the corresponding computations of dose allocations can be easily carried out using WinBugs. We are currently working on extensions of this methodology to accommodate more than one continuous covariate, utilization of categorical covariates, and ordered groups with respect to their susceptibility to treatment.

References

Babb, J.S., and Rogatko, A. 2001. Patient specific dosing in a cancer Phase I clinical trial. *Statistics in Medicine* **20**:2079–2090.

Babb, J.S., Rogatko, A., and Zacks, S. 1998. Cancer Phase I clinical Trials: efficient dose escalation with overdose control. *Statistics in Medicine* **17**:1103–1120.

Cheng, J., Langer, C., Aamdal, S., Robert, F., Engelhardt, L.R., Fernberg, O., Schiller, J. et al. (2004). Individualized patient dosing in Phase I clinical trials: The role of EWOC in PNU-214936. *Journal of Clinical Oncology* **22**:602–609.

Decoster, G., Stein, G., and Holdener, E.E. 1989. "Responses and toxic deaths in Phase I clinical trials," in *Sixth NCI-EORTC Symposium on New Drugs in Cancer Therapy*, Amsterdam, pp. 175–181.

Durham, S.D., and Flournoy, N. 1994. "Random walks for quantile estimation," in *Statistical Design Theory and Related Topics V* (Gupta, S.S., and Berger, J.O., editors), New York: Springer, pp. 467–476.

Eichhorn, B.H., and Zacks, S. 1973. Sequential search of an optimal dosage, I.*Journal of the American Statistical Association* **68**:594–598.

Gasparini, M., and Eisele, J. 2000. A curve-free method for Phase I clinical trials. *Biometrics* **56**:609–615.

Gatsonis, C., and Greenhouse J.B. 1992. Bayesian methods for Phase I clinical trials. *Statistics in Medicine* **11**:1377–1389.

Grieve, A.P. 1987. A Bayesian approach to the analysis of LD50 experiments. *Technical Report 8707*, CIBA-GEIGY AG, 1987.

Hudes, G., Schol, J., Babb, J., Rogatko, A., Bol, C., Horak, I., Langer, C., Goldstein, L. J., Szarka, C., Meropol, N. J., and Weiner, L. 1999. Phase I clinical and pharmacokinetic trial of the Farnesyltransferace inhibitor R115777 on a 21-day dosing schedule (meeting abstract). *American Society of Clinical Oncology*, 1999.

Haines, L.M., Perevozskaya, I., and Rosenberger, W.F. 2003. Bayesian optimal designs for Phase I clinical trials. *Biometrics* **59**:591–600.

Hastings, W.K. 1970. Monte Carlo Sampling Methods using Markov Chains and their Applications. *Biometrika* **57**:97–109.

Metropolis, N., Rosenbluth, A. W., Rosenbluth, M. N., Teller, A. H., and Teller, E. 1953. Equation of State Calculations by Fast Computing Machines. *Journal of Chemical Physics* **21**:1087–1092.

O'Quigley, J., Pepe, M., and Fisher, L. 1990. Continual reassessment method: A practical design for Phase 1 clinical trials in cancer. *Biometrics* **46**:33–48.

Racine, A., Grieve, A.P., Fluhler, H., and Smith, A.F.M. 1986. Bayesian methods in practice: Experiences in the pharmaceutical industry. *Applied Statistics* **35**:93–150.

Ratain, M.J., Mick, R., Schilsky, R.L., and Siegler, M. 1993. Statistical and ethical issues in the design and conduct of Phase I and II clinical trials of new anticancer agents. *Journal of the National Cancer Institute* **85**:1637–1643.

Rogatko, A., Tighiouart, M., and Xu, Z. 2005. *EWOC User's Guide Version 2.0.* Winship Cancer Institute, Emory University, Atlanta, GA. http://www.sph.emory.edu/BRI-WCI/ewoc.html

Rosenberger, W.F., and Haines, L.M. 2002. Competing designs for Phase I clinical trials: A review. *Statistics in Medicine* **21**:2757–2770.

Spiegelhalter, D.J., Thomas, A., and Best, N.G. 1999. *WinBUGS Version 1.2 User Manual.* MRC Biostatistics Unit.

Storer, B.E. 1989. Designs and analysis of Phase I clinical trials. *Biometrics* **45**:925–937.

Tighiouart, M., Rogatko, A., and Babb, J.S. 2005. Flexible Bayesian Methods for Cancer Phase I Clinical Trials: Dose escalation with overdose control. *Statistics in Medicine* **24**:2183–2196.

Tsutakawa, R.K. 1972. Design of experiment for bioassay. *Journal of the American Statistical Association* **67**:584–590.

Tsutakawa, R.K. 1980. Selection of dose levels for estimating a percentage point on a logistic quantal response curve. *Applied Statistics* **29**:25–33.

Whitehead, J., and Brunier, H. 1995. Bayesian decision procedures for dose determining-experiments. *Statistics in Medicine* **14**:885–893.

Wooley, P.V., and Schein, P.S. 1979. *Methods of Cancer Research*, New York: Academic Press.

6
Dose Response: Pharmacokinetic–Pharmacodynamic Approach

NICK HOLFORD

6.1 Exposure Response

Almost all clinical trials include responses measured over time. It is valuable to understand how these responses arise as a function of treatment dose and time. It is particularly important in planning and interpreting Phase IIB ("dose response") and Phase III ("confirmation of effectiveness") trials. This chapter describes how the dose–response relationship can be understood in pharmacological terms. It reviews the basic principles of clinical pharmacology (pharmacokinetics, pharmacodynamics, and disease progress) and shows how they can be used to describe the time course of response both with and without drug.

6.1.1 How Dose Response and Exposure Response Differ

A fundamental difference between dose response and exposure response arises because individuals differ in their responses when given the same dose. Exposure response methods explicitly recognize this and try to describe individual differences as well as the average dose–response relationship.

6.1.2 Why Exposure Response is More Informative

The exposure response approach is capable of describing and explaining the time course of response after a single dose or multiple doses. Unlike the usual dose response approach, which is usually defined by a primary endpoint at a single time, the concept of time is a necessary and fundamental part of understanding pharmacological effects and therapeutic responses to a drug. Dose response can be considered as the least informative form of exposure–response relationship. The time course of exposure can be inferred even if no concentration data are available (Holford and Peace, 1992a).

6.1.3 FDA Exposure Response Guidance

An important step was taken by the United States Food and Drug Administration (FDA) when it issued its Exposure Response Guidance (Food and Drug

Administration, 2003). This document clearly distinguished the pharmacokinetic and pharmacodynamic sources of variability in response to a dose and offers practical advice for implementation of exposure response analysis. Unfortunately, it only hints at incorporation of the time course of response and focuses on the use of simple pharmacokinetic statistics (AUC, C_{max}, C_{min}) as exposure variables rather than considering drug effects and responses as a consequence of the continuous time course of drug concentration.

6.2   Time Course of Response

6.2.1   Action, Effect, and Response

It is helpful to describe the pharmacological and pathophysiological consequences of drug exposure with three terms that are often considered synonyms (Holford and Peck, 1992).

Action—Refers to the mechanism at the primary target for the drug molecule, usually a receptor or enzyme, e.g., stimulation of an adrenergic beta-receptor in bronchial smooth muscle.

Effect—Describes the pathophysiological consequence of the drug action. There are typically several effects that might be observed, e.g., increase in cyclic AMP in bronchial tissue, relaxation of bronchial smooth muscle, increase in airway conductance, and increase in peak expiratory flow rate. These effects are frequently referred to as biomarkers (Lesko and Atkinson, 2001).

Response—This is the clinical outcome that the patient experiences by changes in how he/she feels, functions or survives, e.g., decreased difficulty breathing, reduced frequency of asthma attacks, shorter hospital stay, increased survival.

6.2.2   Models for Describing the
Time Course of Response

The guiding principle for exposure response is the belief that drug concentration is the primary causal factor in generation of a response (Holford and Sheiner, 1981). This differs from the apparent belief expressed by statisticians who analyze dose response as if the dose was the primary causal factor whether allopathic (response increases with increasing dose) or homeopathic (response decreases with increasing dose).

The concentration belief system leads to a simple partition of processes determining the dose–response relationship into pharmacokinetics and pharmacodynamics (Figure 6.1).

The dose-concentration process is described by pharmacokinetics. In almost all instances, this involves the time course of drug concentration in plasma. Frequently this is simplified to consider only the average steady-state concentration with consequent loss of information about the time course of concentration driving the response. The concentration–effect relationship is described by

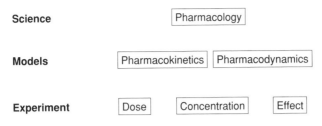

Figure 6.1. The components of the exposure–response relationship.

pharmacodynamics. The time course of effect subsequent to changes in drug concentration (e.g., in plasma) usually requires a further linking model to account for delays in effect.

In addition to changes produced by drug treatment, the time course of response also depends on the underlying progress of the disease, giving rise to the response and the placebo response in a clinical trial. Simple models for describing disease progress and placebo response can be useful for describing and interpreting the action of drugs.

6.3 Pharmacokinetics

6.3.1 *Review of Basic Elements of Pharmacokinetics*

The time course of drug concentration in plasma and other tissues of the body is determined by rates of input, distribution and elimination.

The input process will vary with the route of administration but most often can be adequately described by a single first-order or zero-order mechanism (sometimes with a lag time before the onset of appearance of drug at the site of measurement, e.g., plasma). It is helpful to distinguish between the extent of absorption, or bioavailability, of a dose and the rate of input of the bioavailable fraction. First-order input is described by the absorption half-life (typically 10 to 20 minutes for small molecules but may be much longer for pegylated molecules or monoclonal antibodies) while a zero-order input (for a given dose) is defined by the duration of input. The input duration is nominally under the control of the prescriber when the dose is given as an infusion. A constant rate of input may also be used to describe an oral formulation which may be largely determined by gastric emptying if the formulation dissolves rapidly (with an input duration of 30 to 60 minutes) or by the formulation itself if it is a controlled release product (with input durations measured in hours).

Distribution from the plasma (2.5 L/70 kg) to other tissues involves perfusion of the organ and diffusion from vessels into the extravascular space (18 L/70 kg) and in many cases into cellular water (35 L/70 kg total body water). Equilibration with tissues such as brain and heart typically takes place in minutes while adipose tissues may take hours and bone may take days to weeks. The rate of equilibration is often parameterized in terms of one or more intercompartmental clearances (see below). The apparent volume of distribution is defined by the ratio of the amount of drug in the body to drug concentration (Eq. (6.1)). The apparent volume is initially small and increases with time until the so-called steady-state volume of distribution is achieved when a pseudoequilibrium is reached between plasma and tissue concentrations. The initial volume of distribution is determined by rapidly equilibrating tissues such as plasma and extracellular fluid while the steady-state volume reflects partitioning and binding to extravascular tissues. Apparent volumes at steady state may range from a few liters (e.g., heparin) to several hundred liters (e.g., digoxin).

$$\text{Volume} = \frac{\text{Amount of drug in body}}{\text{Concentration}} \qquad (6.1)$$

Elimination occurs via excretion of unchanged drug through the kidneys, bile or gut and via metabolism primarily in the liver, but the gut wall also plays a key role for some drugs in reducing oral bioavailability. The concept of drug clearance is used to describe all processes of elimination (and can also be used to describe distribution). Clearance is defined by the ratio of elimination rate to drug concentration (Eq. (6.2)). When used to describe the ratio of distribution rate between compartments to the compartment concentration it is known as intercompartmental clearance:

$$\text{Clearance} = \frac{\text{Rate of Elimination}}{\text{Concentration}} \qquad (6.2)$$

6.3.2 Why the Clearance/Volume Parameterization is Preferred

Pharmacokinetic models can be expressed in a variety of parameterizations, e.g., volumes and half-lives or volumes and clearances. From a mechanistic perspective, the volume and clearance parameterization is preferable because the parameters can be directly linked to structural and functional properties of the body. Half-lives (e.g., of drug elimination) should be considered as secondary or derived parameters dependent on the more fundamental parameters of clearance and volume (Eq. (6.3)).

$$\text{Half-life} = \frac{\ln(2) \bullet \text{Volume}}{\text{Clearance}} \qquad (6.3)$$

Changes in half-life alone cannot be readily attributed specifically to changes in elimination or distribution. The cause of half-life changes can only be determined by looking at differences in clearance or volume.

6.4   Pharmacodynamics

6.4.1   Review of Basic Elements of Pharmacodynamics

Pharmacodynamics describes the concentration–effect relationship. The concentration is usually considered to be at the site of action and drug effects occur immediately in proportion to concentration. Delayed effects in relation to concentrations at other sites (e.g., plasma) are discussed below.

The law of mass action predicts the equilibrium occupancy of a receptor by a drug binding to the receptor-binding site with affinity defined by Kd, the equilibrium dissociation constant (Eq. (6.4)). The driving force for binding is the unbound drug concentration, Cunbound.

$$\text{Occupancy} = \frac{\text{Cunbound}}{\text{Kd} + \text{Cunbound}} \tag{6.4}$$

Occupancy leads to a stimulus in proportion to the intrinsic efficacy of the drug. Antagonists have an intrinsic efficacy of zero whereas agonists have intrinsic efficacy up to 1 (called a full agonist). The stimulus–response relationship (f) is typically nonlinear reaching half-maximum effect with a stimulus defined by S50 (Eq. (6.5)). Stimulus is a dimensionless quantity and f has an upper bound of 1.

$$f = \frac{\text{Stimulus}}{\text{S50} + \text{Stimulus}} \tag{6.5}$$

The drug effect, E, is defined by f and a scaling factor, efficacy or $E_{\max}$:

$$E = E_{\max} \cdot f \tag{6.6}$$

This leads to the common $E_{\max}$ model of drug action: $E_{\max}$ is directly related to intrinsic efficacy while EC50, the concentration at 50% of $E_{\max}$, is determined by Kd and S50 (Eq. (6.7)).

$$E = \frac{E_{\max} \cdot \text{Cunbound}}{\text{EC50} + \text{Cunbound}} \tag{6.7}$$

The nonlinear stimulus–response relationship means that most commonly EC50 is less than Kd, often by a factor of 10 or more. In vitro binding studies, which estimate Kd can only give limited guidance for the effective concentrations in vivo with an intact receptor–response system. This may be because in vitro and in vivo binding site conditions are different in terms of physiological substances near the binding site or feedback mechanisms that may affect binding.

6.5   Delayed Effects and Response

From a practical viewpoint drug pharmacokinetics are usually described in terms of plasma concentration because plasma is the most readily sampled site to obtain observations of concentration and thus develop models and estimate parameters. However, with very few exceptions (e.g., heparin effects on blood coagulation) drug actions and consequent effects are not exerted in plasma but in extravascular fluids or within cells. It is therefore naïve to expect that plasma concentrations would themselves be related directly to drug action and attempts to use simple correlation between plasma concentration and response are often doomed. It is not infrequent to find a statement such as "there was no correlation found between plasma concentration and effect." This kind of conclusion indicates the need to consider the basic mechanisms of clinical pharmacology and to separate fixed and random effects in an appropriate fashion.

A clear approach to understanding exposure and response requires thought about the necessary physical and physiological processes that are involved when using plasma concentration time course to predict drug action, effect, and response.

6.5.1   Two Main Mechanism Classes for Delayed Effects

There are two qualitatively different mechanisms linking plasma concentration time course to subsequent actions, effects, and responses. First, the drug molecule must be distributed to the site of action, e.g., at the cell surface in the extracellular fluid adjacent to a receptor. Second, a chain of events involving turnover of physiological mediators such as cyclic AMP, gene transcription factors, and proteins is required before the action is translated into an effect or clinical response. In almost all cases, both of these mechanisms are operative but the rate-limiting step will vary depending on the class of drug.

6.5.1.1   Distribution Delay

Distribution of a drug molecule to its site of action typically occurs quite rapidly and extracellular sites of action can be expected to be reached in minutes. This pharmacokinetic phenomenon of drug distribution may occasionally share a similar time course to the predicted tissue concentration derived from a compartmental pharmacokinetic model. However, in general, the concentration time course at the site of drug action is not reflected in the gross average of tissue and organ distribution predictable from observations of plasma concentration profiles. Direct measurement of concentrations in tissue samples gives a false sense of being "closer" to the site of action. Concentrations measured after homogenization of tissue are only gross mixtures of fine extracellular and intracellular compartments that truly reflect the site of action.

A solution to describing distribution delays comes from making two assumptions. First, that unbound drug concentrations in plasma and at the site of action are the same when distribution equilibrium occurs. This is quite plausible for passive diffusion of unbound unionized molecules. Second, that the observed effect is related to the concentration at the site of action according to some pharmacodynamic model, e.g., linear, E_{max} (Holford and Sheiner, 1981). This second assumption is harder to justify a priori but can often be rationalized by the adequacy of the model to describe the time course of effect and make acceptable predictions.

These assumptions are used to describe the time course of concentrations in an effect compartment driven by plasma concentrations. The time course of equilibration of the effect compartment is determined by a single parameter—the equilibration half-life. This model was originally parameterized in terms of the rate constant corresponding to this half-life (Segre, 1968; Sheiner et al., 1979), but the half-life parameterization is conceptually easier to grasp and relate to the observed effect or response.

Thiopental is a short acting barbiturate used to induce anesthesia. It is given intravenously usually by a short injection over a few seconds. The depth of anesthesia can be related to the frequency of electrical activity in the electroencephalogram (EEG). The EEG frequency changes lag behind changes in plasma thiopental concentration but can be easily linked using the effect compartment model. The delay in EEG effect will be determined by distribution to the brain, activation of GABA receptors and subsequent changes leading to altered electrical activity. It seems plausible that the rate limiting step is pharmacokinetic distribution and this is compatible with the short equilibration half-life of about 1 minute (Stanski, 1992a; Figure 6.2).

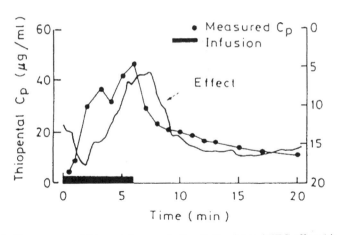

Figure 6.2. Time course of thiopental concentration (left axis) and EEG effect (right axis).

The EEG effect is a biomarker, which gives useful insight into the factors controlling individual response. These include the maximum effect (efficacy), sensitivity (EC50) and speed of onset (equilibration half-life). The slower onset of midazolam compared to similar drugs such as diazepam was responsible for substantial morbidity and mortality. Eventually the slow equilibration was identified as a key factor and a slower rate of administration and lower dose was introduced (Stanski, 1992).

6.5.1.2   Mediator Turnover

The role of mediator turnover as a major determinant of delay in drug effect was first identified by Nagashima and co-workers (Nagashima et al., 1969). This physiological alternative to the effect compartment model was described more generally and was subsequently classified into four basic mechanisms (Dayneka et al., 1993; Holford, 1991). These mechanisms have been termed indirect effects but it is more insightful to recognize that they demonstrate effects of drugs on the turnover of physiological mediators. PK PD models (often including an effect compartment model) can describe the drug action on the turnover process but it is the mechanistic understanding that comes from an appreciation of the mediator of the effect in a physiological sense that allows robust predictions of drug response.

Warfarin is an anticoagulant used to prevent morbidity and mortality associated with vascular thrombosis. Its action is to inhibit the recycling of vitamin K epoxide back to the active reduced form of vitamin K. Reduced vitamin K is a necessary cofactor for the synthesis of coagulation factors collectively termed the prothrombin complex. Inhibition of prothrombin complex synthesis leads to the slow elimination of these factors reaching a new lower steady state and decreased blood coagulability (Holford, 1986). The turnover half-life of these factors averages about 14 hours and it is the rate-limiting step in the onset of warfarin effects.

Delayed effects with apparent effect-compartment half-lives of hours rather than minutes should always raise the possibility that the delay is due to mediator turnover and is not due to pharmacokinetic distribution delay. Physiological mediator turnover (physiokinetic) delay is often substantial and frequently ignored in traditional dose response analyses. This leads to underestimation of the true treatment effect size and failure to properly account for carryover effects in crossover designs.

6.6   Cumulative Effects and Response

6.6.1   The Relevance of Considering Integral of Effect as the Outcome Variable

The most obvious applications of PK PD are to describe the time course of a drug effect or clinical response such as changes in blood pressure or pain. However, many clinical responses are more closely related to the cumulative effects of the drug. For example, the healing of a peptic ulcer is the consequence of cumulative inhibition of gastric acid secretion and increase in pH allowing tissue repair. The time course of changes after each dose may be important for acute symptomatic relief of pain, but it is the cumulative effect that leads to the healing response. Another example would be the use of a diuretic to treat acute pulmonary edema. The clinical benefit arises from the cumulative loss of fluid and is not determined by the effect of the drug at particular times after the dose.

6.6.2   Why Area Under the Curve of Concentration is not a Reliable Predictor of Cumulative Response

Many drugs are used at doses which reach concentrations above the EC50. Because of the nonlinear relationship of concentration to effect the integral of concentration with respect to time will not be proportional to the integral of the effect. When the clinical response is related to cumulative effect (i.e., its time integral) then summary measures of drug exposure such as area under the concentration time curve (AUC) will not properly predict the response.

6.6.3   Schedule Dependence

There is no clearly recognized definition of what constitutes schedule dependence. One way it might be defined is if the same total dose is given with different dosing schedules and the cumulative response varies then this is schedule dependence. On the other hand if the time of peak drug effect changes with dose then this would not be usually called schedule dependence. Nevertheless, changes in the timing and magnitude of neutropenia with different dosing schedule of anticancer drugs have been referred to as schedule dependent (Friberg et al., 2000).

The time course of furosemide concentration and its effect on renal sodium excretion is shown in Figure 6.3. Two dosing schedules are illustrated—a single dose of 120 mg and three doses of 40 mg given every 4 hours. The cumulative excretion of sodium (and thus the cumulative fluid loss) is 50% greater when three smaller doses are given over a 12-hour period. The total dose and the area under the concentration time curve (AUC) over 12 hours is the same for both dosing schedules but the cumulative effect is very different.

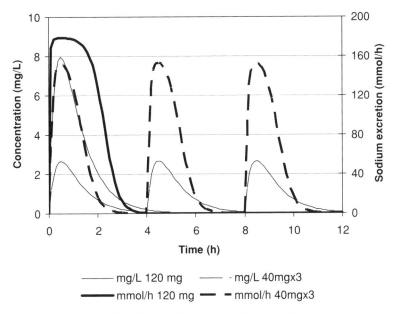

Figure 6.3. Furosemide concentrations and effects.

6.6.4   Predictability of Schedule Dependence

When cumulative drug effect determines clinical response then schedule dependence should be expected. Schedule dependence occurs because of the nonlinear concentration–effect relationship and also requires that the action of the drug is rapidly reversible.

There are two situations when cumulative effect and clinical response may not be schedule dependent. If the doses do not reach concentrations above the EC50 then the concentration–effect relationship will be essentially linear and schedule dependence will not occur. The other case is for drugs, which bind irreversibly to the site of action. Proton pump inhibitors bind irreversibly (e.g., omeprazole) and would be expected to have the same cumulative effect on acid suppression irrespective of the dosing schedule in one day because the turnover and regeneration of new pump molecules takes several days.

6.7   Disease Progress

All diseases have a time course of evolution and the clinical response to a drug will be dependent on this time course. Although experienced clinicians and patients will often have a good idea of this time course, it is unusual to find quantitative descriptions of disease progression.

6.7.1   The Time Course of Placebo Response and Disease Natural History

In the analysis of clinical trials, it is usual to consider the placebo response as if it was indistinguishable from the natural history of the disease. However, it is often plausible to assume that the disease and the placebo response will have different time courses. Slowly progressive diseases, e.g., those that change 10 to 20% over the time course of the trial can be approximated by a linear function even if the profile over longer periods has a more complex shape. It is also reasonable to assume that the disease progression continues at a constant rate. On the other hand, the response to a placebo might be expected to increase initially, reach a peak then fade away with time. The placebo response may be triggered by entry to a trial and be more or less independent of the timing of placebo dose administration or it may be triggered by each dose especially if the dosing event is very recognizable, e.g., placement of a transdermal patch every few days.

The overall response due to natural history and placebo can then be described by the sum of two functions which are separately identifiable (Holford and Peace, 1992a,b). This is illustrated in Figure 6.4 by a linear decline in response due to the natural history with an additional transient placebo response. The placebo response is defined empirically by the sum of two exponentials similar to the model used to describe drug concentrations with first order absorption and elimination. This is sometimes referred to as the Bateman function.

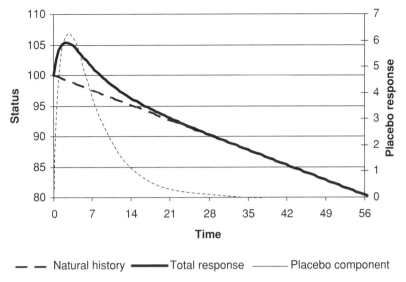

Figure 6.4. Natural history and placebo response (time units are arbitrary but could be interpreted as days).

6.7.2 Two Main Classes of Drug Effect

For any disease progress model, there are two distinct ways that a drug may affect the natural history of the disease. The first simply shifts the natural history curve producing an offset to the untreated time course of disease status. The second is to change the rate of progression of the disease. This is illustrated in Figure 6.5.

6.7.2.1 Symptomatic

The offset pattern of drug effect may also be called symptomatic because it is typically associated with responses that relieve a patient's symptoms (e.g., pain) without any permanent effect on the disease. The response is transient and when treatment is stopped, the effect washes out and the disease state returns to the natural history curve.

The use of cholinesterase inhibitors such as tacrine to treat Alzheimer's disease has had limited success. The effects appear to be purely symptomatic with no evidence that the rate of progression of the disease is slowed (Holford and Peace, 1994) by treatment.

6.7.2.2 Protective

Effects on the rate of disease progression can be considered to be protective. If the direction of progression is reversed, they may even be called curative. When treatment is stopped, it would be expected that treatment effects persist. In

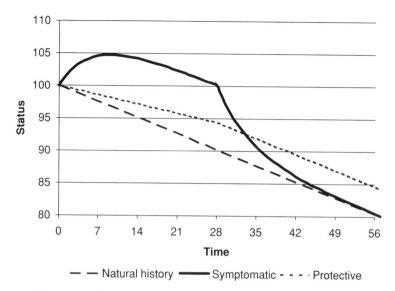

Figure 6.5. Symptomatic and protective drug effects during and after treatment for 28 units of time (units are arbitrary but could be interpreted as days).

practice, it can be hard to demonstrate protective effects by attempting to detect this persistent benefit after stopping treatment. This is because the worsening of the disease after treatment withdrawal is typically unacceptable to patients and effects are only observable over short withdrawal intervals.

Attempts to demonstrate a protective effect of levodopa to slow down the progression of Parkinson's disease have produced controversial results (The Parkinson Study Group, 2004). In part, this is because of the slow washout of symptomatic benefit. It also arises from the use of an experimental design and analysis method that was unable to distinguish protective from symptomatic effects.

6.8   Modeling Methods

Mathematical models describing pharmacokinetics, pharmacodynamics, and disease progression are helpful for understanding dose–response because they can incorporate the mechanistic underlying processes thought to be responsible for observations of disease state. Descriptions of these models and their applications in clinical drug development have been reviewed elsewhere (Chan and Holford, 2001; Holford and Ludden, 1994; Sheiner and Steimer, 2000).

6.8.1   Analysis

The analysis of dose–response relationships based on PK PD models typically requires the use of nonlinear regression. Although linear models, e.g., quadratic, can be used to describe curvi-linear dose–response relationships, there are usually other nonlinear components of the model, e.g., using exponential functions to describe the time course of onset and loss of effect.

Sometimes doses are coded in sequential categories that lose information about the size of the dose, e.g., doses of 0, 50, 100, 200, 400 might be coded as 1, 2, 3, and 4. This recoding should be avoided when trying to understand dose–response relationships in pharmacological terms.

6.8.2   Mixed Effect Models

Many clinical trials will include multiple observations of the response variable in the same subject. This usually means that between subject variability (and sometimes within subject variability) in parameters of the dose–response model can be estimated. The ability to describe both fixed and random effect sources of variability is essential for prediction of effects and responses, e.g., when used in clinical trial simulation.

Statistical software systems such as SAS or S-Plus provide mixed effect modeling procedures but do not provide support for pharmacokinetic predictions based on the often complex and irregular actual doses taken in a clinical trial. NONMEM (Beal et al., 1999) and WinBUGs with the PKBUGs extension (Best et al., 1995) include pharmacokinetic model libraries capable of describing almost any real dosing data pattern which is usually necessary to undertake a mixed effects model analysis of dose–response data. Duffull et al. (2005) provide a discussion of the advantages and disadvantages of these two programs.

6.8.3   Simulation

It can be argued that the primary purpose of undertaking a dose–response analysis is not just to describe results, but to be able to predict responses to future doses. This typically involves simulation using a simple deterministic description of the time course of effects and responses after different doses. A more complex stochastic simulation can be used to explore trial design properties and construct prediction intervals for the likely range of outcomes.

6.8.4   Clinical Trial Simulation

The purposes and methods of clinical trial simulation have been reviewed by Holford et al. (2000). Numerous applications in clinical trial simulation have been reported in recent years (Anderson et al., 2003; Bonate, 2000; Chabaud et al., 2002; Girard et al., 2004; Gomeni et al., 2002; Jumbe et al., 2002; Kimko et al, 2000; Lockwood et al., 2003; Veyrat-Follet et al., 2000). Almost all of these have been concerned with evaluating dose–response relationships in drug development programs. Further examples can be found in Chapter 8.

6.9   Conclusion

The quantitative description of dose–response relationships can be approached from a scientific basis by the application of principles of clinical pharmacology. These recognize the central role of concentration as the explanatory variable linking dose to effect. It is not necessary to measure concentrations or develop a formal pharmacokinetic model in order to describe the effects of drugs (Holford and Peace, 1992; Pillai et al., 2004), but recognition of the separate contributions of pharmacokinetic and pharmacodynamic sources of variability is important for accurate description and informative predictions.

References

Anderson, J.J., Bolognese. J.A., and Felson, D.T. 2003. Comparison of rheumatoid arthritis clinical trial outcome measures: A simulation study. *Arthritis and Rheumatism* 48(11):3031–3038.

Beal, S.L., Boeckmann, A.J., and Sheiner, L.B. 1999. *NONMEM Users Guides*, NONMEM Project Group, University of California at San Francisco, San Francisco.

Best, N.G., Tan, K.K., Gilks, W.R., and Spiegelhalter, D.J. 1995. Estimation of population pharmacokinetics using the Gibbs sampler. *Journal of Pharmacokinetics and Biopharmaceutics* 23(4):407–435.

Bonate, P.L. 2000. Clinical trial simulation in drug development. *Pharmaceutical Research* 17(3):252–256.

Chabaud, S., Girard, P., Nony, P., and Boissel, J.P. 2002. Clinical trial simulation using therapeutic effect modeling: Application to ivabradine efficacy in patients with angina pectoris. *Journal of Pharmacokinetics and Pharmacodynamics* 29(4):339–363.

Chan, P.L.S., and Holford, N.H.G. 2001. Drug treatment effects on disease progression. *Annual Review of Pharmacology and Toxicology* 41:625–659.

Dayneka, N.L., Garg, V., and Jusko, W.J. 1993. Comparison of four basic models of indirect pharmacodynamic responses. *Journal of Pharmacokinetics and Biopharmaceutics* 21(4):457–478.

Duffull, S.B., Kirkpatrick, C.M.J., Green, B., and Holford, N.H.G. 2005. Analysis of population pharmacokinetic data using NONMEM and WinBugs. *Journal of Biopharmaceutical Statistics* 15(1):53–73.

Food and Drug Administration. 2003. *Guidance for Industry Exposure-Response Relationships—Study Design, Data Analysis, and Regulatory Applications.* Rockville.

Friberg, L.E., Brindley, C.J., Karlsson, M.O., and Devlin, A.J. 2000. Models of schedule dependent haematological toxicity of 2′-deoxy-2′-methylidenecytidine (DMDC). *European Journal of Clinical Pharmacology* 56(8):567–574.

Girard, P., Cucherat, M., and Guez, D. 2004. Clinical trial simulation in drug development. *Therapie* 59(3):287–295, 297–304.

Gomeni, R., Dangeli, C., and Bye, A. 2002. In silico prediction of optimal in vivo delivery properties using convolution-based model and clinical trial simulation. *Pharmaceutical Research* 19(1):99–103.

Holford, N.H.G. 1986. Clinical pharmacokinetics and pharmacodynamics of warfarin. Understanding the dose-effect relationship. *Clinical Pharmacokinetics* 11:483–504.

Holford, N.H.G. 1991. "Physiological alternatives to the effect compartment model," in *Advanced Methods of Pharmacokinetic and Pharmacodynamic Systems Analysis* (D'Argenio, D.Z., editor), New York: Plenum Press. pp. 55–68.

Holford, N.H.G., Kimko, H.C., Monteleone, J.P., and Peck, C.C. 2000. Simulation of clinical trials. *Annual Review of Pharmacology and Toxicology* 40:209–234.

Holford, N.H.G., and Ludden, T. 1994. "Time course of drug effect," in *Handbook of Experimental Pharmacology* (Welling, P.G., and Balant, L.P., editors), Heidelberg: Springer-Verlag.

Holford, N.H.G., and Peace, K. 1994. The effect of tacrine and lecithin in Alzheimer's disease. A population pharmacodynamic analysis of five clinical trials. *European Journal of Clinical Pharmacology* 47(1):17–23.

Holford, N.H.G., and Peace, K.E. 1992a. Methodologic aspects of a population pharmacodynamic model for cognitive effects in Alzheimer patients treated with tacrine. *Proceedings of the National Academy of Sciences of the United States of America* 89:11466–11470.

Holford, N.H.G., and Peace, K.E. 1992b. Results and validation of a population pharmacodynamic model for cognitive effects in Alzheimer patients treated with tacrine. *Proceedings of the National Academy of Sciences of the United States of America* 89(23):11471–11475.

Holford, N.H.G., and Peck, C.C. 1992. "Population pharmacodynamics and drug development," in *The In Vivo Study of Drug Action* (Boxtel, C.J., Holford, N.H.G., and Danhof, M., editors), New York: Elsevier Science. pp. 401–414.

Holford, N.H.G., and Sheiner, L.B. 1981. Understanding the dose-effect relationship: Clinical application of pharmacokinetic-pharmacodynamic models. *Clinical Pharmacokinetics* 6:429–453.

Jumbe, N., Yao, B., Rovetti, R., Rossi, G., and Heatherington, A.C. 2002. Clinical trial simulation of a 200-microg fixed dose of darbepoetin alfa in chemotherapy-induced anemia. *Oncology* (Huntingt) 16(10 Suppl 11):37–44.

Kimko, H.C., Reele, S.S., Holford, N.H., and Peck, C.C. 2000. Prediction of the outcome of a phase 3 clinical trial of an antischizophrenic agent (quetiapine fumarate) by simulation with a population pharmacokinetic and pharmacodynamic model. *Clinical Pharmacology and Therapeutics* 68(5):568–577.

Lesko, L.J., and Atkinson, A.J. 2001. Use of biomarkers and surrogate endpoints in drug development and regulatory decision making: Criteria, validation, strategies. *Annual Review of Pharmacology and Toxicology* 41:347–366.

Lockwood, P.A., Cook, J.A., Ewy, W.E., and Mandema, J.W. 2003. The use of clinical trial simulation to support dose selection: Application to development of a new treatment for chronic neuropathic pain. *Pharmaceutical Research* 20(11):1752–1759.

Nagashima, R., O'Reilly, R.A., and Levy, G. 1969. Kinetics of pharmacologic effects in man: The anticoagulant action of warfarin. *Clinical Pharmacology and Therapeutics* 10:22–35.

Pillai, G., Gieschke, R., Goggin, T., Jacqmin, P., Schimmer, R.C., and Steimer, J.L. 2004. A semimechanistic and mechanistic population PK-PD model for biomarker response to ibandronate, a new bisphosphonate for the treatment of osteoporosis. *British Journal of Clinical Pharmacology* 58(6):618–631.

Segre, G. 1968. Kinetics of interaction between drugs and biological systems. *Farmaco* 23:907–918. Author: Please check the journal name for correctness.

Sheiner, L., and Steimer, J-L. 2000. Pharmacokinetic/Pharmacodynamic Modeling in Drug Development. *Annual Review of Pharmacology and Toxicology* 40:67–95.

Sheiner, L.B., Stanski, D.R., Vozeh, S., Miller, R.D., and Ham, J. 1979. Simultaneous modeling of pharmacokinetics and pharmacodynamics: Application to D-tubocurarine. *Clinical Pharmacology and Therapeutics* 25(3):358–371.

Stanski, D.R. 1992a. "Pharmacodynamic measurement and modelling of anesthetic depth," in *The In Vivo Measurement of Drug Action* (Van Boxtel, C.J., Holford, N.H.G., and Danhof M., editors), New York: Elsevier Science.

Stanski, D.R. 1992b. Pharmacodynamic modeling of anesthetic EEG drug effects. *Annual Review of Pharmacology and Toxicology* 32:423–447.

The Parkinson Study Group. 2004. Levodopa and the Progression of Parkinson's Disease. *The New England Journal of Medicine* 351(24):2498–2508.

Veyrat-Follet, C., Bruno, R., Olivares, R., Rhodes, G.R., and Chaikin, P. 2000. Clinical trial simulation of docetaxel in patients with cancer as a tool for dosage optimization. *Clinical Pharmacology Therapeutics* 68(6):677–687.

7
General Considerations in Dose–Response Study Designs

NAITEE TING

7.1 Issues Relating to Clinical Development Plan

As mentioned in Chapter 1, one important step in early clinical development of a new drug is to draft a clinical development plan (CDP). Various clinical studies are designed and carried out according to this plan, and the CDP is updated over time based on newly available information. Estimation of dose–response relationship should be one of the very important components in CDP.

Considerations and plans regarding dose finding should be in place starting from the nonclinical development stage. Across all phases of clinical development, information to help with dose selection is needed. The key stage for finding the appropriate range of doses should be around Phase II. But critical information to help design Phase II studies are obtained from nonclinical, and Phase I studies. In certain situations, the drug candidate belongs to a well-established drug class in which information from other drugs of the same class is available. Clinical scientists need to make best use of that available information to help design Phase II studies. Hence, one of the primary objectives in the earlier part of CDP should be to deliver useful data to help designing dose ranging and dose selection studies in Phase II. Based on information collected from Phase I clinical studies, a number of Phase II studies should be planned and carried out—proof of concept (POC), dose ranging, and dose-finding studies. Some of these studies are carried out to measure the clinical endpoints, while some others are implemented to characterize biomarkers. Choice of appropriate endpoints for each study should be considered in the CDP. Criteria to measure success should also be clarified in the CDP.

After the multiple dose pharmacokinetics (PK) is established for a drug candidate from Phase I studies, there is often an estimated Maximally Tolerated Dose (MTD). With the PK and MTD information available, a typical step to progress the drug development is to conduct a POC study. A commonly used POC study usually has two parallel treatment groups—a control (often placebo) group and a test treatment group using a high dose very close to MTD, or the MTD itself. In some situations, the test treatment group allows dose titration up to the MTD. The reason a very high dose (very close to MTD) is used for

POC is that the highest dose may provide the best hope to demonstrate drug efficacy.

Dose ranging studies usually include a placebo group, plus a few doses of the test drug—e.g., low dose, medium dose, and high dose. An ideal dose ranging study should cover a wide range of doses from low to high. Typically, these studies are parallel group with fixed doses. The main objective of a dose ranging study is to estimate the dose–response relationships for efficacy, and possibly for safety. Hence, in analyzing results from these studies, various dose–response models are often applied to help understand the underlying dose–response relationship.

On the other hand, dose selection studies or dose finding studies are mainly designed to confirm the efficacy of one or several doses. Although the design of a dose selection study is very similar to a dose ranging study (with placebo or active control, plus a few test doses), the data analysis tends to be hypothesis testing of each test dose against the control.

In the CDP, considerations should be made to determine whether studies could be conducted simultaneously or sequentially. In other words, in trials designed to study PK, this study can also provide safety information to help estimate MTD. Meanwhile, another study can be designed to learn the food effect. In these situations, we should try to maximize the amount of information that can be collected in each study, and minimize the time to achieve these objectives. On the other hand, a POC study or a dose ranging study cannot be designed without MTD information. Hence, these studies should be conducted after MTD information can be obtained from earlier studies. Therefore, the CDP needs to lay out the sequence of studies to be designed and executed over time. Estimation of the starting time of a new study should be based on critical information available to help design that study. In some cases POC and dose ranging studies are combined and in others dose ranging studies and dose selection studies are combined. All of these strategies need to be discussed while drafting the CDP.

Section 7.2 introduces some general considerations in designing clinical trials (not just for dose finding purposes). Section 7.3 discusses design considerations specifically for dose finding trials, and Section 7.4 provides concluding remarks.

7.2   General Considerations for Designing Clinical Trials

Figure 7.1 illustrates data collected from a typical dose–response study, often referred to as a "randomized, double-blind, placebo-controlled, fixed dose, parallel group, and dose–response design". In such a study, patients are randomized into predetermined dose groups (often including a placebo, a low dose, one or several medium doses and a high dose). Patients take the randomized dose for the planned study duration. The efficacy and safety data obtained are analyzed to evaluate the dose–response relationships. Note that "parallel group", "fixed dose", and "placebo-controlled" are some important features of this design. Each asterisk in Figure 7.1 represents the efficacy measurement from one subject. Suppose a higher

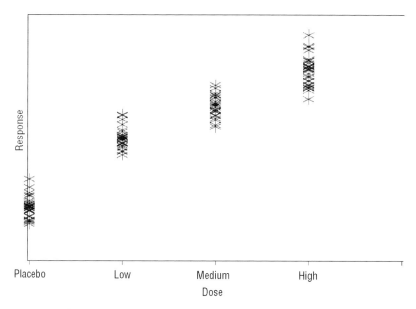

Figure 7.1. Observations from a simulated dose response study.

value indicates a better efficacy response, then Figure 7.1 indicates that as the dose of the test drug increases, the efficacy response improves.

Dose–response trials are typically conducted in Phase II, although occasionally they are done earlier or later. They are designed to explore a range of doses and to characterize the dose–response relationship. In this chapter, we will discuss some of the important clinical study design considerations for dose–response studies. Many of these points focus on Phase II (exploratory) study design, although some may be applicable to Phase III (confirmatory) studies, also.

7.2.1   Subject Population and Endpoints

Every clinical trial starts with a clinical question. Based on this question, clinical trial team members work together to draft a clinical trial protocol. This protocol serves as the design document for the trial. The results obtained from a clinical trial will help address the key clinical question. Hence, the most important study design consideration is to understand the objective(s) of the given study, and the trial is designed to collect the necessary clinical data to help answer these important clinical questions.

In designing a clinical trial, it is always important to collect and analyze data to address the primary objective. Typically, the primary objective can be studied by analyzing one or a few specific clinical variables (endpoints) from a well-defined study population. Hence, it is critical that in every study design, the subject population and the clinical endpoints be prespecified in the protocol. Primary and secondary objectives should be aligned with the primary and secondary endpoints and populations.

As discussed in Chapter 1, clinical development is divided into four general phases (Phase I, II, III, and IV). In most of the Phase I studies, the purpose is to estimate pharmacokinetics (PK), pharmacodynamics (PD), and MTD. In Phase I, healthy and normal volunteers are recruited for trials to study drug candidates developed to treat non-life-threatening diseases. Endpoints used in Phase I include PK and PD parameters, as well as safety endpoints. Safety endpoints typically include adverse events, laboratory values and other measurements collected from examination equipment such as electrocardiogram (ECG). In all of the clinical studies, safety endpoints are collected, regardless at which phase the study is designed. This is because drug safety should be monitored closely in every stage of drug development.

In drugs developed for non-life-threatening diseases, a Phase II clinical trial is usually the first one to recruit patients with the disease under study. Patients for Phase II trials are recruited so that these patients may be most likely to benefit from the drug candidate and least likely to be exposed to potential toxicities. Endpoints used in Phase II studies include efficacy and safety endpoints. The efficacy endpoints may be clinical endpoints such as blood pressure, time to disease relapse, number of painful joints, visual acuity or surrogate markers such as white blood cell count, bone mineral density, among others.

Phase III studies are usually designed to recruit a wider patient population. This population could be very similar to the actual patients with the target disease. Clinical efficacy and safety endpoints are collected so that they are similar to the real world situation. Results obtained from Phase III studies are analyzed and reported to regulatory agencies for drug approval. In Phase III, we tend to have more relaxed inclusion/exclusion criteria with a hope to generalize well to clinical practice, but the heterogeneity of patient characteristics may reduce power of the trial.

The primary endpoint should be selected based on clinical relevance, directly related to study objectives. Other considerations may include the choice of scale (continuous, dichotomous, categorical), its potential impact on how analysis will be done, its impact on power, and its impact on interpretation.

In many situations, more than one efficacy endpoints are used to address the primary objective. When this is the case, it creates a multiple comparison issue in statistical analysis. Let the prespecified Type I error rate be α (usually a two-sided α is set at 0.05, or a one-sided α set at 0.025), then how should this α be spent for these multiple endpoints? What analysis should be performed so that the experiment-wise error rate (the Type I error is prespecified for the entire experiment) is controlled? All of these considerations will need to be addressed in the protocol and in the statistical analysis plan.

Often times, these multiple endpoints can be prioritized according to their importance in the clinical study. In this case, a stepwise test procedure can be applied to address the multiple endpoint issue by testing the most important endpoint first. If this null hypothesis is not rejected, stop. Otherwise, continue to test for the second most important endpoint; then continue in this fashion until all prespecified endpoints are tested (please refer to Chapters 11 and 12 of this book). On the other hand, if two or three endpoints are equally important, then it is possible to combine these endpoints into a single score, and the primary analysis is performed on this composite score. It is also possible to apply multiple comparison adjustment to these equally important endpoints.

7.2.2 Parallel Designs versus Crossover Designs

In a fixed-dose parallel group design, a patient receives the same treatment for the duration of the trial. In contrast, in a crossover design, each patient receives a sequence of treatments during two or more study phases. Multiple sequence groups are used. Each has a different order of treatments, to account for any trends (such as disease progression or seasonal variation). For instance, in a 2×2 crossover design, a subject is randomized into one of two sequences. For one sequence, the subject takes treatment A in the first study period and treatment B in the second period, usually after washout period between treatments. The treatment order is reversed for the other sequence. Sometimes more complicated crossover designs are utilized.

In many cases, drug efficacy takes some time to demonstrate. A trial designed to study efficacy may need each patient to go through several weeks to several months of double-blind treatment. With this length of treatment, it is often difficult to use crossover designs. Hence, a parallel study design is used in many of the Phase II/III clinical trials.

7.2.3 Selection of Control

Three types of treatment controls can be considered in clinical trial designs: (1) historical control, (2) placebo control and (3) active control. Historical controls are based on data from other studies or the published literature, and they are usually less credible than placebo or active controls. Hence, historical controls are rarely used in clinical trials for new drug development. An active control is a treatment that is already on the market. Usually this is the standard treatment available for the disease under study. Active control group may be more useful in later phase studies. The advantages and disadvantages of using an active control group depend on the disease under study, characteristics of the drug candidate being developed, and specific clinical inferences of interest (ICH E10, 2001). Studies with an active control, but without a placebo group, suffer from the additional burden of demonstrating that the treatment groups are effective (assay sensitivity), either through superiority to the active control or on the basis of some type of historical control information (Temple and Ellenberg, 2000; Ellenberg and Temple, 2000). An active control, however, may provide a reference from a treatment of 'known' effectiveness. In practice, the use or not use of an active control mainly depends on objectives of the study. However, in certain cases, it may also depend on clinical budget considerations.

In the early stage of clinical development of a new drug, it is a common practice (if deemed ethical) to compare the test drug with a placebo. This is important since detecting positive signals of effectiveness beyond that achieved with placebo is an important milestone for continuing development of this drug candidate. Accordingly, placebo plays an important role in a dose–response study—it represents a zero dose in the study. Patient response at zero dose is a basic standard for comparison with active doses. In typical dose–response studies, a few fixed doses (usually two, three or four) would be chosen. These doses plus placebo constitute the treatment groups for a randomized dose–response trial.

The basic principle is that the design needs to cover a range of doses, as wide as possible in most cases. Generally, the low end will be placebo (at dose 0), but sometimes the lowest dose may exceed zero (e.g., for ethical concerns). This raises at least two issues: (1) a narrower dose range reduces the power to detect a relationship, all other things being equal; (2) even if there is a significant dose–response slope in the right direction, we need to be able to argue that this slope reflects an improvement in all groups (rather than the case where a higher dose may be worse than placebo).

An active control group can be useful, for example, if the test drug did not show a difference from placebo, but the active control group demonstrates a superiority response compared with placebo. This provides evidence that the study drug did not work. However, if the active control does not show a difference from placebo, then one of two possibilities can be contemplated: either the placebo response is too high, or the conduct of the study was flawed so that nothing can be differentiated.

7.2.4   Multiple Comparisons

In typical dose–response studies, more than two treatment groups are included in a clinical trial. When this is the case, it is important to understand the questions related to the objectives of the study:

- To show a trend such that higher doses tend to have better responses? or
- To show a particular dose is better than placebo?

Depending on the objective of a study, appropriate multiple comparison adjustment need to be made so that the probability of making a Type I error can be controlled under α. In most Phase II studies, the objective is to estimate a trend of dose–response relationship. A modeling approach is commonly applicable for this purpose. Commonly used dose–response models include linear, quadratic, E_{max}, logistic or others. Chapters 9 and 10 of this book discuss the modeling approach in analyzing dose–response data. In certain situations, a preplanned dose–response test with a positive slope can be considered as one of the pivotal proof of efficacy trials.

For Phase III, it is critical that during the study design stage, a multiple comparison procedure be prespecified. This is similar to the multiple endpoint issue: e.g., How is the Type I error α (or one-sided $\alpha/2$) controlled when more than one comparison is made? A number of multiple comparison procedures are available.

Commonly used procedures include Dunnett, Bonferroni, Hochberg, stepwise, and others (Hsu, 1996). Choice of procedures to be used for a particular study depends on the objective(s) of the study, the background disease for treatment, and how much prior knowledge is available at the time when the study is designed. Multiple comparison procedure is one of the most important statistical concerns in design and analysis of dose–response studies. This will be discussed in Chapters 10–13.

7.2.5 Sample Size Considerations

During the design stage of any clinical trials, one important question is always How many subjects will be needed for this study? Generally, for a continuous variable, four important quantities are used to estimate the sample size: namely α, β, δ, and σ. Here α and β represents the probability of making a Type I error and a Type II error, respectively. These two quantities are prespecified probabilities to control for false positive and false negative rate, respectively. The quantity δ is the clinically important difference we want to detect from this study (often this is postulated as minimally clinically important difference), and σ is the common standard deviation for each treatment group (usually obtained from previous studies). Depending on the type of data to be used for analysis (continuous data, categorical data, time-to-event data), various formulas are available to calculate sample sizes using these four quantities.

When designing a dose–response study, the main concern in sample size calculation is how to handle multiple group comparisons. This issue is dictated by the objective of the study. A few examples of the objective of a dose–response study may be as follows:

- Testing to see if a specific dose of the study drug is different from placebo
- Finding the minimum effective dose
- Differentiating efficacy between active doses
- Checking to see if there is an increasing dose trend
- Demonstrating noninferiority between a particular dose and the active control

As a good clinical practice, it is important to keep a single and clear primary objective for a single study. Hence, the above examples can be considered mutually exclusive. The appropriate statistical method used to perform data analysis should be aligned with the primary objective. Sample size estimation, in turn, should be consistent with the data analysis method.

In the first example, if the trial were designed to differentiate a specific dose of test drug from placebo, then the sample sizing method would be similar to performing a two-sample t-test comparing the test drug against placebo. In most situations when analyzing dose–response studies, multiple comparison adjustments will be needed. Depending on the type of multiple comparison to be used for data analysis, sample sizes should be estimated based on the chosen method. For example, if a pre-determined stepwise multiple comparison adjustment will be used for analysis, then the two-sample t test at level α could be appropriate. On the other hand, if the Bonfferoni adjustment is proposed for data analysis, then the appropriate α adjustment will have to be made prior to sample size estimation. In Phase II dose–response studies, the main purpose is to estimate a monotonic relationship and hence the sample size and power will help demonstrating a significant slope in a regression model.

There is another angle of sample size estimation: a study is powered to achieve a required amount of precision for an estimated quantity using a confidence interval approach (rather than testing Ho: effect = 0). The quantity could be an accepted range of responses at a given dose—or, more usefully, the dose to give a required range of response. This angle is not covered in this book.

A general discussion regarding sample size determination and power can be found in the (*Encyclopedia of Biopharmaceutical Statistics*, 2003). These considerations specifically for dose–response clinical trials will be covered in Chapter 14 here in this book.

7.2.6 Multiple Center Studies

Clinical trials are commonly conducted at a number of different investigator sites or centers. The main reason for this practice is to ensure timely enrollment of sufficient number of patients. Another benefit of multiple center studies is that results obtained from these studies can represent a wider variety of patient background. This means that a multiple center study including various type of centers are more desirable, and the conclusion is not heavily dependent on one single center. In other words, the conclusion of multiple center studies is more "generalizable", so that the interpretation of these results is more likely to be applied to a broader patient population.

Different centers may have different recruitment rates. As a result, this can cause an imbalance in the number of patients recruited from various centers. If this happens, some centers may fail to provide enough patients to be randomized to each treatment group, and the treatment-by-center interaction may become nonestimable. Therefore, we tend to limit the number of treatment groups in order to minimize the imbalance problem.

For example, in a dose–response study, there is often a need to include many doses in one study. As demonstrated in Figure 7.1, a typical dose–response study would include a placebo and three test doses (a total of four treatment groups). When this is the case, in a multiple center study, it is desirable to include at least four patients (one in each treatment group) from each center. However, in some cases, the center may fail to recruit up to four patients and this will cause imbalance in data analyses. There can also be situations where one particular dose is over (or under) represented in many centers. Then, when all centers are pooled together, the data causes another type of imbalance.

7.3   Design Considerations for Phase II Dose–Response Studies

Dose–response studies are usually carried out in Phase II. At this point, there is often a considerable amount of uncertainty regarding any hypothetical dose–

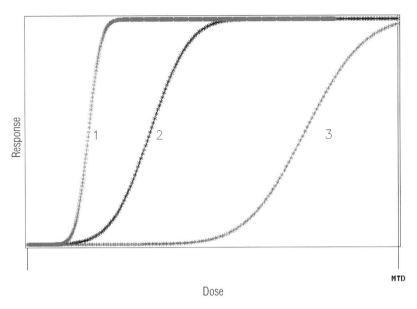

Figure 7.2. Several possible dose–response curves.

response curves. It is typical at this time that the MTD is known from Phase I studies, and it may also be assumed that efficacy is nondecreasing with increasing doses. Even so, the underlying dose–response curve can still take many possible shapes. Under each assumed curve, there are various strategies of allocating doses. For example, in Figure 7.2, the population dose–response curve can be assumed to take a variety of shapes. If we select doses to detect the ascending part of curve 3, then the planned doses should be on the higher range. On the other hand, if we need to select doses to detect the activities of curve 1, then the doses should be chosen on the lower end. Thus, the dose allocation strategy can be very different depending on the underlying assumed dose–response curves.

In general, when designing a Phase II dose–response clinical trial, we need to consider the following important points: dose frequency, dose range, number of doses, dose spacing, use of control (or lack of), sample size for each treatment, fixed dose or dose titration, and others. Some of these points are discussed in the subsections below.

7.3.1   Frequency of Dosing

In designing dose–response clinical studies, we need to know how often should a patient take the test drug (e.g., once a day, twice a day, or dose every 4 hours during the day). This is a question about dosing frequency, and it is usually guided by the Phase I PK–PD findings. One of the PK parameters is the half-life of a drug. The estimated half-life helps to estimate how long the drug will stay in human body. Using this information, we can propose a dosing frequency to be used for dose–response study design. In certain cases, we may study more than one dosing frequency in a single study. When this is the case, a factorial design (dose, frequency, dose × frequency) can be considered.

However, in some drugs, the PD response may be different from PK. Recall that PD measures how the drug works in human body while PK measures how the body do to the drug. In this case, even from the PK half-life data, we think there is insufficient drug in the body after several hours of dosing, but there may still be enough drug in the tissue to help with PD responses. On the other hand, the PK may indicate that there are still plenty of drug in the body, but these drugs may not cause any effective PD responses. In some drugs, the concentrations for PD activities can be very different from that for PK activities. Hence, the dose frequency derived from PK may either overestimate or underestimate the concentration needed for PD response. In some cases, the best dose frequency may be derived in later phases of the drug development.

Another important guiding principle in selecting dosing frequency is based on the market assessment. For example, if the market requires a once daily dosing treatment, but the drug candidate under development has a twice-a-day PK profile, then some formulation change may be necessary. Figure 7.3 presents time–concentration curves of this situation. The horizontal line that is above the x-axis represents the efficacy concentration level (often based on PD information). Theoretically speaking, we need to keep the drug concentration staying above this line all the time for the drug to work. In order to achieve this concentration, two strategies are possible: we can either dose the subject twice-a-day (BID) with low dose (Figure 7.3), or once-a-day (QD) with the high dose (which is twice the

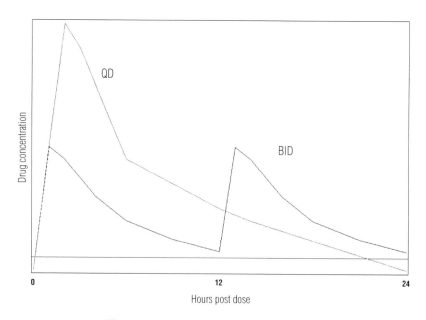

Figure 7.3. Once a day vs twice a day dosing.

dosage of the low dose, Figure 7.3). Note that in the first few hours post dosing, the high dose may result in a very high concentration, which could potentially cause severe adverse events. When this is the case, re-formulation of the drug may be needed so that when dosed as once a day, the C_{max} would not be too high, while the efficacy concentration can be maintained throughout a 24-hour period.

In designing the first few Phase I trials to study PK, there is very limited information about how will the human body metabolize this drug candidate. At this stage, data observed from preclinical studies and animal experiments on this drug candidate are used to help guide designing these Phase I trials. In case the drug candidate belongs to a certain drug class where other drugs of the same class were already on the market, information obtained from these other drugs can be used to help guiding the study designs for this drug candidate.

During the development of a drug candidate, sometimes reformulation may be needed. There can be many different reasons why there is a need for drug reformulation, including to help absorption, and to change the half-life. It is critical to understand that after reformulation, the PK–PD properties of the drug candidate are different from what they were prior to reformulation. Hence, all of the dosing information and drug regimen obtained from studies before the reformulation will need to be changed and re-studied. This can potentially cause major re-work. Rework in drug research and development delays the development process and results in additional amount of investment.

In studying the PK–PD relationship, we should realize that the main point is whether C_{min}, C_{max}, or AUC drives the PD. This is a fertile area for collaboration between statisticians and pharmacokineticists. Models based on prior trial data (e.g., from preclinical data, clinical data of the drug candidate under study, other compound of the same class) can be developed to inform the decision.

7.3.2   Fixed-Dose versus Dose-Titration Designs

A fixed-dose design is in contrast to a dose-titration design. In a fixed-dose design, once a patient is randomized to a dose group, the patient would take the same dose of study drug throughout the entire dosing period. In a dose titration design, a patient is randomized to a dose regimen with a starting dose, then the dose for a patient can be changed over time. In a dose-titration study, subjects are randomized to start with a low dose, and depending on either patient's response to the drug, or a predetermined schedule, the dose is gradually increased until a suitable dose level is found. For example, in a "titration to response" design, each subject can receive more than one dose. A patient who responds to a low dose may stay on this low dose, and a patient who does not respond to a low dose after a prespecified treatment period may receive the next highest dose of the drug. This procedure is repeated until some designed criteria are satisfied. There are at least two ways of analyzing data obtained from this design:

1. If patients are titrated until a response occurs (e.g., sufficient efficacy or a tolerable level of adverse events), the response measure is the dose achieved

and the study generates an estimate of the distribution of doses required for a response. This can be useful—but it's not a dose–response relationship per se.

2. This same data (assuming multiple measurements of some parameter prior to response) can be analyzed with a mixed effects model in an attempt to tease out the dose–response relationship. This is based on the assumption that individuals vary in their dose–response parameters and we observe a censored set of data.

In this design, the time effect versus dose effects complicate matters.

In addition to the titration-to-response design, there are other types of titration designs. One example is a fixed titration design: doses are changed on a fixed schedule without regard to response. The time on dose is confounded with dose, so that either a model-based analysis is needed or preferably the dose groups are split at the titration times, keeping some patients on the same dose to allow estimation of the time effect. Another example is dose–response cross-over design—this can be considered as a type of titration design—with the sequence groups taking care of the time effect mentioned for the fixed titration design.

There are some advantages of a titration design. For example, a study with this design will allow a patient to be treated at the optimum dose for the patient; this dose allocation feature reflects the actual medical practice. However, the disadvantage of a titration design is the difficulty in data analysis. For example, if a patient responded to the test drug after doses are escalated, it is unclear whether the higher dose or the accumulation of the lower dose caused the response. In titration designs with multiple treatment groups, there may be overlapping doses—e.g., one treatment group is 10 mg escalating to 20 mg, while another group is 20 mg escalating to 40 mg. When this is the case, it is difficult to make inferences about the 20 mg dose group.

In some rare cases, instead of a dose–response study, a concentration response study is designed. A concentration response study assesses efficacy and safety measurements observed from subjects according to the plasma concentration of the study drug, but not the doses of the study drug. There are many practical limitations in using this type of designs, these include, among others, how to blind the patient and the physician, and how and when to measure the blood concentration.

Because of the issues with dose titration designs and concentration response designs, the parallel, fixed dose designs are, in general, the more commonly used designs for dose–response studies. Therefore, in many of the dose–response studies, patients are randomized to a few fixed dose groups and are compared with one or more control treatment groups.

7.3.3   Range of Doses to be Studied

As discussed earlier, drug efficacy can only be studied from patients with the target disease. Hence, at the beginning of Phase II there is no efficacy information on these patients to help define the dose range for study. It is desirable to obtain information that helps describing the efficacy and safety dose–response curves. Studies should be designed to help estimate MaxED, MinED, and possibly to obtain additional information to support MTD. Although estimates regarding MTD should have been available prior to Phase II, more information will be helpful to re-confirm or to adjust MTD estimates obtained from previous trials. If the budget and timeline are permissible, the first dose ranging study should cover a wide dose range in a hope that this study will help identify the doses where most of the activities exist. The next study will then be designed to capture the dose–response relationship using information obtained from the first study.

Note that nonclinical information on the candidate and perhaps both clinical and nonclinical data for related compounds often provide a minimum drug concentration profile that is expected to be required for efficacy and safety. Together with the PK profile, this provides a target dose range, which we would want to explore, and possibly, a minimum dose expected to have little or no efficacy that we might want to include.

In a dose–response design with placebo, low dose, high dose and several doses in between, the dose range is defined as the range between the lowest and the highest dose. Dose range can be expressed as the ratio of highest dose over lowest dose—as a rule of thumb, in the first dose ranging study, the range should be at least 10-fold. In many cases, when the dose range is too narrow, the dose–response study failed to deliver the necessary information for efficacy or safety, and re-work will be needed after these studies. Costs of re-work can be tremendous at times. These costs may include costs of additional studies and costs of delaying the drug get to the market, in addition to all the resources foregone in conducting the current studies.

7.3.4   Number of Doses to be Tested

In order to cover a wide range of doses, it is desirable to study as many doses as possible. However, the number of doses that can be tested in a given study is limited. There are practical constraints in determining the number of treatment groups. Most trials with sufficient number of patients are multicenter trials. As mentioned earlier, different centers may have different recruitment rates, and imbalance in number of patients between treatment groups may exist. If this happens, the treatment-by-center interaction may become nonestimable. By increasing the number of treatment groups, the risk of imbalanceness increases. In order to minimize this risk, we tend to limit the number of treatment groups in each study. If we need to have more dose groups in a Phase II setting, we can prespecify that the primary model for data analysis is a main effect model, and that the treatment-by-center interaction is not to be tested or estimated.

Another practical issue is dosage form. Sometimes there are only limited dosage forms available in the early stage of clinical development. When this is the case, the number of doses to be used in a study may also be restricted. For example, if the tablet strengths are 10, 20, and 50 mg, respectively, then it is very difficult to study doses of 1, 3, or 25 mg, respectively. For some studies, the technique to achieve blinding is to produce matching placebos for each treatment group. The more doses that are included in a study, the more matching placebos may be needed. For example, if 1 mg tablets, 5 mg tablets and 10 mg tablets are used in the same study and these three types of tablets look different, then a placebo for each dose will be needed; i.e., three types of matching placebo to be used in this study. The number of dose groups may also be limited by practical considerations of how many pills we might reasonably expect a subject to take for any given dose. For these reasons and others, clinical studies designed with more than six or seven treatment groups are rare.

7.3.5   Dose Allocation, Dose Spacing

As depicted in Figure 7.2, with very limited information about the drug candidate, after allocating a placebo control, a high dose that is close to MTD, it will be very difficult to select the medium or low doses. The challenge is that at an early stage, there is no information as to what the underlying dose–response curve should be. Is it curve 1, curve 2, curve 3 or some other form? When there is very limited data to help allocating doses, we may consider the potential use of other information such as preclinical and related compounds. This is much more than an issue for statisticians, we should preferably work with the pharmacokineticists, clinicians, and pharmacologists. Dose allocation also depends upon the primary question: detecting an effect, estimating the slope near the MTD, finding the lowest dose with effect of at least some minimally clinically important difference, fitting a specific type of model, and so forth.

   After the number of dose groups is chosen, it is still a challenge to determine the high dose, low dose, and spacing between test doses. Typically, the high dose is a dose selected around or below the MTD, but choices of lower doses are often challenging. Wong and Lachenbruch (1996) introduce cases using equal dose spacing from low to high doses; that is to divide the distance from placebo to highest dose by the number of active doses, then use that divided distance as the space between two consecutive doses (e.g., 20, 40, 60 mg, respectively). Others may consider some type of log dose spacing; e.g., 1, 3, 10, and 30 mg, respectively, for the design.

   Hamlett et al. (2002) proposed to use binary dose spacing (BDS) design for dose allocation. If the study includes two test doses and placebo, BDS suggests to pick a mid-point between placebo and MTD, then allocate a dose above the midpoint and another dose below. If the study uses three test doses and placebo, BDS suggests to keep the high dose as the one selected in the two-dose case. Then pick a second midpoint between placebo and the first mid-point, allocate the low dose below the second midpoint, and the medium dose between the two mid-points. When more doses are used, BDS picks more mid-points to the lower end and allocates doses accordingly. BDS provides a wide dose range, helps identify MinED, avoids allocating doses too close to the MTD, allows a log-like dose spacing, it is flexible, and easy to implement.

7.3.6   Optimal Designs

The dose levels and the number of subjects at each level can be chosen mathematically (using mathematical theory, simulation, or some other tools) in order to optimize a statistical criterion such as small errors of estimation. This set of dose levels and number of subjects at each level is called the statistically optimal experimental design, and the design depends on the chosen criterion and the underlying model for the dose–response curve.

The statistical principles of optimal experimental design can be applied to many studies. Optimal design techniques can be used with various statistical models. For a given study objective and a reasonable model, optimization techniques allow one to determine the statistically best set of doses and number of subjects to be used at each dose. These designs help to estimate the parameters of the model; for example, slope and ED50 (the dose which achieves 50% of efficacy response) in logistic regression models, and intercept and slope in linear regression models. The doses used might not necessarily be those intended for use in the label, but they provide a basis for estimation of the dose–response curve so that the response at any dose can be predicted with validity and precision. Depending on the optimality criteria chosen, the doses studied may not necessarily be equally spaced or have equal numbers of subjects at each dose. Information on the shape of the dose–response curve should be attained where possible from PK–PD studies and early Phase II studies, which can help the design of the late Phase II studies.

Pukelsheim (1993) proposes a comprehensive set of statistical approaches to optimal experimental design. Wong and Lachenbruch (1996) review dose–response designs and use optimal design criteria for linear and quadratic regression. They also use simulation to illustrate the effect of optimal design criteria on spacing of doses and the numbers of subjects at each dose.

The key to optimizing a design is availability and use of prior information—based on candidate information and related compounds. A second key is to take into account the uncertainty in an a priori model. A goal might be to obtain a design that will work adequately no matter where the dose–response curve sits on the dose scale (over the range deemed most likely). On the other hand, the focus may be on average success—weighted average success, integrated over the prior distribution of the dose location uncertainty. Clinical simulation can be a useful tool here.

7.4   Concluding Remarks

Dose finding or dose selection happens mostly during Phase II or Phase III clinical development. The primary challenge for designing a Phase II dose–response clinical study is the lack of knowledge about how the drug works because this is the first time the test drug is studied in patients with the target disease. Again, Phase II studies are designed primarily for exploratory purposes and hence the main statistical method is estimation, and scientists tend to use model approaches in analyzing data collected from these studies. The main challenge in Phase III is to guess the correct dose or range of doses and be able to demonstrate it. Phase III studies are for confirmatory purposes. Multiple comparison procedures are commonly used to test statistical hypotheses for each dose comparing with placebo. This chapter introduced some considerations and difficulties in designing dose–response clinical trials.

A changing environment is pushing scientists, especially statisticians, to be more creative in designing dose-finding studies. Recently, FDA discusses the Critical Path initiative, which pressure the sponsors to reduce the development cost and speed up the time line. Within many pharmaceutical companies, there is a strong push to do more creative Phase II programs, aimed at assessing the dose response for safety and efficacy so that the drug candidate enter Phase III with the right dose range (or to stop developing compounds in Phase II if they're not likely to measure up). The potentially more creative designs and analyses serve a role in the regulatory review—for justifying the dose selection and possibly even for Phase III pivotal trials. Hence we hope to encourage readers to think about some of the newer strategies based on considering a wider range of potential designs, using prior information to inform the design, and basing at least some of the interpretation on model-based analyses that can take advantage of prior information and pharmacologically-reasonable assumptions about the underlying dose–response relationship.

At the end of Phase III, in the preparation of an NDA, the sponsor drafts summary of clinical efficacy (SCE) and summary of clinical safety (SCS). Traditionally, this often includes simple pooling of similar studies and side-by-side presentation of results. There is much more that can be done. One objective is to perform dose–response oriented meta-analyses of individual patient data, to combine all the relevant information about dose response and in particular, how it depends upon the indication, concomitant disease conditions, patient demographics, as well as time factors to accommodate different trial lengths. These were useful in the FDA discussions. This sort of meta-analysis can be built prospectively into the clinical development plan. In this regard, we hope to promote the collaboration of statisticians with PK–PD scientists, as natural 'partners in quantification'. This means broadening the perspective and understanding the difference between 'learning' and 'confirming' objectives for design and analysis of trials (and the entire programs).

Clinical trial simulation is a very useful tool to help with dose–response study designs. Simulation can be used to examine the impact of dose spacing, number of groups, and method for data analysis. There's not one right answer about number of groups as it depends upon the specific trial objectives, the data characteristics, and the dose–response relationship itself. An example of a clinical trial simulation is provided in Chapter 8.

References

Ellenberg, S.S., and Temple, R. 2000. Placebo-controlled trials and active-control trials in the evaluation of new treatments (Part 2). *Annals of Internal Medicine* 133(6):464–470.

Chow, S. 2003. *Encyclopedia of Biopharmaceutical Statistics*. 2nd ed. New York: Marcel Dekker.

Hamlett, A., Ting, N., Hanumara, C., and Finman, J.S. 2002. Dose spacing in early dose response clinical trial designs. *Drug Information Journal* 36(4):855–864.

Hsu, J.C. 1996. *Multiple comparisons—Theory and methods*. New York: Chapman-Hall.

ICH E10. 2001. Choice of control group and related issues in clinical trials. *Harmonized Tripartite Guideline*. http://www.fda.gov/cder/guidance/index.htm

Pukelsheim, F. 1993. *Optimal Design of Experiments*. New York: Wiley.

Temple, R., and Ellenberg, S.S. 2000. Placebo-controlled trials and active-control trials in the evaluation of new treatments (Part 1). *Annals of Internal Medicine* 133(6):455–463.

Wong, W.K., and Lachenbruch, P.A. 1996. Tutorial in biostatistics: Designing studies for dose response. *Statistics in Medicine* 15:343–359.

8
Clinical Trial Simulation—A Case Study Incorporating Efficacy and Tolerability Dose Response

WAYNE EWY, PETER LOCKWOOD, AND CANDACE BRAMSON

8.1   Clinical Development Project Background

This case study is based on an early clinical development project we conducted. Details that identify the candidate compound have been obscured for confidentiality reasons, but the situation described is not uncommon in early clinical development.

An important feature of the setting is that the candidate drug belongs to a class that shares a similar mechanism of action and for which considerable clinical and nonclinical information is available. This is a benefit because this information can be used to inform the clinical program design. But the challenge is also greater because the key question becomes differentiation from the class relatives, and not simply finding a safe and efficacious dose. This is historically a Phase III type of question, but in the increasingly cost-constrained development environment, there is a great advantage if inadequately active candidates can be identified and terminated early in Phase II.

The therapeutic setting is symptomatic treatment of a chronic condition, where efficacy is assessed by one primary and other secondary measures. Based on available information (including Phase I data for the candidate), we were confident that we would be working within a safe dose range, so that for trial design we could ignore the unlikely possibility that an entire dose group might need termination due to safety issues. The main safety-related concern was tolerability as reflected by the incidence and severity of a particular class of adverse events (AE). Clinical trial efficacy and tolerability data in the same indication were available for a related compound. A head-to-head comparison trial with this reference agent was not possible, so historical data would provide the performance target for the candidate.

An overall development goal was to identify a dose range of the candidate that is clinically noninferior to the "best dose" of the reference agent, considering both efficacy and tolerability. *Clinical noninferiority* means that the candidate is not *worse than the reference agent by more than a clinically relevant amount;* i.e., it is *clinically similar or better.* If a noninferior dose were not found, there would be no commercial or medical value in continued development. If a qualifying dose were found, additional development decisions would be based on the potential for superior efficacy, tolerability, or regimen.

8.1.1   Clinical Trial Objectives

An obvious objective for the first Phase II trial is to confirm the candidate's basic pharmacology (efficacy and safety). This *proof of concept* (POC) objective could be achieved by a simple two-group study, using some relatively high dose (near the maximally tolerated dose, MTD) versus placebo, with a sample size appropriate to the measures' variability and anticipated effect sizes. However, based on prior knowledge about the compound class, it is almost certain that the candidate will have the predicted pharmacological effects, so proving this need not be the major focus of the first trial. Rather, the design goal for this trial was to provide a basis for an early Go/No Go decision and to select the doses for subsequent registration trials.

More specifically, the trial objective is to estimate the dose–response relationship (DRR) for each measure, allowing estimation of the dose expected to give a response comparable to the reference agent's best dose and identification of a dose range with sufficient potential for continued development. These estimates will be imprecise relative to what a Phase III trial would provide. Nevertheless, there might be sufficient information to at least broadly determine if the candidate has useful potential, with some inevitable gray range for which this first study cannot provide a Go/No Go decision. Simulation helped us to evaluate different trial designs and analysis methods and to set expectations about how successful the trial might be (Bonate, 2000; Holford et al., 2000; Kimco and Duffull, 2003).

8.1.2   Uncertainties Affecting Clinical Trial Planning

Three major uncertainties about the DRRs were relevant to trial planning.

(1) *The DRRs for the reference agent.* The reference agent could not be included in this trial, for reasons beyond the scope of this discussion. Thus, the trial needed to be based on the strong (and to a large extent untestable) assumption that the reference and proposed trials' patient populations, methods, etc., would be similar enough to justify comparison of the placebo-adjusted results. The prior reference agent trial (with sample size of approximately 500) provided an estimated DRR and the associated uncertainty for each endpoint, as well as target values (TV), the estimated responses at the best dose, to be met by the candidate. The TVs will be considered as constants in the candidate trial analysis.

(2) *The relative potency (RP) for tolerability, for the candidate compared to the reference agent.* The relative potency for tolerability can be defined as the ratio (mg of reference/mg of candidate), where mg of reference is simply the reference drug's best dose and mg of candidate is the candidate dose that produces an identical AE incidence. Both pharmacokinetic and pharmacodynamic

differences are reflected in this RP value. An initial RP estimate and its uncertainty were based on nonclinical data, and updated estimates would become available at the completion of the Phase I trials.

(3) *The therapeutic index (TI) of the candidate compared to the reference agent.* The TI can be defined as the ratio (*RP for efficacy/RP for tolerability*), where the RP for efficacy is defined similarly to the RP for tolerability. The TI is a more convenient parameterization than considering the efficacy and tolerability RPs separately. The same best-dose value for *mg of reference* is used in both definitions, while the *mg of candidate* can differ for the two endpoints. A true TI = 1 implies the compounds have identical performance at their respective best doses (and all other doses if the DRRs have similar shapes). A TI > 1 implies superiority and TI < 1 inferiority; a value "sufficiently close" to 1 implies clinical similarity. The trial's objectives can be viewed, in effect, as estimation of the TI from the first (human) estimate of the efficacy RP and an updated estimate of the tolerability RP.

These uncertainties play different roles in the trial design, as elaborated below.

8.2   The Clinical Trial Simulation Project

The planning for the Phase II trial began prior to the candidate entering Phase I. Because the proposed dose-finding objectives were much more ambitious than those of a typical Phase IIa POC trial, we also began planning a clinical trial simulation (CTS) project to support the design process. A colleague who was not a regular clinical project team member led the CTS project. This administrative arrangement was necessary because the regular team members could not devote sufficient time, within the project schedule, to conduct a project of the proposed scope. In addition, a secondary project goal was a more general exploration of the usefulness of the methodology and of the performance characteristics of some novel (for us, at least) criteria for optimizing trial design in early clinical development.

One of the first steps, continued iteratively during the project, was to develop a written CTS project plan (Holford et al., 1999). This plan described the CTS project objectives, which are quite distinct from the clinical trial objectives. The plan described the range of trial designs that would be considered, the range of data models to be employed, the specific clinical trial objectives for which the design was to be optimized, and the performance criteria upon which alternative designs would be compared. Specific analysis methods were defined for each endpoint, comprising three alternatives from which we planned to select the best for inclusion in the trial protocol; time constraints eventually allowed CTS implementation of only two. We also developed the overall evaluation plan (decision criteria) by which a simulated trial's conclusions are obtained from its data— e.g., the steps to estimate a clinically noninferior dose range. For the simulations to be relevant, these methods and criteria must be consistent with those eventually used for the actual trial. This all amounts to developing and implementing a

Table 8.1. Selected acronyms

AE	Adverse event (the tolerability measure)
ANCOVA	Analysis of covariance (includes analysis of variance)
CI, LCL, UCL	Confidence interval, lower and upper confidence limits, for a difference from placebo, often used with the % as a suffix: e.g., 80% CI: LCL80, UCL80
CTS	Clinical trial simulation
DR, DRR	Dose response, dose–response relationship
LCSL, UCSL	Lower (efficacy) and upper (tolerability) clinical similarity limits
MCID	Minimal clinically important difference (from TV)
MTD	Maximally tolerated dose (for extended therapy)
N	Total sample size in a trial (not per group)
NI, NI region	Non-inferiority, NI dose region
RD, ED, TD	Reference, efficacy, and tolerability doses
RP	Relative potency (efficacy or tolerability)
TI	Therapeutic index (ratio of RPs)
TV	Target response value (efficacy or tolerability)

complete statistical analysis plan for each proposed design and alternative analysis method. Clearly, this situation has the potential for exponentially expanding complexity, which must be managed against the available personnel time and project timelines.

Table 8.1 lists some of the acronyms used in this chapter.

8.2.1   Clinical Trial Objectives Used for the CTS Project

For the CTS project work, the following clinical trial objectives were adopted:

(1) Confirm that the candidate is efficacious on the primary efficacy measure.
(2) Estimate the target doses—the candidate doses expected to give the target response levels (TVs) for efficacy and tolerability.
(3) Estimate a dose range that is "potentially clinically noninferior" to the reference agent for efficacy and tolerability.

A fourth trial objective, not covered due to space limitations, related to evaluating potential superiority to the reference agent.

Objective 3 is the key for subsequent development decisions, so that if a "potentially clinically noninferior" dose range were identified, this would provide a "Go signal" for the project (which would need to be further interpreted within the broader development context), while failing to identify a range would be a "No Go signal".

- *Definitions and assumptions related to the clinical trial objectives*: Noninferiority is a more complex concept in a multidimensional DR context than in the case of a simple comparison on a single endpoint of one candidate dose to a reference agent dose. Prerequisite definitions, conventions, and basic assumptions are presented in the remainder of this section, as a basis for describing the decision criterion in Section 8.2.4. While perhaps cumbersome initially, the terminology does allow a concise operational statement of the decision criteria.

- *Conventions*: Tolerability is measured by AE incidence, so that lower values are desired, while efficacy is scored so that increased values are desired. The true efficacy and tolerability DRRs are assumed to increase monotonically with dose. The terms "confirm", "potentially", and "clinically noninferior" in the objectives statement must be interpreted in the context of Phase IIa, during which the results are used for internal decision-making regarding the candidate's development. Such decisions can be based on a lower degree of certainty than would be necessary, for instance, for a regulatory filing.

- *Tolerability*: The tolerability target value (tolerability TV—the estimated AE incidence at the reference's best dose) and a clinical indifference margin (tolerability MCID, minimal clinically important difference) define the highest true AE incidence rate that would be considered clinically noninferior (the upper clinical similarity limit or tolerability UCSL). In the simulated trials, the candidate's true DRR determines the dose (the true tolerability dose or true TD) with an AE incidence equal to this UCSL; lower doses are clinically noninferior and higher are clinically inferior. From this perspective, the key question is not whether the candidate is noninferior, but what the highest noninferior dose is. Inference is based on an upper confidence limit for the AE incidence difference at a dose compared to placebo (tolerability UCL). If UCL $\leq$ UCSL, the dose is judged noninferior. The highest noninferior dose is designated the estimated TD.

- *Efficacy*: For efficacy, an efficacy TV and an efficacy MCID set the lower clinical similarity limit (efficacy LCSL). The true DRR defines a true efficacy dose (True ED) that divides the dose range into inferior (lower) and noninferior (higher) regions. The estimated ED is the lowest dose satisfying two criteria—significantly better than placebo (LCL > 0) and not significantly worse than the target value (UCL $\geq$ TV). (An alternative to the LCL > 0 element could be LCL > LCSL, analogous to the estimated TD definition. For this particular case, this was determined to be an unrealistic standard, based on the sample sizes being considered.)

- *Noninferior Dose Range*: The true NI dose range is the True ED to the True TD, surrounding the target or reference dose (RD). For a candidate with a TI of 1, the width of the NI range depends upon the efficacy and tolerability MCIDs, as well as the shapes of the DRRs in the RD region. For this project, the RD was 75% of the MTD, and the True ED and True TD were 62.5 and 87.5% MTD, respectively, based on clinical and statistical review of the reference data (rounded for presentation purposes). For a candidate with TI > 1, the interval is wider, while for a candidate with a sufficiently low TI, True ED > True TD and there is no dose that is truly noninferior. The inference for the noninferiority objective (Objective 3) has two logical steps.

(1) The trial gives a Go signal if the estimated ED $\leq$ the estimated TD, otherwise the result is No Go signal. A Go signal is correct if True ED $\leq$ True TD, for the DRRs being simulated, while a No Go signal is correct when the DRRs have True ED > True TD.

(2) In the case of a Go signal, the estimated NI dose range is (estimated ED, estimated TD). Scoring this estimated dose range for correctness might be done in a variety of ways. Our method is based on whether the estimated and true dose ranges at least partially overlap.

These definitions are revisited in Section 8.2.4. The key message, however, is that we attempted to mimic the decision process for recommending a Go/No Go decision and a dose range for further study, based on the key efficacy and tolerability measures, in contrast to, for instance, simply providing hypothesis tests of efficacy for each dose group against placebo. Of course, with the actual trial data in hand, these recommendations would be integrated with all other information for making the overall development decisions.

8.2.2 The Simulation Project Objective

The main objective of the CTS project was to compare the performance of alternative trial designs and analysis methods for correctly assessing candidate drugs across a range of candidate efficacy and tolerability DR profiles which might be encountered in the actual trial and among which we want to discriminate, while taking into account our current uncertainty about the response profile for the reference drug and the relative potency for tolerability for the candidate versus reference, resulting in design and analysis recommendations.

8.2.3 Simulation Project Methods 1: Data Models and Design Options

The key step of a clinical trial simulation is to simulate a single trial, analyzing and drawing conclusions from it just as one would do in a real-life trial. This requires using patient data models to populate the particular trial design being considered and applying the proposed statistical methodology and decision rules. From the trial's statistical results, conclusions are drawn for each study question, mimicking the logical process that will be used in the real-life trial. Based on the correct answer (which is known from the simulation set-up), the trial's inferences can be scored for accuracy. A simple "correct"/"incorrect" scoring is natural and convenient for many trial questions; for scoring point estimates, it is convenient to reduce the assessment of bias and precision to a single dichotomy, based on whether the estimate is "close enough" to the true value (Lockwood et al., 2003). Somewhat arbitrarily, we used ±25% for this project. The percentage of correct trials can easily be calculated (for each question), based on a series of replicate randomized trials (e.g., 1000) conducted under identical conditions. This percentage becomes a single data point in the evaluation of the impact of design features on trial performance.

Preparation for the CTS project includes decisions on the range of designs to be investigated and numerous other aspects of the data models for generating patient data in the context of each design. Analysis methods and decision rules must be implemented for each design. The entire process is akin to planning, executing, and analyzing a series of related (but not identical) clinical trials, and then comparing their results. While this may require a substantial investment of effort, it is almost certainly less expensive than doing a trial that fails to achieve its objectives because of incomplete planning.

The remainder of this section describes some of the key elements of the simulation process and models employed in this project.

Endpoints: For simplicity in this presentation, we focus on the primary efficacy measure (a change from baseline) and one tolerability indicator (occurrence of the most important adverse event). Other measures were included in the full CTS project; of these, one important secondary efficacy measure appears in the data models, but is not otherwise discussed in this chapter.

Candidate profiles and data models: Four distinct candidate profiles are considered, spanning a range of TIs among which it would be important to distinguish. We use the same tolerability DRR model for all candidate profiles, while shifting the efficacy DRR model to achieve the desired TI. The models were based on the reference data for a single trial, but because that trial used a narrower dose range than will be available for the candidate's POC trial, we needed to extrapolate this model based on assumptions grounded in knowledge of this compound class. For tolerability, we imposed a gradually increasing DR slope for AE incidence. The reference efficacy data had a linear DRR in the tested dose range, while our extrapolation included a plateau approached with a steadily decreasing slope.

Our base model (TI = 1) has this assumed shape, with the candidate dose scale related to the reference agent dose scale by a relative potency factor.

- The profile with TI = 0.5 ("inadequate efficacy") has less efficacy, for the same level of tolerability, compared to TI = 1. It reaches the same plateau, but the dose required to reach a given response is double that for the TI = 1 profile.
- The profile with TI = 2.0 ("superior efficacy") has more efficacy conditional on tolerability. As with TI = 0.5, the same plateau is reached, but it requires just half the TI = 1 dose to reach any particular response level.
- The profile with TI = 0 ("inactive") has a flat DR relationship. Its purpose was for verifying that our analysis methods had the desired Type 1 error rate for Objective 1.

Additional data model details are provided following the discussion of trial designs.

Designs: The designs considered are all parallel group, placebo-controlled, with no positive control. The comparison to the reference agent is indirect, through the differences from placebo in the current and historical trials. The trial length is a fixed number of weeks, based on regulatory requirements and the anticipated time course of therapeutic response. The data models are based on the reference trial data for this period, thereby incorporating the impact of dropouts. The following design alternatives reflect a focus on Objective 3 more than 1.

- *Total trial sample size (N)*: The total trial sample size varied from 100 to 600 in steps of 100. Viewed as a surrogate for trial cost, the impact of the other design factors are examined conditional upon size.
- *Number of candidate dose groups*: The number of candidate dose groups varied from three to seven including placebo.
- *Allocation of total trial sample size to groups*: Two patterns for allocating the total sample size (N) among the groups are considered—equal allocation to all groups and "end-weighting" in which the placebo and highest dose groups are twice the size of the other groups. The end-weighting scheme was proposed on the basis that, for a linear regression, the minimum variance for the slope is obtained when dose values are spaced as widely as possible. (In retrospect, considering the regression analysis model used, described below, an allocation pattern favoring the placebo, low dose and high dose might have been a better choice. However, pragmatically, in the early stages of drug development, in our experience, the scientists' strong preference is to study the doses expected to be of clinical value, so that a convincing performance benefit would be needed to justify a plan emphasizing the placebo and lowest dose.)
- *Dose spacing pattern*: Four patterns of dose assignment are evaluated for designs with two to six groups (plus placebo). The *intended dose* for each group is expressed as a fraction of the true (but unknown) MTD. As described below, the *actual dose assignment* is based on an estimated MTD, available at the start of a (real or simulated) trial.
  (1) *"High-narrow 50%" spacing*: Equally spaced doses from 50 to 100% of MTD, respectively (e.g., for five groups: 0, 50, 66.7, 83.3, 100%).
  (2) *"High-narrow 40%" spacing*: Equally spaced doses from 40 to 100% of MTD, respectively (e.g., 0, 40, 60, 80, 100%).
  (3) *"Wide" spacing*: Equally spaced doses over the full MTD range, from 0 to 100 (e.g., 0, 25, 50, 75, 100%).
  (4) *"Narrow-middle" spacing*: Equally spaced doses centered around 50% of MTD (e.g., 0, 20, 40, 60, 80%).
  These patterns were created arbitrarily to provide a range of feasible alternatives. The rationale for emphasizing the range above 40% MTD was based on experience with the class of compounds; otherwise including doses as low as 5 or 10% MTD would have been prudent. The lowest target doses in these designs are 17 and 14% MTD in the wide and narrow-middle patterns, respectively, with six groups. Because of uncertainty about the tolerability RP and considerable uncertainty in the TI and the DRR shape over the extended dose range, we saw no firm basis for fine-tuning the dose spacing based on theoretical optimality criteria.

Location of the dose groups relative to the data model: The dose levels for a trial are assigned on the candidate scale, while the data models are based on the reference scale. An estimated RP for tolerability can be calculated from the MTD estimates for the candidate and reference agent, which allows an approximate mapping between the candidate and reference dose scales. However, error in MTD estimation results in the assigned doses differing from their intended location on the reference agent dose scale. As a further complexity, the dose level finally assigned to a group is the intended dose rounded down to an available dosage size, based on a set of candidate tablet sizes available (e.g., 0, 10, 50, and 200 mg, respectively) and a maximum number of tablets per dosage administration (e.g., ≤3). The resulting available dosage levels are not uniformly spaced over the entire range.

To reflect the uncertainty in the relative potency for tolerability, the MTD for each simulated trial is selected randomly from a lognormal distribution. The clinical project team determined the distribution parameters, based on nonclinical and ultimately Phase I tolerability data for the candidate. The variance of this distribution is particularly important because the larger the variance, the more the realized dose range placement can vary, trial to trial, from the intended location—one trial might have multiple doses on the efficacy plateau while another might have none. The mean for the lognormal distribution was also estimated from the available information—the impact of this choice is through the uneven spacing of the available dosage levels. Doses higher than the true MTD can be given in a particular trial. We did not consider the impact of discontinuing groups due to safety concerns.

Figure 8.1 shows the intended dose spacing for the four design patterns, for two to six groups; the placebo group at 0% MTD is not shown. The reference line at 75% MTD indicates the TI = 1 target reference dose.

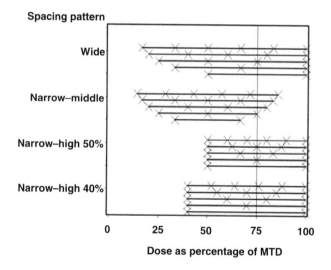

Figure 8.1. The intended dose spacing patterns.

Figure 8.2 illustrates the impact of candidate MTD uncertainty on the realized dose range, for a sample of 40 typical trials having an intended nonplacebo dose range from 25 to 100% MTD. Each line corresponds to a single trial, with its endpoints showing the lowest nonplacebo and highest doses assigned. The highest assigned doses range from approximately 80 to 120%, around the 100% target.

Trial

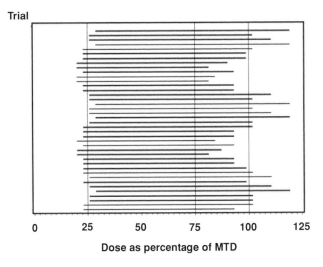

Dose as percentage of MTD

Figure 8.2. Variation in assigned doses levels (40 sample trials).

Data models for efficacy endpoints: Following exploratory analyses of the reference efficacy data, we selected a model for efficacy change from baseline that included terms for the intercept, a drug versus placebo indicator, linear dose, and the baseline values for the primary and secondary efficacy measures. There was no apparent departure from linearity over the dose range studied, so no nonlinear dose term was needed. The estimated parameters and covariance matrix from this analysis provided the starting point for creating the efficacy data model.

- To reflect our uncertainty about the true DRR, the model coefficients used for each simulated trial were randomly selected from a multivariate normal distribution, with mean and covariance matrix as estimated from the reference data.
- Some adjustments, on a trial-to-trial basis, are needed to produce a more reasonable model over the entire dose range. First, since we believe the true DRR monotonically increases, any negative DR slope obtained is set to zero. In addition, since our chosen model structure is discontinuous as the dose approaches zero, linear interpolation is used in those rare trials having an assigned dose between 0 and 12.5% MTD. Based on an estimated theoretical maximum response, a plateau is imposed at dose levels above 75% of MTD, by gradually decreasing the dose slope to zero.
- For each patient, the baseline efficacy values are drawn from a distribution based on the reference trial population.
- A random residual variate is added to complete each patient's efficacy response. Based on reference data patterns, the residual variance linearly increases with dose, with a unique set of regression coefficients randomly selected for each trial.

The base TI $= 1$ model is modified to provide models for the other TIs—for TI $= 0$, the DR slope is set to zero. An "adjusted" dose is used in the calculations

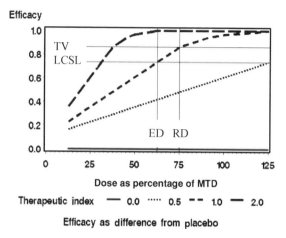

Figure 8.3. Efficacy data models for the four TI profiles.

for TI = 0.5 (half the assigned) and TI = 2 (double). Figure 8.3 shows the four efficacy data models, without between-patient and between-trial variation. The reference lines on the dose scale at the ED (62.5%) and RD (75%) cross the TI = 1 line at the efficacy LCSL (about 0.75) and the efficacy TV (about 0.86), respectively.

Figure 8.4 shows the efficacy DRRs (without patient variability) for 10 sample trials (TI = 1). Note especially the locations relative to the target value TV. For four of these trials, the expected response does not reach the target (at doses ≤125% MTD), including one with a flat line at about 0.6 (for it, the sampled slope was negative, so it was reset to zero). For two trials, the target level is reached at about 50% of the MTD.

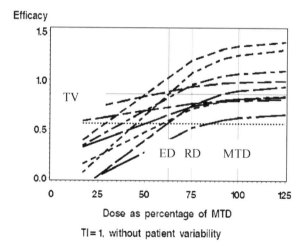

Figure 8.4. Sample data models for efficacy (10 trials).

Data models for tolerability endpoints: Following a similar model building process, the probability of an AE event is calculated as a logistic function, with terms for intercept, drug versus placebo indicator, dose, the secondary efficacy measure baseline, and the observed response on the primary efficacy measure. Above 75% MTD, the DR slope for a trial is made increasingly steep, reflecting our expectation for these extrapolated doses. Because the patient's observed efficacy response is in the model, there is a correlation between the efficacy and tolerability endpoints, as observed in the reference data, presumably reflecting that some patients' good efficacy is accompanied by increased risk of adverse events.

The same tolerability DR model is used for all TIs, as shown in Figure 8.5 (without patient and trial variability). The reference lines at 75 and 87.5% MTD intersect the model line at the tolerability target and UCSL levels, respectively.

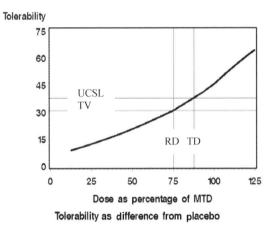

Figure 8.5. Tolerability data model (% adverse event incidence).

Figure 8.6 shows the tolerability DRR (without patient variability) for 10 sample trials, again demonstrating the range of data models that are consistent with the data from the reference agent trial.

8.2.4   Simulation Project Methods 2: Analysis and Evaluation Criteria

The evaluation criteria for the trial objectives are described in this section. Both linear regression and analysis of variance methods were implemented, to allow a better method (as measured by the percentage of correct trials) to be identified for proposed inclusion in the trial protocol.

Analysis of covariance (ANCOVA): Based on an ANCOVA of the change from baseline for the efficacy measure (with baseline as covariate) and an ANOVA of the AE incidence (no covariate), the key statistics are the least squares adjusted

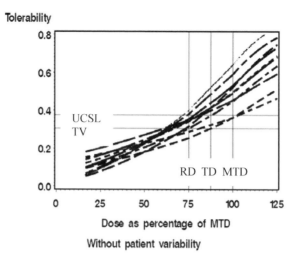

Figure 8.6. Sample data models for tolerability (10 trials).

mean (LSMean) differences between each dose group and placebo, each with an associated 80% confidence interval (CI) comprising upper and lower limits (LCL80, UCL80). Linear interpolation between adjacent groups is used for dose estimation based on the mean response, but criteria based on the CI are evaluated only at the tested doses.

Linear regression: A linear regression model is used to calculate the predicted difference from placebo at all dose levels up to the highest tested dose, with an associated (nonsimultaneous) 80% CI band. The model terms include an intercept, drug versus placebo indicator (1 or 0), and linear dose; if ≥ 3 nonplacebo groups, a quadratic dose term is also included. For efficacy, the baseline observation is a covariate. The discontinuity of this model at dose $= 0$ has little practical impact for estimation in the higher dose regions of primary interest. The quadratic dose term provides some flexibility to fit the underlying nonlinear data patterns; in an actual trial, it would be a matter of judgment as to whether this term realistically improves the estimation.

A third planned set of methods could not be implemented in the CTS due to project time constraints—nonlinear regression for efficacy using an "E_{max}" model, which would likely match more closely the true DRR, and logistic regression for AE incidence, to avoid the clear violation of the variance homogeneity assumption in the ANOVA and linear regression methods.

8.2.4.1 Data Evaluation Criterion for Trial Objective 1: Confirming Efficacy

We set the experiment-wide significance criterion at 10% (one-sided) to limit the false positive risk when the efficacy response is flat (TI = 0). The trial success criterion for this objective is based on the correct answers of "no efficacy" when TI = 0 and "efficacy" when TI > 0.

ANCOVA: A 10% one-sided Dunnett's test for the two highest doses compared to placebo is used as the first step in a modified step-down approach. If either of these groups meets the significance criterion, the trial is judged to have confirmed efficacy; and if so, the remaining groups are separately tested at the 10% level without further multiplicity adjustment. A monotonic true DRR is expected, with the possibility that the higher doses are on a plateau, so that this procedure focuses the first test on the two groups most likely to have the biggest effect. With the caveat that the LCL80 is multiplicity-adjusted for the two highest doses, we can, as shorthand, say that any group deemed significantly better than placebo has passed the "LCL80 > 0" criterion. The lowest dose passing this criterion is used in Objective 3. Note that it is possible that only the highest and lowest doses in a trial pass LCL80 > 0; the lowest dose would be used in Objective 3, despite the nonsignificance of the intermediate groups.

Regression: A contrast of the dose coefficients is tested at the 20% 2-tailed level. If this contrast is statistically significant, the LCL80 band is examined to find the lowest dose in the tested range, if any, for which LCL80 > 0. The trial is deemed to have confirmed efficacy if such a dose is found. The lowest LCL80 > 0 dose, possibly between two tested dose levels, is the lowest significant dose used in Objective 3.

8.2.4.2 Data Evaluation Criterion for Trial Objective 2: Estimated Target Doses for Efficacy and Tolerability

The fitted model is used to find the dose corresponding to the target response. If not achieved in the tested dose range, the conclusion is that the target dose is "above the top tested dose". For the ANCOVA, the "fitted model" is a linear interpolation between adjacent group LSMeans. The trial success criterion is based on whether the estimated dose is "close enough" to the true dose. For the TI $= 1$ and two candidates, the estimate is judged correct if it is within 25% of the true value, while a larger error or an estimate "above the top tested dose" is incorrect. For TI $= 0$ or 0.5, the correct answer is "above the top tested dose".

8.2.4.3 Data Evaluation Criterion for Trial Objective 3: Estimated Dose Range Potentially Clinically Noninferior to the Reference Agent for Efficacy and Tolerability

This is the key objective for the trial and the most complex to define, calculate, and score. The basic logic, definitions, and abbreviations were introduced in Section 8.2.1. The estimated efficacy dose (estimated ED) is defined as the higher of two dose values—the lowest dose with significant efficacy (LCL80 > 0) and for which the UCL80 $\geq$ target, i.e., with no evidence of inferiority to the target level, based on a nonmultiplicity-adjusted 1-tailed 10% level test of Ho: Effect $=$ target or better. The estimated tolerability dose (estimated TD) is the highest dose with UCL80 < UCSL. The trial success criterion for Objective 3 consists of two sequentially evaluated components.

(1) *Go signal*: A Go signal results from a finding that estimated ED $\leq$ estimated TD. Correspondingly, when estimated ED $>$ estimated TD, the No Go signal reflects that no potentially acceptable dose range was found. The correct answer for TI $= 1$ or 2 is "Go" and for TI $= 0$ or 0.5, "No Go".

(2) *Dose range estimate*: The dose range estimate (applicable only when there is a Go signal) is from estimated ED to estimated TD. We employ a relatively weak success criterion: "Correct" if the estimated range at least partially overlaps the true clinical NI range (True ED, True TD); otherwise "Not correct".

A trial's answer for Objective 3 is correct if both the Go/No Go signal and dose range are correct.

The designs are compared on the percentage of correct trials, for each objective.

8.3   Simulation Results and Design Recommendations

The various design features and data models combine to give a large number of simulation "scenarios", each yielding a percentage of correct estimates for each trial objective. The complete set of results is complex, with no single design being obviously superior on all criteria under all circumstances. The selected results presented below illustrate the basis for our design recommendations; it is certainly possible that others reviewing the results could come to different recommendations.

In each case, 1000 replicate trials were conducted for each specific trial scenario. This provides a resolution of about 2 to 4 percentage points for the design comparisons, depending upon the overall levels of percentage success.

8.3.1   Objective 1: Power for Confirming Efficacy

For the TI $= 0$ candidate (no efficacy), the percentages of correct trials were approximately 90% for all design and analysis combinations, confirming that the 10% Type 1 error rate was preserved as desired.

For the active candidates (TI > 0), the percentage of positive trials (i.e., the power for confirming efficacy) generally increased with larger total trial size (N) and decreased as the selected number of patients was spread over more groups. Table 8.2 shows results for the TI $= 1$ data model, for selected size and number of groups combinations, based on end-weighted allocation and the narrow-high 40% dose spacing, using the ANCOVA analysis.

Table 8.2. Power (%) for Objective 1

Groups\N	100	200	400
3	72	90	97
5	69	85	95
7	64	81	93

There was little difference among the three dose-spacing patterns that included a group at the MTD, while the narrow-middle pattern, with its doses centered around 50% MTD and with highest dose always less than the MTD, had lower power. The end-weighted allocation was somewhat superior to equal weighting—for the Table 8.2 scenarios, regression success ranged from about 1% lower with total $N = 400$ in three groups to about 9% lower with 100 in seven groups. The regression analysis tended to be inferior to ANCOVA, ranging from almost identical with 400 in three groups to about 8% lower with 100 in five or seven groups.

8.3.2   Objective 2: Accuracy of Target Dose Estimation

8.3.2.1   Tolerability Target Dose

Because the same data models for tolerability were used for all TI, only random differences were seen among the four TI. There was essentially no impact of allocation strategy on estimation success, as measured by the percentage of trials with a "close enough" estimate ($\pm 25\%$). Similarly, the differences between the regression and ANCOVA-based estimation were small. There were negligible differences among the three dose spacing patterns including an MTD group, while the narrow-middle pattern was inferior—for $N = 400$ in five groups, the three MTD designs had approximately 74% success compared to about 50% for the narrow-middle pattern. There was a gradual improvement in estimation with increased sample size (e.g., for five groups—about 55% at $N = 100$ and 78% at $N = 600$). The number of groups had little impact (given a fixed total N). Based on these results, the narrow-middle dose spacing pattern is not recommended.

8.3.2.2   Efficacy Dose Estimation

For TI $= 0$ (inactive), all design scenarios had a high success rate for correctly declaring the target dose to be above the top tested dose (e.g., $>99\%$ for $N = 400$ in five groups for all scenarios). For TI $= 0.5$ (e.g., with $N = 400$ in five groups), there was about 70% successful declaration that the target dose is above the top tested dose for the designs including the MTD and around 80% for the narrow-middle design. The modest advantage of the narrow-middle spacing here derives from its lower tested range, leading to more "above top tested dose" findings. For the TI $= 1$ and 2 profiles, the "close enough" success rates were quite small (e.g., 20 to 30% for $N = 400$, five groups, TI $= 1$), with no marked advantage for any scenario.

8.3.3   Objective 3: Estimation of a Potentially Clinically Noninferior Dose Range

For the inactive (TI $= 0$) profile, the 10% type 1 error rate used for Objective 1 provides a minimum Objective 3 success rate of 90%, with these 90% of trials correctly declaring the efficacy dose to be above the top tested dose. The other two criterion components further improve the success rate, e.g., to approximately 95% with $N = 400$ in five groups.

Trial

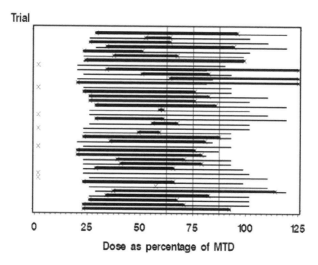

Dose as percentage of MTD

Figure 8.7. Assigned dose levels and estimated NI ranges for 40 sample trials.

(1) For TI $\geq$ 1: Recall that for TI $\geq$ 1, a correct trial provides a Go signal (i.e., estimated ED $\leq$ estimated TD) and this estimated dose range at least partially overlaps the true NI dose region (which for TI = 1 is 62.5 to 87.5% MTD). Figure 8.7 illustrates the regression method Objective 3 results for the same 40 TI = 1 trials displayed in Figure 8.1. As before, each light gray line depicts a trial's tested dose range. For the 33 trials correctly finding estimated ED $\leq$ estimated TD, a darker overlaid line depicts the (estimated ED, estimated TD) interval; when estimated TD is "above top tested dose", the overlay extends, arbitrarily, to 125% MTD in this figure. The seven trials giving an incorrect No Go signal (i.e., estimated ED > estimated TD) have a single X at the left margin of the plot and no overlay, as in the 8th trial from the top. The three vertical reference lines indicate the reference target dose (75% MTD) and the surrounding NI dose region (62.5%, 87.5%). The first four trials, for example, are scored as correct for Objective 3, while the 5th is not, since it gives a Go signal but has its estimated range somewhat below the 62.5% mark.

Recall that a key purpose for the estimated (ED, TD) range is to suggest dose levels for subsequent trials. Considering the ranges observed in the successful trials in Figure 8.7, a strategy such as selecting three doses (at ED, TD, and an intermediate dose) would be necessary to have a good chance to have at least one dose in the targeted range. Picking either the midpoint or the two ends might miss the target range.

Returning to the design feature impact on Objective 3 success for the active candidate profiles (TI > 0), the impact of dose spacing pattern and allocation balance appears to be minor, using the regression method. The regression method has a considerable advantage over ANCOVA. For example, for TI = 1 with the total $N = 400$ using end-weighted allocation and narrow-high 40% spacing, regression had 60% correct with three groups, increasing monotonically to 68% with seven groups. The corresponding AN-COVA results were in the much lower 10–36% range. The key to this better performance is that the regression method interpolates between tested doses using the regression model's CI bands, whereas at least one of the tested dose groups in the ANCOVA must meet all criterion elements.

The impact of the total sample size and number of groups on Objective 3 success is complex. In part, this is because the success for both correctly declaring No Go for TI ≤ 0.5 and Go for TI ≥ 1 are considered. Design features that increase the likelihood of recommending Go will increase the error rate for TI ≤ 0.5 and the success rate for TI ≥ 1. Of course, there will always be the region just below TI $= 1$ where "not quite adequate" candidates have a high risk of getting a mistaken "Go". Beyond that, however, the interplay of the factors is complex.

- Since the estimated TD is the highest dose satisfying the tolerability UCL < UCSL criterion, any design feature that narrows the CI will increase the TD (and the likelihood of a Go).
- Since the estimated ED is the maximum of two dose estimates, the design impact on the larger of these two will determine whether a design feature decreases or increases the estimated ED (and the likelihood of a Go or No Go). The LCL > 0 dose will be higher than the UCL > TV dose when the DR curve is relatively flat, with a wide CI band and/or a relatively low TV. Correspondingly, the UCL > TV dose will be the higher of the two when there is a steep DR curve, narrower CI, and/or a relatively high TV. As the CI narrows, due to increased N or other design features, an LCL-dominant situation becomes UCL-dominant.

Table 8.3 illustrates the impact of total sample size (200 or 400) and number of groups (3 or 5) for candidates with TI $= 0.5$, 1, and 2. It provides the percentages of successful trials for detecting efficacy (Objective 1), for a correct Go/No Go signal and for an acceptable dose range estimate (Objective 3), based on

Table 8.3. Success percentages for selected sample sizes and numbers of groups

N\groups	TI $= 0.5$		TI $= 1$		TI $= 2$	
	3	5	3	5	3	5
Any efficacy						
200	60	48	85	76	90	81
400	80	70	97	91	98	94
Go /No Go						
200	57	62	72	65	87	77
400	63	50	72	80	90	91
Dose range						
200	57	62	52	42	72	77
400	63	50	64	64	82	91

the regression method for designs using the dose spacing pattern from 40 to 100% MTD with balanced allocation.

(2) For TI = 0.5: The success rates for correctly declaring "No Go" vary somewhat (50–63%) among these four configurations. The best are 400/3 and 200/5, so that increasing total N from 200 to 400 in five groups degrades performance, while performance is improved by larger sizes in three groups. In general, the success rate versus sample size relationship is nonmonotonic when TI < 1, reaching a low point when the sample size is large enough to detect efficacy but not large enough to declare it as inferior to the target value.

(3) For TI ≥ 1: For the complete Objective 3 success metric (Go + successful dose range estimation), the larger sample sizes improve performance for both three and five group designs. But for just "Go" component, three group designs with $N = 200$ and 400 perform similarly; for five groups, the larger size improves success about 15%. The impact of using more dose groups (keeping total sample size constant) depends somewhat upon the sample size, with no clear pattern evident with just selected sample sizes and numbers of groups, but none of the comparative rates differ by more than 10%.

Perhaps the most notable finding is how well the 200/3 design performs relative to the 400/3 and 400/5 designs. Consider the 200/3 versus 400/5 comparison—for TI = 0.5, the 200/3 design does 7% *better* for the Go decision (57% vs. 50%). For TI = 1, 400/5 has the expected advantage over 200/3 (80% vs. 72% for Go and 64% vs. 52% for dose range). If we focus on the Go decision only, and if our a priori expectation were that the TI = 0.5 and 1.0 candidates are equally likely to be encountered (and ignoring other TI levels), the average success rates, over TI = 0.5 and 1.0, for the four design configurations are quite similar—the 200/3 average is 64.5% (from 57 and 72), 400/5 has 65% (from 50 and 80), 200/5 has 63.5%, and 400/3 has 67.5%, all within the simulation margin of error. From this specific, limited perspective, there would be little or no gain from doubling the sample size, when measured by the success for correctly stopping or proceeding with development.

8.3.4 Trial Design Recommendations

Based on a review of all the simulation results, and considering the stated trial objectives and assumptions, we made these design recommendations:

- *Analysis method*: Regression-based estimation should be used, except for the confirmation of efficacy, where ANCOVA has a modest advantage.
- *Allocation of patients to dose groups*: There was no consistent advantage to either equally balanced or end-weighted allocation, so either could be used.
- *Dose spacing*: An MTD group should be included in the design -i.e., do not use the "narrow-middle" design - but there was no consistent advantage noted for any of the three spacing patterns with an MTD group.

- *Sample size and number of groups*: As discussed, the interplay of these factors' impact on trial performance is complex, particularly when considering both correct "Go" and "No Go" decisions. Over the full range of N, a larger N will, of course, be better. However, the false Go rate is not monotonic in N for TI < 1, so that a larger N, over a limited range, can lead to poorer performance. Our judgment, in the end, was to give two recommendations, one for each of two levels of investment:

  (1) For an N in the 300 to 400 range, use five or six groups. There was little advantage to using more than 400, and four to seven groups performed similarly (and better than 3 groups).

  (2) For an N around 200, 3 groups would be slightly preferable, especially if a TI $= 1$ is expected, when 3 groups has about a 10% advantage. Of course, this would sacrifice the ability to evaluate the degree of linearity for the DR relationships, but could be reasonably successful for the stated objectives, as long as the assumed DR models used were close to the truth.

8.4 Conclusions

CTS can be viewed as an extension of conventional statistical power analysis for selecting and adequately sizing a design. CTS allows us to consider a richer set of drug development decisions and design optimization criteria than simply "is there evidence for efficacy?" A full-scale simulation project, such as the one we describe, requires a larger investment of time than a simple power analysis, so it will not be the best choice for all drug development programs. The analysis methods used for the simulated trial data were candidates for the actual trial's formal analysis plan. Further, the more difficult task of integrating the analysis results into an evaluation framework for drug development decisions was attempted. The simulations helped set expectations about the likelihood of success for these more complex decisions.

Despite efforts to be as realistic as possible in the models and criteria, this work just provides an approximation to reality. Inevitably, design questions will be asked that stretch the limits of the models' relevance. For instance, when design factors have opposing impacts (as with the total sample size and number of groups), the models might predict a specific configuration to be optimum. However, different model assumptions might move this optimal performance to another configuration, begging the question of how literally the simulation results should be taken. Thus the simulation results must be integrated with everything else known about the design and the scientific setting to develop a trial plan that has the best chances for success.

Both the interdisciplinary planning and the review of the simulation results contributed to the progress of the clinical program development. This helped to focus discussion upon the specific trial goals and decisions to be made, while also helping us to incorporate, in a coherent manner, the knowledge available from prior clinical and nonclinical sources.

Acknowledgments

David Hermann, Raymond Miller, Ken Kowalski, and other members of the Pharmacometrics group are recognized for their guidance in formulating the simulation plan and their critique of the emerging results.

References

Bonate, P.L. 2000. Clinical trial simulation in drug development. *Pharmaceutical Research* 17:3252–3256.

Holford, N.H.G., Kimko, H.C., Monteleone, J.P.R., and Peck, C.C. 2000. Simulation of clinical trials. *Annual Review of Pharmacology and Toxicology* 40:209–234.

Holford, N.H.G., Hale, M., Ko, H.C., Steimer, J-L., Sheiner, L.B., Peck, C.C., Bonate, P., Gillespie, W.R., Ludden, T., Rubin, D.B., and Stanski, D. 1999. *Simulation in Drug Development: Good Practices.* Draft Publication of the Center for Drug Development Science (CDDS), Georgetown University, http://cdds.georgetown.edu/research/sddgp723.html.

Kimco, H.C., and Duffull, S.B. 2003. *Simulation for Designing Clinical Trials.* New York: Marcel Dekker.

Lockwood, P., Cook, J., Ewy, W., Mandema, J. 2003. The use of clinical trial simulation to support dose selection: Application to development of a new treatment for chronic neuropathic pain. *Pharmaceutical Research* 20:1752–1759.

9
Analysis of Dose–Response Studies—E_{max} Model

James MacDougall

9.1 Introduction to the E_{max} Model

The E_{max} model is a nonlinear model frequently used in dose–response analyses. The model is shown in Eq. (9.1)

$$R_i = E_0 + \frac{D_i^N \times E_{max}}{D_i^N + ED_{50}^N} \tag{9.1}$$

where

i	= The patient indicator
R_i	= The value of the response for patient i
D_i	= The level of the drug for patient i, the concentration may also be used in many settings
E_0	= The basal effect, corresponding to the response when the dose of the drug is zero
E_{max}	= The maximum effect attributable to the drug
ED_{50}	= The dose, which produces half of E_{max}
N	= The slope factor (Hill factor), measures sensitivity of the response to the dose range of the drug, determining the steepness of the dose–response curve ($N > 0$)
ε_i	= The random error term for patient i. A standard assumption, adopted here, is that the ε_i terms are independent identically distributed with a mean of 0 and variance σ^2. An additional standard assumption is that the error terms are normally distributed.

The E_{max} model dose–response curve shown in Eq. (9.2) is the expected value of the E_{max} model.

$$R = E_0 + \frac{D^N \times E_{max}}{D^N + ED_{50}^N} \tag{9.2}$$

The E_{max} model dose–response curve can be either increasing or decreasing relative to an increase in dose. If the response is decreasing, the value of the E_{max}

parameter will be negative. Figure 9.1 illustrates the E_{max} model dose–response curve where the response increases with increasing dose. Note the difference between E_{max}, the maximal effect attributable to the drug, and $(E_0 + E_{max})$, the asymptotic response with increasing dose. This difference is particularly relevant when the drug of interest is being administered along with concurrent therapy, as the response at maximum dose includes both the maximal effect of the drug (E_{max}) plus the effect of the concurrent therapy (E_0).

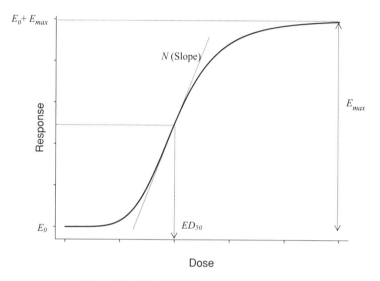

Figure 9.1. E_{max} Model dose–response curve.

Salient features of the model are:

- The E_{max} model has four parameters: E_0, E_{max}, ED_{50}, and N.
- The E_{max} model predicts the maximum effect a drug can have (E_{max}).
- The E_{max} model predicts a zero-dose effect (E_0) when no drug is present.
- The E_{max} model follows the "law of diminishing returns" at higher doses.
- The E_{max} model parameters are readily interpretable.

A particular case of the E_{max} model is given by Eq. (9.3):

$$R_i = E_0 + \frac{D_i \times E_{max}}{D_i + ED_{50}} + \varepsilon_i \tag{9.3}$$

Here the slope factor, N, is not included in the model and as such has an implicit value of one. The E_{max} model without the slope factor parameter is sometimes referred to as the hyperbolic E_{max} model, while the model including the slope factor is referred to as the sigmoidal E_{max} model. Although both the hyperbolic and sigmoidal E_{max} models can be justified on the relationship of drug-receptor interactions (Boroujerdi, 2002), they are primarily used for empirical reasons.

Another common modification of the $E_{\max}$ model is to not include the E_0 parameter if the response at the no drug level is known to be zero.

The $E_{\max}$ model is a common descriptor of dose–response relationships. However, as in all modeling, there are situations where it may not be appropriate to apply. These scenarios include:

- Where the dose–response relationship is not monotonic. The $E_{\max}$ model assumes a monotonic dose response.
- Where the number of different doses for the model is small. As the $E_{\max}$ is a four-parameter model, it desirable to have at least five different doses across the effective dose–response range.
- When the response should not be modeled as a continuous outcome.

Dose estimates other than ED_{50} are often of interest in dose–response analysis. For example ED_{90}, the dose which produces 90% of $E_{\max}$, is sometimes used as an estimate of the maximal effective dose (MaxED). From the $E_{\max}$ model, the ED_{90} is estimated by the formula in Eq. (9.4) where p $(0 < p < 1)$ is the percentile of interest. For example if the slope factor N is 0.5, the estimate of ED_{90} is $(ED_{50} \times 81)$.

$$ED_p = ED_{50} \left(\frac{p}{1-p} \right)^{(1/N)} \tag{9.4}$$

9.2   Sensitivity of the $E_{\max}$ Model Parameters

This section reviews the sensitivity of the $E_{\max}$ model dose–response curve to changes in its four parameters: E_0, $E_{\max}$, ED_{50}, and N. In addition, study design criteria based on these parameters will be reviewed.

9.2.1   Sensitivity of the E_0 and $E_{\max}$ Parameters

As described in Section 9.1, the E_0 parameter is the response when there is no drug present, and the $E_{\max}$ parameter is the maximum attributable drug effect. These two parameters define the upper and lower asymptotic values for the dose–response curve. Changes in the E_0 parameter affect the "starting value" of the dose–response curve (i.e., when there is no drug present). Changes in the $E_{\max}$ parameter affect the range of the dose–response curve.

Figure 9.2 illustrates the change in response as the E_0 and $E_{\max}$ parameters vary. In Figure 9.2, the dotted line illustrates the change in the $E_{\max}$ model curve relative to the solid line when the E_0 and $E_{\max}$ parameters are increased from 0 to 10 and 100 to 110, respectively.

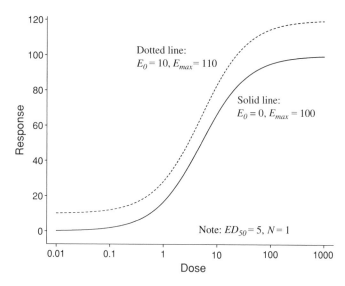

Figure 9.2. E_{max} Model dose–response curves with differing E_0 and E_{max} values.

9.2.2   Sensitivity of the ED_{50} Parameter

The ED_{50} parameter is the dose of the drug which produces half the maximal effect. A higher ED_{50} value indicates a higher dose is needed to produce an effect. Figure 9.3 illustrates the effect of changes in the ED_{50} parameter on the E_{max} dose–response curve.

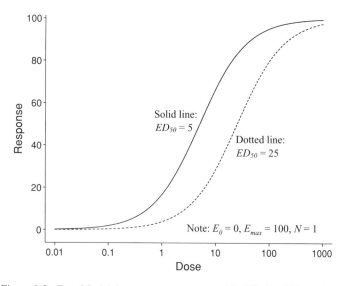

Figure 9.3. E_{max} Model dose–response curves with differing ED_{50} values.

9.2.3   Sensitivity of the N Parameter

The slope factor (Hill factor), determines the steepness of the dose–response curve. As the slope factor N increases, the dose range, defined as the ratio of ED_{90} to ED_{10} tightens. Hence, the larger the value of N, the more sensitive the response is to changes in the dose of the drug. Figure 9.4 illustrates the effect of a change in the slope parameter N from 1 to 3 on the E_{max} model dose–response curve. Figure 9.5 illustrates the dose range (ED_{90}/ED_{10}) as a function of the slope factor based on the E_{max} model.

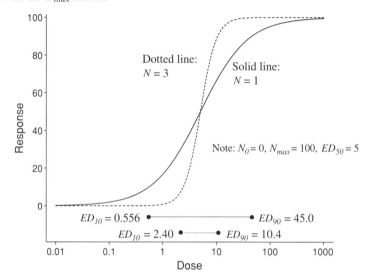

Figure 9.4. E_{max} Model dose–response curves with differing N values.

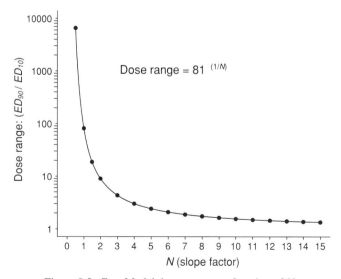

Figure 9.5. E_{max} Model dose range as a function of N.

A useful approximation for the slope factor is given by Eq. (9.5), where DR is the dose range, (ED_{90}/ED_{10}),

$$N \approx \frac{1.91}{\log_{10}(DR)} \qquad (9.5)$$

As the hyperbolic E_{max} model in Eq. (9.3) implicitly has the slope factor parameter set to one, when using this model the implied dose range is 81, meaning the ED_{90} is 81 times the value of the ED_{10}.

9.2.4   Study Design for the E_{max} Model

In the design of a dose–response analysis study, the decision of which dose levels to include is a critical step. For the E_{max} model, having a placebo dose provides an estimate of response when there is no drug present which corresponds to the E_0 parameter. For the three other parameters in the E_{max} model: E_{max}, ED_{50}, and N, one method for determining the active dose levels is the D-optimality criterion. The D-optimality criterion is a method of choosing the dose levels such that the parameters are estimated in an optimal fashion (Seber and Wild, 2003; Bates and Watts, 1988). Figure 9.6 illustrates the results of applying the D-optimality criterion to each of the E_{max} parameters individually for an E_{max} model with parameter values $E_0 = 0$, $ED_{50} = 5$, $E_{max} = 100$, and $N = 1$. For each of the three curves, the maximum value indicates the optimal dose for that parameter based on the D-optimality criterion.

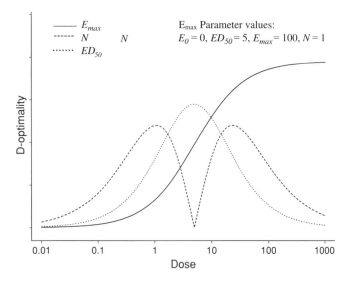

Figure 9.6. D-Optimal design criteria for the E_{max} model parameters ED_{50}, E_{max}, and N.

The curve for the E_{max} parameter is monotonically increasing with respect to dose, indicating that for this parameter a high dose should be utilized. For the ED_{50} parameter, the curve is maximized at ED_{50}. For the slope parameter N, there are two maximums, at approximately ED_{20} and ED_{80}.

The D-optimality criterion can also be used in a multivariate setting, optimizing the design criterion over multiple parameters. For example, in the scenario where a placebo group and four different active dose levels are planned, applying the D-optimality criterion for the E_{max} model with parameter values of $E_0 = 0$, $ED_{50} = 5$, $E_{max} = 100$, and $N = 1$ yields the four active dose levels at: (1) $ED_{15} - ED_{25}$, (2) $ED_{35} - ED_{65}$, (3) $ED_{70} - ED_{80}$, and (4) a maximum dose. This method has the limitation that the E_{max} model parameter values are used in the calculations, which, as they are unknown prior to the dose–response study, would need to be estimated. In addition, this method implicitly assumes that the E_{max} model is an appropriate model for the dose–response data.

In situations where the study design does not include dose values that produce close to a maximal effect, the resulting parameter estimates may be poorly estimated. The results of Dutta et al. (1996) demonstrated that when the highest dose in the study was less than ED_{95} the parameter estimates for E_{max}, ED_{50}, and N are poorly estimated with a high coefficient of variation and bias. However, within the range for which the data were available, the fit of the E_{max} model to the data was quite good. As it is not uncommon for a circumstance to arise where it may not be reasonable or ethical to include a high dose in the study design (e.g., safety issues), care should be taken in the interpretation of the parameter estimates when an E_{max} model is applied.

9.2.5 Covariates in the E_{max} Model

In a dose–response setting there is the possibility that one or more covariates could significantly account for patient variation in the response to a drug. In a situation where a covariate may influence the response, it can be beneficial to incorporate that covariate in the E_{max} model. For example, if it is desired to allow for gender differences in the ED_{50} parameter, the E_{max} model can be modified as in Eq. (9.6),

$$R_i = E_0 + \frac{D_i^N \times E_{max}}{D_i^N + (ED_{50} + (Z_i \times ED_{50M}))^N} + \varepsilon_i \qquad (9.6)$$

In Eq. (9.6), a fifth parameter is added to the E_{max} model, ED_{50M}, and an indicator variable, Z_i, equal to 0 if the patient is female, 1 if the patient is male. For females the estimate of the dose achieving half E_{max} is ED_{50}; for males the estimate is $ED_{50} + ED_{50M}$.

9.3   Similar Models

The four-parameter logistic model as described in O'Connell et al. (1993) is given by the following equation

$$R_i = \beta_2 + \frac{(\beta_1 - \beta_2)}{1 + (D_i/\beta_3)^{\beta_4}} + \varepsilon_i \tag{9.7}$$

where

i = The patient indicator
R_j = The value of the response for patient i
D_i = The level of the drug for patient i
β_1 = The response when there is no drug present
β_2 = The maximal attributable effect of the drug $+ \beta_1$
β_3 = The dose, which produces the response halfway between β_1 and β_2
β_4 = This parameter is related to the steepness of the slope
ε_i = The random error term for patient i.

As can be seen from Eq. (9.7), the four-parameter logistic model is nonlinear. As applied in O'Connell et al. (1993), the β_4 parameter is set to be >0. There are similarities between the four-parameter logistic model and the $E_{\max}$ model. When the β_4 parameter is set to be >0, the four-parameter logistic model is equivalent to an $E_{\max}$ model with an inverse transformation on the dose (see the Appendix). When the β_4 parameter is set to be <0, then the four-parameter logistic model is equivalent to the $E_{\max}$ model (see the Appendix).

Other models used in dose–response analysis are described in Chapter 10 and in Ruberg (1995). The books by Seber and Wild (2003) and Bates and Watts (1988) provide information on the theory and applications of nonlinear regression. Texts on nonlinear regression for repeated measures include Davidian and Giltinan (1995), and Vonesh and Chinchilli (1997).

9.4   A Mixed Effects $E_{\max}$ Model

Equation 9.8 describes a mixed effects $E_{\max}$ model as presented in Girard et al. (1995). This model is useful when there are multiple observations per patient as it accounts for the correlation of the within-patient responses and can be used to describe individual dose–response curves,

$$R_{ij} = E_{0i} + \frac{D_{ij}^N \times E_{\max i}}{D_{ij}^N + ED_{50i}^N} + \varepsilon_{ij} \tag{9.8}$$

where

i	=	The patient indicator
j	=	The observation number for a patient
R_{ij}	=	The response of patient i, observation j
D_{ij}	=	The dose of the drug for patient i, observation j
E_{0i}	=	The zero-dose response for patient i
E_{maxi}	=	The maximum attributable drug effect for patient i
ED_{50i}	=	The dose, which produces half of E_{maxi}
N	=	The slope factor
ε_{ij}	=	The random error term for patient i, observation j.

This model assumes individual variation in E_0, ED_{50}, and E_{max}. However, the slope factor parameter, N, does not vary among patients. This restriction of having the slope parameter only as a fixed effect is not a requirement of a mixed-effect E_{max} model and there may be scenarios where the data is suitable and it is desired to allow patient variation in the slope factor.

Discussions on the optimal study design to obtain repeated measures on a patient for a dose–response study is beyond the scope of this chapter. However, discussions on the design of clinical trials for obtaining multiple observations on a patient are provided in Chapter 7 of this volume and also in Girard et al. (1995), ICH-E4 Guidelines (1998), Senn (1997); Sheiner et al. (1989), Sheiner et al. (1991), and Temple (1982, 2004).

9.5 Examples

The data analyses for these two examples were performed using SAS with the corresponding analysis code presented in the Appendix. In particular, Proc NLIN and Proc NLMIXED in SAS were used for estimating the E_{max} model parameters. It should be noted, however, that there are other available software packages as well, such as NONMEM and S-PLUS, which are both utilized for E_{max} modeling in dose–response analyses.

9.5.1 Oral Artesunate Dose–Response Analysis Example

The following example is based on a study by Angus (2002). The objective of the study was to characterize the dose–response of oral artesunate on falciparum malaria. Forty-seven adult patients were randomized to a single dose of oral arte-sunate varying from 0 to 250 mg together with a curative dose of oral mefloquine. A patient could receive a dose of either: 0, 25, 50, 75, 100, 150, 200, or 250 mg.

Figure 9.7 illustrates patients' parasite clearance time (the time required for a patient to reach a count of <1 parasite per 200 white blood cell nuclei) versus their dose of artesunate divided by the patient's weight (in units of mg/kg). An E_{max} model curve and smoothing spline both fit to the data are also shown. The

Table 9.1. Oral artesunate example: E_{max} model parameter estimates

	Sigmoidal E_{max}	Hyperbolic E_{max}
E_0 (s.e.)	70.2 (4.5)	72.8 (7.0)
ED_{50} (s.e.)	1.4 (0.14)	3.19 (4.18)
E_{max} (s.e.)	−28.4 (5.8)	−54.0 (27.7)
N (s.e.)	12.9 (23.9)	—

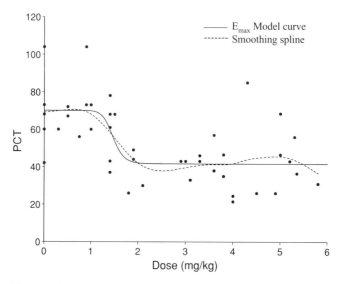

Figure 9.7. Parasite clearance time (PCT) versus dose of artesunate (mg/kg).

smoothing spline fit to the data illustrates that an E_{max} model may be appropriate to characterize the dose–response of parasite clearance time. Table 9.1 presents the corresponding estimated E_{max} model parameters.

The results of this analysis of the example data indicate a MaxED of less than 2.0 mg/kg ($ED_{90} = 1.7$), indicating limited additional benefit in the reduction of parasite clearance time (PCT) with doses of artesunate higher than 2.0 mg/kg.

In this example the slope factor N is fairly high, corresponding to a steep dose–response curve and a dose range of approximately 1.4. However, the slope parameter is estimated with poor precision (standard error: 23.9).

Given the poor precision of the slope parameter N, the hyperbolic E_{max} model was fit to the data. Figure 9.8 illustrates the contrast in fitting the hyperbolic E_{max} model (which has the slope parameter N fixed equal to one) to the oral artesunate malaria data versus the sigmoidal E_{max} model. As the estimated dose range for oral artesunate is 1.4 using the sigmoidal E_{max} model and the dose range for hyperbolic E_{max} model is set at 81, it is not surprising that the two curves look markedly different. The suitability of the hyperbolic E_{max} model is questionable

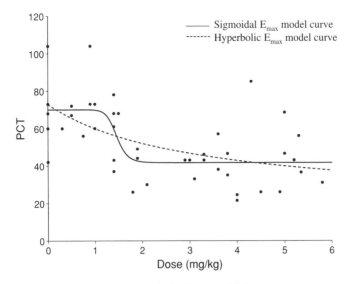

Figure 9.8. Sigmoidal and hyperbolic E_{max} model dose–response curves.

as two of the three parameters have relatively large standard errors. In addition, the estimate of ED_{90} from the hyperbolic E_{max} model is 28.7 mg/kg, well outside the dose range being investigated. An F-test to compare these two nested E_{max} models (Bates and Watts, 1988) indicates that the slope parameter, N, should be retained in the model ($p = 0.013$).

9.5.2   Estimation Methodology

Iterative methods are used to estimate the parameters in the E_{max} model based on minimizing the residual sum of squares. In SAS Proc NLIN, the residual sum of squares is initially determined by using the starting values for the parameters. Then new values of the parameters are chosen based on an iterative technique such that the sum of squares is reduced. The five iterative method options in SAS Proc NLIN are: steepest-descent (gradient), Newton method, Modified Gauss-Newton, Marquardt, and the multivariate secant method. The iterative estimation procedure stops when the convergence criterion is met. In the example presented in Section 9.5.1, the Marquardt iterative method (recommended as a method which works well in many situations by Draper and Smith, 1966) was used. However, other methods were tried as well with essentially no difference in the parameter estimates, except for the steepest-descent method, which failed to converge after 1000 iterations (the slow convergence of the steepest-descent method is described in Draper and Smith, 1966). Further details on the estimation methodology and iterative methods used in Proc NLIN are found in *SAS/STAT Users Guide* (1999), Bates and Watts (1988), and Draper and Smith (1966).

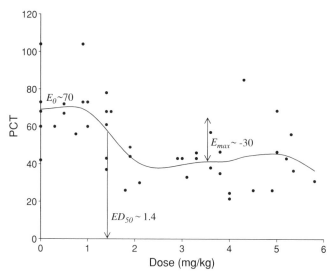

Figure 9.9. Estimation of starting values for E_0, E_{max}, and ED_{50} using a smoothing spline.

9.5.3   Initial Parameter Values for the Oral Artesunate Dose–Response Analysis Example

As discussed in Section 9.5.2, starting values for the parameters are required for Proc NLIN. Figures 9.9 and 9.10 illustrate fitting a smoothing spline to the data to provide initial estimates of E_{max} model parameters.

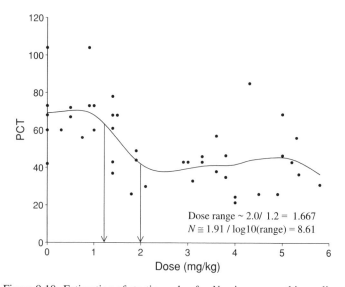

Figure 9.10. Estimation of starting value for N using a smoothing spline.

Figure 9.10 illustrates the use of Eq. (9.5) in estimating a starting value for the slope parameter N. Based on Figures 9.9. and 9.10, the starting parameter values are $E_0 = 70$, $E_{max} = -30$, $ED_{50} = 1.4$, and $N = 8.61$. In many cases, the parameter estimates from the E_{max} model are fairly robust to the starting parameter values. For example, modifying the starting values given above to: $E_0 = 50$, $E_{max} = -50$, $ED_{50} = 2.0$, and $N = 3$ yields essentially the same parameter estimates using SAS Proc NLIN (albeit more iterations were needed to reach the convergence criteria).

A discussion on other methods of determining starting values for parameters in nonlinear models can be found in Bates and Watts (1988).

9.5.4 Diastolic Blood Pressure Dose–Response Example

The following example is based on a simulation study by Giradet al. (1995). This example considers the effect of an anti-hypertensive drug administered to patients with a diastolic blood pressure over 95 mmHg. The data are simulated as follows: 40 patients with doses of 0, 10, 20, 40, and 80 given to all patients (each patient takes multiple doses). The E_{max} model is used to simulate the data.

The model used to simulate the data is given by Eq. (9.9):

$$R_{ij} = E_{0i} + \frac{D_{ij}^N \times E_{max\,i}}{D_{ij}^N + ED_{50i}^N} + \varepsilon_{ij} \tag{9.9}$$

where

i	= Patient number $i = 1, \ldots, 40$
j	= Observation number for a patient $j = 1, \ldots, 5$ corresponding to doses of 0, 10, 20, 40, and 80
R_{ij}	= The diastolic blood pressure for patient i at observation j
D_{ij}	= The dose of the drug for patient i, observation j
E_{0i}	= The baseline diastolic blood pressure for patient i; normally distributed ($\mu = 80, \sigma = 15$)
$E_{max\,i}$	= The maximum effect of the drug (relative to the baseline response) for patient i; normally distributed ($\mu = -12, \sigma = 6$)
ED_{50i}	= The dose which produces half of the maximum response for patient i; normally distributed ($\mu = 10, \sigma = 3.5$)
N	= The slope factor; set to a value of 2
ε_{ij}	= The error term; normally distributed ($\mu = 0, \sigma = 2$).

The first 40 simulated patients with an E_{0i} of 95 mmHg or greater were included in the analysis. Figure 9.11 illustrates the simulated dose–response data for 3 of the 40 patients across the five doses. Figure 9.12 illustrates the individual dose–response curves for these three patients. Table 9.2 illustrates the population level parameter estimates.

Table 9.2 displays the mean and standard deviation estimates for the parameters based on the forty patients' actual values and the values estimated from the mixed

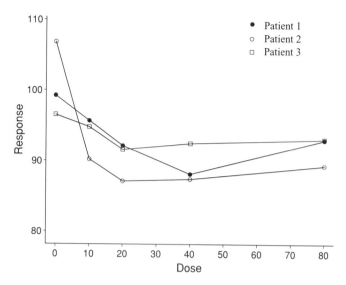

Figure 9.11. Simulated diastolic blood pressure data for three patients.

effects $E_{\max}$ model. As can be seen from Table 9.2, the analysis of the simulated data produced estimates similar to the values used in the simulation. The mean and standard deviation estimates of E_{0i} are different from the initial simulation model values ($\mu = 80$, $\sigma = 15$) due to the constraint that a patient have an E_{0i} value 95 mmHg or greater.

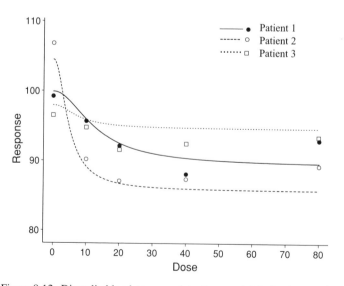

Figure 9.12. Diastolic blood pressure data $E_{\max}$ model fit for three patients.

Table 9.2. Blood pressure example: E_{max} model parameter estimates

	E_{0i}	ED_{50i}	E_{maxi}	N
Actual: μ (σ)	104.3 (8.4)	9.9 (3.3)	−12.1 (6.0)	2 (−)
Estimated: μ (σ)	104.8 (8.5)	9.1 (2.8)	−12.8 (6.2)	1.7 (−)

Note: The slope factor, N, was included as a fixed effect.

Proc NLMIXED uses a different method of parameter estimation than Proc NLIN; maximizing an approximation to the likelihood integrated over the random effects. Details on the estimation methodology can be found in *SAS/STAT Users Guide* (1999), Davidian and Giltinan (1995), and Pinheiro and Bates (2000).

9.6 Conclusions

This chapter reviewed the E_{max} model for dose–response analyses in clinical trials. The model was introduced, parameters interpreted, and sensitivities of the E_{max} model curve to changes in the parameters reviewed. Study design considerations, estimating starting values, and data analysis examples using the E_{max} model were also reviewed.

Understanding the dose response is a fundamental part of the choosing the right dose. The E_{max} model is flexible, the parameters are readily interpretable, and software packages make the implementation straightforward. The utility of the E_{max} model has been demonstrated by its use over a wide variety of therapeutic areas and stages of drug development including pre-clinical, PK/PD, and Phase II studies. The decision to consider an E_{max} model as part of a dose–response analysis ideally should be made prior to the start of the study. In doing so, the response of interest, number of patients/observations, number of doses, and design of the study can be evaluated to ensure the suitability of the E_{max} model. When appropriately applied, the results of an E_{max} model analysis can be a fundamental part of the dose-selection process.

References

Angus, B.J., Thaiaporn, I., Chanthapadith, K., Suputtamongkol, Y., and White, N.J. 2002. Oral artesunate dose-response relationship in acute falciparum malaria. *Antimicrobial Agents and Chemotherapy* 46(3):778–782.

Bates, D.M., and Watts, D.G. 1988. *Nonlinear Regression Analysis and Its Applications*. New York: Wiley.

Boroujerdi, M. 2002. *Pharmacokinetics: Principles and Applications*. New York: McGraw Hill.

Davidian, M., and Giltinan, D. M. 1995. *Nonlinear Models for Repeated Measurement Data*. New York: Chapman and Hall.

Draper, N., and Smith, H. 1966. *Applied Regression Analysis*, 2nd ed. New York: Wiley.

Dutta, S., Matsumoto, Y., and Ebling, W.F. 1996. Is it possible to estimate the parameters of the sigmoid E_{max} model with truncated data typical of clinical studies? *Journal of Pharmaceutical Sciences* 85(2):232–239.

Girard P., Laporte-Simitsidis S., Mismetti P., Decousus H., and Boissel J. 1995. Influence of confounding factors on designs for dose-effect relationships estimates. *Statistics in Medicine* 14:987–1005.

ICH-E4 Guideline. 1998. *Dose–Response Information to Support Drug Registration, Step 4.* Web-site: http://www.ich.org/cache/compo/276-254-1.html

O'Connell M.A., Belanger, B.A., and Haaland, P.D. 1993. Calibration and assay development using the four-parameter logistic model. *Chemometrics and Intelligent Laboratory Systems* 20:97–114.

Pinheiro, J.C., and Bates, D.M. 2000. *Mixed-Effects Models in S and S-PLUS.* New York: Springer-Verlag.

Ruberg, S.J. 1995. Dose–response studies II. Analysis and interpretation. *Journal of Biopharmaceutical Statistics* 5(1):15–42.

SAS/STAT User's Guide Version 8 Volumes 1–3. 1999. Cary NC: SAS Publishing.

Seber, G. F., and Wild, C.J. 2003. *Nonlinear Regression.* New Jersey: Wiley.

Senn, S. 1997. *Statistical Issues in Drug Development.* West Sussex, England: Wiley.

Sheiner, L.B., Beal, S.L., and Sambol, N.C. 1989. Study designs for dose-ranging. *Clinical Pharmacology and Therapeutics* 46:63–77.

Sheiner, L.B., Hashimoto Y., and Beal, S.L. 1991. A simulation study comparing designs for dose ranging. *Statistics in Medicine* 10:303–321.

Temple, R. 1982. Government viewpoint of clinical trials. *Drug Information Journal* 16:10–17.

Temple, R. 2004. *Where protocol design has been a critical factor in success or failure.* Presentation at the DIA Annual Meeting June 14, 2004.

Vonesh, E.F. and Chinchilli,V.M. (1997) *Linear and Nonlinear Models for the Analysis of Repeated Measurements.* New York: Marcel Dekker.

Appendix

Comparison of the Four-Parameter Logistic Model to the E_{max} Model: When $\beta_4 > 0$

Given the four-parameter logistic model:

$$R = \beta_2 + \frac{(\beta_1 - \beta_2)}{1 + (D/\beta_3)^{\beta_4}} \tag{9.10}$$

Re-arranging the terms yields:

$$R = \beta_2 + \frac{(\beta_1 - \beta_2)}{1 + (D \times \beta_3^{-1})^{\beta_4}} \tag{9.11}$$

$$R = \beta_2 + \left(\frac{D^{-\beta_4}}{D^{-\beta_4}}\right) \times \frac{(\beta_1 - \beta_2)}{1 + (D \times \beta_3^{-1})^{\beta_4}} \tag{9.12}$$

$$R = \beta_2 + \frac{(D^{-1})^{\beta_4} \times (\beta_1 - \beta_2)}{(D^{-1})^{\beta_4} + (\beta_3^{-1})^{\beta_4}} \tag{9.13}$$

Setting

$$
\begin{aligned}
X &= D^{-1} \\
\beta_2 &= E_0 \\
(\beta_1 - \beta_2) &= E_{\max} \\
\beta_3^{-1} &= ED_{50} \\
\beta_4 &= N
\end{aligned}
\tag{9.14}
$$

yields an $E_{\max}$ model with an inverse dose transformation:

$$R = E_0 + \frac{X^N \times E_{\max}}{X^N + ED_{50}^N} \tag{9.15}$$

Note that due to the inverse transformation of the dose, the $E_{\max}$ model parameters are interpreted in terms of the inverse dose. For example, E_0 would be the response when the inverse dose is zero.

Comparison of the Four-Parameter Logistic Model to the $E_{\max}$ Model: When $\beta_4 < 0$

The following demonstrates the equivalence of the $E_{\max}$ model and the four-parameter logistic model when $\beta_4 < 0$.

Given the four-parameter logistic model:

$$R = \beta_2 + \frac{(\beta_1 - \beta_2)}{1 + (D/\beta_3)^{\beta_4}} \tag{9.16}$$

Re-arranging the terms yields:

$$R = \beta_2 + \frac{D^{-\beta_4} \times (\beta_1 - \beta_2)}{D^{-\beta_4} + \beta_3^{-\beta_4}} \tag{9.17}$$

Setting

$$
\begin{aligned}
\beta_2 &= E_0 \\
(\beta_1 - \beta_2) &= E_{\max} \\
\beta_3 &= ED_{50} \\
-\beta_4 &= N
\end{aligned}
\tag{9.18}
$$

yields the $E_{\max}$ model:

$$R = E_0 + \frac{D^N \times E_{\max}}{D^N + ED_{50}^N} \tag{9.19}$$

SAS Code Used for $E_{\max}$ Model Parameter Estimation

Proc NLIN and NLMIXED in SAS were used to estimate the $E_{\max}$ model parameters. Further details on Proc NLIN and NLMIXED can be found in the SAS/STAT Users Guide (1999).

Core SAS Code for the E_{max} Model Analysis of the Oral Artesunate Example Data in Section 9.5

```
proc nlin data=malaria method=marquardt hougaard;
  parms e0=70 ed50=1.4 emax=−30 n = 8.61;
  if dose=0 then
    model pct=e0;
  else
    model pct=e0 + ((dose**n)*emax)/((ed50**n) + (dose**n));
  ods output parameterestimates=ests;
run;
```

Comments on this SAS code are:

- malaria was the name of the SAS data set used, containing dose (mg/kg) and parasite clearance time.
- The method option specifies the iterative technique NLIN uses to estimate the parameters (method = marquardt) was used.
- pct is the dependent variable, the parameters in the model are e0, emax, ed50 and n.
- The hougaard option provides a skewness measure, assessing if the parameters have properties similar to linear regression estimates: unbiased, normally distributed (|values| >1 nonlinear behavior is considerable).
- The parm option specifies the initial values for the parameters.
- The if dose = 0 code was used because Proc NLIN calculates the partial derivatives for the four parameters and the partial derivative with respect to the slope factor involves log(dose). Hence a separate equation when the dose = 0 was used, however when the dose = 0 the E_{max} model simplifies to $R = E_0$.

Core SAS Code for the E_{max} Model Analysis of the Blood Pressure Example Data in Section 9.5

```
proc nlmixed data=bp_01;
  parms e0=100 ed50=10 emax=−12 n=2 s2e0i=225 s2emaxi=36
s2ed50i=12.25 err=4;
  e0_=(e0 + e0i);
  if dose=0 then do;
    pred=e0_;
  end;
  else do;
    numer = (dose**n)*(emax+emaxi);
```

```
    denom = ((ed50+ed50i)**n) + (dose**n);
    pred = e0_ + numer/denom;
  end;
  model dbp ~ normal(pred, err);
  random e0i emaxi ed50i ~ normal([0, 0, 0],[s2e0i, 0, s2emaxi, 0,
0, s2ed50i])
    subject=patid;
  run;
```

Comments on this SAS code are:

- bp_01 was the name of the SAS data set used. The dataset contained the patient's dose values and their corresponding diastolic blood pressure (mmHg).
- The parm option specifies the initial values for the population parameters (e0, ed50, emax, n); the variance parameters for random effects (s2e0i, s2emaxi, s2ed50i), and error term (err).
- Similar to the NLIN SAS code in the previous example, programming statements were used for the dose = 0 case due to log(dose) component of the partial derivative for the slope factor.
- In this code the E_{max} model is defined in two stages, first a numerator (numer) and a denominator (denom) are defined, then the E_{max} model is defined as the ratio with the e0_ term included.
- The model statement is the mechanism for specifying the conditional distribution of the data given the random effects.
- The random statement defines the random effects and their distribution. The variance matrix is defined using the lower triangular method.

10
Analysis of Dose–Response Studies—Modeling Approaches

JOSÉ C. PINHEIRO, FRANK BRETZ, AND MICHAEL BRANSON

10.1 Introduction

Identifying the correct dose is one of the most important and difficult goals in drug development. Selecting too high a dose can result in an unacceptable toxicity profile, while selecting too low a dose decreases the chance of it showing effectiveness in Phase III trials and thus getting regulatory approval. Typically decisions derived from dose–response studies can be divided into two main components: establishing that the treatment has some effect on the outcome under consideration, the so called proof-of-activity (PoA), sometimes also referred to as a proof-of-concept (PoC), and selecting a dose (or doses) that appears to be efficacious and safe, for further development in Phase III, the so-called dose-finding step.

The statistical analysis of dose–response studies can be divided into two major strategies: multiple comparison procedures (MCP) and model–based approaches. The model-based approach assumes a functional relationship between the response and the dose, taken as a quantitative factor, according to a pre-specified parametric model, such as a logistic or an $E_{\max}$ model. The fitted model is then used to test if a dose–response relationship is present (PoA) and, if so, to estimate an adequate dose(s) to achieve a desired response using, for example, inverse regression techniques. Such an approach provides flexibility in investigating the effect of doses not used in the actual study. However, the validity of its conclusions will highly depend on the correct choice of the dose–response model, which is of course a priori unknown. This creates a dilemma in practice, because, within the regulated environment in which drug development takes place, it is required to have the analysis methods (including the choice of the dose–response model) defined at the study design stage.

Multiple comparison procedures, on the other hand, regard the dose as a qualitative factor and make very few, if any, assumptions about the underlying dose-response model. The primary goal is often to identify the minimum effective dose (MED) that is statistically significantly superior to placebo and produces a clinically relevant effect (Ruberg, 1995; ICH E4, 1994). One approach is to evaluate the significance of contrasts between different dose levels, while preserving the family-wise error rate (FWER), i.e., the probability of committing at least one

Type I error. Such procedures are relatively robust to the underlying dose–response shape, but are not designed for inter- and extrapolation of information other than at the observed dose levels. Inferences are thus confined to the selection of the target dose among the dose levels under investigation.

The general framework adopted for this chapter is that a response Y (which can be an efficacy or a safety variable) is observed for a given set of parallel groups of patients corresponding to doses $d_2, d_3, \ldots, d_k$ plus placebo d_1, for a total of k arms. For the purpose of testing PoA and estimating target doses, we consider a one-way layout for the model specification

$$Y_{ij} = \mu_{d_i} + \epsilon_{ij}, \quad \epsilon_{ij} \overset{ind}{\sim} \mathcal{N}(0, \sigma^2), \ i = 1, \ldots, k, j = 1, \ldots, n_i, \qquad (10.1)$$

where the mean response at dose d_i can be represented as $\mu_{d_i} = f(d_i, \boldsymbol{\theta})$ for some dose–response model $f(.)$ parameterized by a vector of parameters $\boldsymbol{\theta}$ and ϵ_{ij} is the error term for patient j within dose group i.

To make things more concrete let us introduce an example of a dose-finding study presented in Bretz et al. (2005), which will also be used in later sections to illustrate different dose-finding methods. This was a randomized double-blind parallel group trial with a total of 100 patients being allocated to either placebo or one of four active doses coded as 0.05, 0.20, 0.60, and 1, with $n = 20$ per group. To maintain confidentiality, the actual doses have been scaled to lie within the $[0, 1]$ interval. The response variable was assumed to be normally distributed and larger values indicate a better outcome. A priori the assumption of monotonicity $\mu_0 \leq \mu_{0.05} \leq \mu_{0.2} \leq \mu_{0.6} \leq \mu_1$ was made. Figure 10.1 shows the estimated difference in response with respect to placebo for each dose, together with the associated 90% confidence intervals.

A fixed sequence test (Westfall and Krishen, 2001) was adopted as an MCP to test the PoA and determine efficacious doses using a 5% one-sided level. In Table 10.1, the pairwise comparisons of treatment to placebo based on the one-way analysis of variance model in Eq. (10.1) are summarized.

Table 10.1. Pairwise comparisons to placebo

Parameter	Estimate	Standard error	t-value	One-sided P-value	Marginal 90% CI
$\mu_1 - \mu_0$	0.6038	0.2253	2.68	0.0044	(0.2296, 0.9780)
$\mu_{0.6} - \mu_0$	0.5895	0.2253	2.62	0.0052	(0.2153, 0.9638)
$\mu_{0.2} - \mu_0$	0.4654	0.2253	2.07	0.0201	(0.0912, 0.8396)
$\mu_{0.05} - \mu_0$	0.1118	0.2253	0.50	0.3103	(−0.2624, 0.4861)

From the results in Table 10.1, it is clear that the formal closed test stopped after having concluded that the top three doses of treatment were statistically significantly different from placebo. The question then arises as the determination of a MED (all doses were well tolerated, so safety was not a concern for the given dose range). The estimation of the MED using a modeling approach will be discussed when this example is re-analyzed in Sections 10.3 and 10.5.

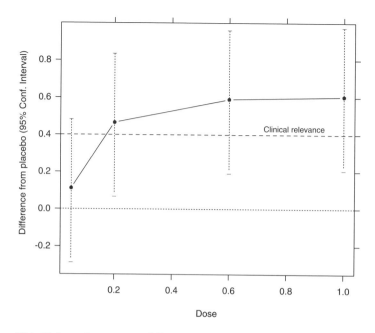

Figure 10.1. Estimated treatment differences with respect to placebo and associated marginal 90% confidence intervals for each dose in the Phase II example.

More complex designs, such as crossover and within-patient dose-escalation designs are also used in practice with dose-finding studies but do not fall into the general framework described by Eq. (10.1). In particular, the assumption of independence among the observations, included in Eq. (10.1), is no longer reasonable for these repeated measures designs. As a consequence, more complex modeling of the dose–response profiles, typically utilizing linear or nonlinear mixed-effects models (Pinheiro and Bates, 2000), is needed. Such designs and models are out-of-scope for this chapter. However, the main ideas about dose response modeling and estimation of target doses presented here remain valid for the more complex cases, with the appropriate modifications.

The rest of this chapter is organized as follows. Section 10.2 describes some commonly used dose–response models, discussing the interpretation of the associated parameters and approaches for deriving starting estimates for determining model contrasts. The estimation of target doses, and the MED in particular, using a modeling approach is the topic of Section 10.3. The important topic of selecting the most appropriate dose–response model within a set of possible candidate models, and the uncertainty associated with it, is discussed in Section 10.4. In Section 10.5, we describe a novel, unified strategy for the analysis of data from dose–response studies which combines multiple comparison and modeling techniques to allow inferences about PoA and dose selection. Our conclusions and suggestions for further research are included in Section 10.6.

10.2   Some Commonly Used Dose–Response Models

In this section, we describe some of the most common models used in practice to represent dose–response profiles. As noted in Section 10.1, the general framework adopted here for (parametrically) modeling the dose–response relationship for a response Y is given by

$$Y_{ij} = f(d_i, \boldsymbol{\theta}) + \epsilon_{ij}, \qquad \epsilon_{ij} \overset{\text{ind}}{\sim} \mathcal{N}(0, \sigma^2) \qquad (10.2)$$

where the dose–response model $f(.)$ may be a linear or nonlinear function of the parameters $\boldsymbol{\theta}$.

The testing of PoA and the selection of target doses using a modeling approach requires the estimation of the model parameters $\boldsymbol{\theta}$. Under the assumption of independent, identically distributed errors ϵ_{ij} adopted here, ordinary least squares (OLS) estimates that minimize the residual sum of squares $\sum_{i=1}^{k} \sum_{j=1}^{n_i} |Y_{ij} - f(\boldsymbol{\theta}, d_i)|^2$ are typically used. In the case of nonlinear dose–response models, nonlinear least squares algorithms are needed to estimate $\boldsymbol{\theta}$. The most popular of these is the Gauss-Newton algorithm (Bates and Watts, 1988; Seber and Wild, 1989), which is an iterative procedure consisting of solving, until convergence, a sequence of linear least squares problems based on a local approximation of the nonlinear model. Such iterative algorithms typically require a starting point, the so-called initial values, for the parameters. Methods for deriving initial estimates for nonlinear models are discussed in Bates and Watts (1988).

The Gauss-Newton algorithm for nonlinear least squares is implemented in mainstream statistical software packages. The functions nls (Chambers and Hastie, 1992) and gnls (Pinheiro and Bates, 2000) implement it in S-PLUS and R, while PROC NLIN (Freund and Littell, 2000) implements it in SAS. Examples on the use of these functions and procedure can be found in the references given above.

The dose-finding methodology combining MCP and modeling techniques described in Section 10.5 requires the determination, at the time of protocol write-up, of model contrasts for model selection. As described in Section 10.5, a model contrast is a function of the corresponding mean response vector $\boldsymbol{\mu} = (\mu_{d_1}, \ldots, \mu_{d_k})$ taken at the planned doses for the study. The mean response vector is itself a function of the unknown model parameters $\boldsymbol{\theta}$. So, in order to utilize the methodology of Section 10.5, initial values for $\boldsymbol{\theta}$ are needed prior to any data is available, which then need to rely on prior information/expectation about the dose–response relationship. This should be contrasted with more traditional methods of deriving initial estimates for fitting nonlinear regression models, described for example in Bates and Watts (1988), which assume that the data to be modeled is already available. Strategies for deriving initial parameter estimates based on prior dose–response assumptions and before data is collected are included with the presentation and discussion of dose–response models below.

For the purpose of determining initial parameter estimates for either model fitting or constructing model contrasts, it suffices to consider a standardized version of the dose–response model. That is, if the model function f in Eq. (10.2) can be written as

$$f(d, \boldsymbol{\theta}) = \theta_0 + \theta_1 f^0(d, \boldsymbol{\theta}^0)$$

then one only needs to consider initial estimates for the parameters $\boldsymbol{\theta}^0$ in the standardized model f^0. In the case of model fitting, given initial estimates for $\boldsymbol{\theta}^0$, initial estimates for the remaining parameters can be obtained via linear regression. Model contrasts can be derived from the response vector corresponding to f^0. The advantages of using the standardized model f^0 instead the full model f will become clear when developing a new method of combining MCP and modeling in Section 10.5.

What follows is a selection of models used frequently in dose–response analysis. The selection given below is not meant to be exhaustive. A graphical display for each of these models is shown in Figure 10.3, included in Section 10.5.3.

10.2.1 $E_{\max}$ Model

In its simplest form, the $E_{\max}$ model is defined, for $\boldsymbol{\theta}' = (E_0, E_{\max}, ED_{50})$ as

$$f(d, \boldsymbol{\theta}) = E_0 + E_{\max} d / (ED_{50} + d) \tag{10.3}$$

E_0 is the basal effect, corresponding to $d = 0$, $E_{\max}$ is the maximum change in effect associated with d (at an infinite dose), and ED_{50} is the dose that gives half of the maximum change. Note that the $E_{\max}$ model can accommodate both an increase in effect ($E_{\max} > 0$), as well as a decrease in effect ($E_{\max} < 0$). Additional parameters can be included to give greater flexibility of shapes to the $E_{\max}$ model, but we will consider herein only the simpler version of Eq. (10.3). We refer to MacDougall (2005), Chapter 9 of this book, for further information about the $E_{\max}$ model.

The standardized $E_{\max}$ model is accordingly defined as

$$f^0(d, ED_{50}) = d / (ED_{50} + d) \tag{10.4}$$

The standardized $E_{\max}$ model represents the percentage of the maximum change from the basal effect associated with dose d. The advantage is that the specification of the single parameter ED_{50} is sufficient to obtain a fully parameterized standardized model f^0. An initial estimate for ED_{50} can be obtained from knowledge of the prior expected percentage of the maximum effect p^* associated with a given dose d^*. By inverting Eq. (10.4) one obtains

$$\widehat{ED}_{50} = d^*(1 - p^*)/p^*$$

If different (d^*, p^*) pairs are available, one can use the average of the corresponding $\widehat{ED}_{50}$ as an initial value, or use different estimates $\widehat{ED}_{50}$ to determine different sets of model contrasts for the $E_{\max}$ model.

10.2.2   Linear in Log-Dose Model

The linear in log-dose model is defined, for $\theta' = (E_0, \delta)$ as

$$f(d, \theta) = E_0 + \delta \log(d + c)$$

where a value $c > 0$ is added to d to avoid problems with the placebo ($d = 0$) arm. E_0 is the basal effect and δ is the slope associated with $\log(d + c)$. As with the E_{max} model, an increasing effect ($\delta > 0$) model will be assumed.

Clearly, the linear in log-dose model is a location-scale model which can be expressed as $f(d, \theta) = E_0 + \delta f^0(d)$, with the standardized model being equal to

$$f^0(d) = \log(d + c) \tag{10.5}$$

so that the determination of the appropriate model contrasts can be done on the basis of the doses alone, and no initial parameter estimates are needed.

10.2.3   Linear Model

Again, the model contrast is shown to be independent of the parameters, as in the linear in log-dose model. The general model formulation and its standardized form are given below, with $\theta' = (E_0, \delta)$,

$$f(d, \theta) = E_0 + \delta d, \quad f^0(d) = d$$

10.2.4   Exponential (Power) Model

This model is intended to capture a possible sub-linear or a convex dose–response relationship. It is defined, for $\theta' = (E_0, E_1, \delta)$ as

$$f(d, \theta) = E_0 \exp(d/\delta) \tag{10.6}$$

As before, E_0 represents the basal level corresponding to $d = 0$ and $\delta > 0$ (< 0) controls the rate of increase (decrease) in the effect.

Because E_0 is a scale parameter in the exponential model in Eq. (10.6), the model contrast can be determined from the standardized model

$$f^0(d, \delta) = \exp(d/\delta) \tag{10.7}$$

being a function of δ alone. An initial estimate for δ can then be obtained from knowledge of the prior expected percentage effect p^* over E_0 associated with a given dose d^*. By inverting Eq. (10.7), and noting that the percentage increase over E_0 is given by $f^0(d, \delta) - 1$, one obtains

$$\hat{\delta} = d^* / \log(1 + p^*)$$

As in the E_{max} model, if different (d^*, p^*) pairs are available, one can use the average of the corresponding $\hat{\delta}$ as initial value, or use different estimates $\hat{\delta}$ to determine different sets of model contrasts for the exponential model.

10.2.5 Quadratic Model

This model is intended to capture a possible non-monotonic dose–response relationship, in either a concave (umbrella or inverted-U) shape, or a convex (U) shape. The full three-parameter model, with $\theta' = (E_0, \beta_1, \beta_2)$, is defined as

$$f(d, \theta) = E_0 + \beta_1 d + \beta_2 d^2 \tag{10.8}$$

If $\beta_2 > 0$, the model corresponds to a U-shape, while $\beta_2 < 0$ gives an umbrella-shape. A simple variation of the model above would result from replacing d with $\log(d)$ in Eq. (10.8).

Since $d_{opt} = -\beta_1/2\beta_2$ is the dose corresponding to the maximum (minimum) response under Eq. (10.8), a necessary assumption in the context described in this chapter is $d_{opt} > 0$, which in turn implies that β_1 and β_2 have opposite signs. The standardized versions of the quadratic model in Eq. (10.8), which will be different for the U- and umbrella-shaped models, are then given by

$$f^0(d, \delta) = \begin{cases} d + \delta d^2, \ \beta_2 < 0 \\ -d + \delta d^2, \ \beta_2 > 0 \end{cases} \tag{10.9}$$

where $\delta = \beta_2/|\beta_1|$. It follows that $f(d, \theta) = E_0 + \beta_1 f^0(d, \delta)$. Without loss of generality, we will restrict ourselves to the umbrella-shape form of the model for the remainder of this section.

Again, an initial estimate for δ can be obtained from knowledge of the prior expected percentage p^* of maximum effect associated with a given dose d^* and whether this d^* is smaller or larger than $d_{opt} = -1/2\delta$. There are two $\hat{\delta}$ corresponding to the pair (d^*, p^*): $\hat{\delta} = (-1 \pm \sqrt{1 - p^*})/2d^*$. The solution becomes unique when conditioning on d_{opt} being greater or smaller than d^*,

$$\delta^* = \begin{cases} -(1 - \sqrt{1 - p^*})/2d^*, \ d^* < d_{opt} \\ -(1 + \sqrt{1 - p^*})/2d^*, \ d^* \geq d_{opt} \end{cases}$$

10.2.6 Logistic Model

The logistic model is a four-parameter model, $\theta' = (E_0, E_{max}, ED_{50}, \delta)$, defined as

$$f(d, \theta) = E_0 + E_{max}/\{1 + \exp[(ED_{50} - d)/\delta]\} \tag{10.10}$$

E_0 is the left-asymptote parameter, corresponding to a basal effect level (not the placebo effect, though), E_{max} is the maximum change in effect from the basal level, and ED_{50} is the dose that gives half of the maximum change in effect. Finally, δ is a parameter controlling the rate of change with dose in the effect and which has a graphical interpretation as the increment over the ED_{50} dose that produces a change in effect of $E_{max}/(1 + \exp(-1)) \approx 3E_{max}/4$, that is, approximately three-quarters of the maximum change in effect. Note that the logistic model can accommodate an increase in effect ($E_{max} > 0$), as well a decrease in effect ($E_{max} < 0$).

Because E_0 and E_{max} are respectively the location and scale parameters in the logistic model in Eq. (10.10), the model contrast can be determined on the basis of the standardized model

$$f^0(d, ED_{50}, \delta) = 1/\{1 + \exp[(ED_{50} - d)/\delta]\} \qquad (10.11)$$

being, therefore, a function of ED_{50} and δ only. As in the E_{max} model, $f^0(d, ED_{50}, \delta)$ represents the percentage of the maximum effect E_{max} associated with dose d. Because two unknown parameters are involved, derivation of initial estimates requires, at a minimum, knowledge of the prior expected percentages of maximum effect p_1^* and p_2^* associated with two given doses d_1^* and d_2^*. Letting $\text{logit}(p) = \log(p/(1-p))$ one obtains from Eq. (10.11)

$$\hat{\delta} = \frac{d_2^* - d_1^*}{\text{logit}(p_2^*) - \text{logit}(p_1^*)}, \qquad \widehat{ED}_{50} = \frac{d_1^* \text{logit}(p_2^*) - d_2^* \text{logit}(p_1^*)}{\text{logit}(p_2^*) - \text{logit}(p_1^*)}$$

If more than two (d^*, p^*) pairs are available, one can obtain estimates for ED_{50} and δ by regressing $\text{logit}(p^*)$ on d^*: letting b_0 and b_1 represent the corresponding intercept and slope estimates, one could use $\widehat{ED}_{50} = -b_0/b_1$ and $\hat{\delta} = 1/b_1$. Alternatively, different estimates for ED_{50} and δ could be obtained to determine different sets of model contrasts for the logistic model.

10.3   Estimation of Target Doses

Once an adequate dose–response model has been chosen and successfully fitted to the data, one may proceed to estimate the target dose(s) of interest. In this chapter, we restrict our attention to the estimation of the minimum effective dose (MED), although the ideas are equally applicable when estimating other target doses. Following Ruberg (1995), the MED is defined as the smallest dose, which shows a clinically relevant and a statistically significant effect. Let Δ denote the clinically relevant difference, i.e., the smallest relevant difference, by which we expect a dose to be better than placebo. Note that Δ does not depend on the particular dose–response model under consideration, but only on the objectives of the drug development program.

Two definitions of the MED are possible, depending on whether the target dose is selected out of the the discrete dose set $\mathcal{D} = \{d_1, \ldots, d_k\}$ under investigation or from the entire dose range $(d_1, d_k]$. In the former case,

$$MED = \text{argmin}_{d_i \in \mathcal{D}}\{\mu_{d_i} > \mu_{d_1} + \Delta\}$$

where argmin of a function, or an expression, denotes the value of the argument that minimizes it. Typically, estimation of $MED \in \mathcal{D}$ in this framework is conducted by applying appropriate multiple testing procedures, see Tamhane et al. (1996). In contrast, model based approaches allow $MED \in (d_1, d_k]$. Given a model $f(., \boldsymbol{\theta})$,

$$MED = \mathrm{argmin}_{d \in (d_1, d_k]}\{f(d, \boldsymbol{\theta}) > f(d_1, \boldsymbol{\theta}) + \Delta\} \qquad (10.12)$$

Note that we restrict the MED to lie within the interval $(d_1, d_k]$ in order to avoid problems arising from extrapolating beyond the dose range under investigation.

In the following paragraphs, we focus on defining Eq. (10.12) and consider three different rules for estimating the true MED proposed by Bretz et al. (2005). Denote by L_d (U_d) the lower (upper) $1 - 2\gamma$ confidence limit of the predicted value p_d at dose d based on the model $f(., \boldsymbol{\theta})$, as computed, for example, by the nls function (Chambers and Hastie, 1992) in S-PLUS and R. Note that the choice of γ is not driven by the purpose of controlling Type I error rates, in contrast to the selection of α for controlling the FWER for the PoA. As discussed below, γ should nevertheless be set reasonably small in order to avoid interpretation problems with the final estimate of the MED. The following alternative estimates are investigated via simulation in Section 10.5.3:

$$\widehat{MED}_1 = \mathrm{argmin}_{d \in (d_1, d_k]}\{U_d > p_{d_1} + \Delta, L_d > p_{d_1}\}$$
$$\widehat{MED}_2 = \mathrm{argmin}_{d \in (d_1, d_k]}\{p_d > p_{d_1} + \Delta, L_d > p_{d_1}\} \qquad (10.13)$$
$$\widehat{MED}_3 = \mathrm{argmin}_{d \in (d_1, d_k]}\{L_d > p_{d_1} + \Delta\}$$

By construction, $\widehat{MED}_1 \leq \widehat{MED}_2 \leq \widehat{MED}_3$ and it is seen from Section 10.5.3 that $\widehat{MED}_2$ tends to be less biased in estimating the true MED than the alternative estimates. Note that a dose obtained through any of the criteria above may not have a significant effect at level α, especially when γ is not small enough. Since γ and Δ are prespecified, it may happen that a MED is obtained which is lower than a dose in the study which had no significant effect. To avoid such problems, γ should be set reasonably small, perhaps even taking multiplicity due to the construction of the confidence bands into account (Scheffé, 1953). An alternative approach to guarantee statistical significance would be to use the confidence bounds L_{d-d_1} for the difference between the response at dose d and placebo d_1. One would then require $L_{d-d_1} > 0$ instead of $L_d > p_{d_1}$ in the estimates above for MED.

Once the MED is estimated using one of the methods above, it is important to assess its precision, for which a confidence interval is generally the most useful tool. Bootstrap methods can be used to derive such a confidence interval. One possibility is to implement a full, nonparametric bootstrap approach, in which the patients within each dose group are re-sampled, with replacement, and the whole dose–finding procedure is repeated, yielding a bootstrap sample of MED values. A simpler, less computationally intensive alternative is to use a parametric bootstrap approach. Let $\widehat{\boldsymbol{\theta}}$ denote the estimated parameter vector for the dose selection model, with corresponding estimated (possibly approximate) covariance matrix $\widehat{\Sigma}$. For the model and data scenarios considered here, $\widehat{\boldsymbol{\theta}}$ is asymptotically normally distributed. The parametric bootstrap approach then consists in re-sampling the parameter vector $\boldsymbol{\theta}$ from its approximate distribution $\mathcal{N}(\widehat{\boldsymbol{\theta}}, \widehat{\boldsymbol{\Sigma}})$ and using these values to derive a bootstrap sample of MED values. In either case, the bootstrap sample of MED values would be used to derive an appropriate confidence interval for the MED.

10.3.1   Estimating the MED in Dose-Finding Example

To illustrate the methods described in this section for estimating the MED from a dose–response model, we consider again the dose-finding study introduced in Section 10.1. The plot of mean responses per dose in Figure 10.1 suggests that an $E_{\max}$ model as described in Section 10.2 can be used to adequately describe the dose–response relationship and is the model that is used here to illustrate the MED estimation methods.

Figure 10.1 can also be used to provide initial estimates for the ED_{50} parameter: it appears that half of the maximum effect is attained at about $d = 0.2$, so we set $\widehat{ED}_{50} = 0.2$. By fixing ED_{50} at its initial value, linear regression can be used to obtain initial estimates for the other two model parameters. We used the lm function in **S-PLUS** to obtain $\tilde{E}_0 = 0.344$ and $\tilde{E}_{\max} = 0.777$. The nls function can then be used with these initial estimates to fit the $E_{\max}$ model to the dose–response data, producing the nonlinear least squares estimates

$$\widehat{E}_0 = 0.321, \quad \widehat{E}_{\max} = 0.746, \quad \widehat{ED}_{50} = 0.142, \quad \text{and} \quad \widehat{\sigma} = 0.706. \quad (10.14)$$

Assuming a clinically relevant difference of $\Delta = 0.4$ and applying the MED estimates defined in Eq. (10.13) with $\gamma = 0.1, 0.2$ we obtain the values in Table 10.2. Figure 10.2 gives a graphical respresentation of the different MED estimates for $\gamma = 0.2$.

Table 10.2. MED estimates for Phase II example

γ	$\widehat{MED}_1$	$\widehat{MED}_2$	$\widehat{MED}_3$
0.1	0.07	0.17	0.34
0.2	0.10	0.17	0.27

Let us assume that the set of active dose levels used in this study ($d = 0.05, 0.2, 0.6, 1$) define the only doses for which it is possible to manufacture the experimental treatment. In this case, we observe that the next highest dose neighboring the selected dose level is 0.2. A pragmatic approach could then be to suggest that the dose 0.2 is determined as the minimum dose which attains the prescribed conditions for selection. In principle, any dose lying above 0.17 (based on $\widehat{MED}_2$) may be defined as an acceptable dose, provided that the gain in efficacy does not result in an unacceptable safety risk. If, on the other hand, this study had been undertaken with the aim of manufacturing a dose as close as possible to that

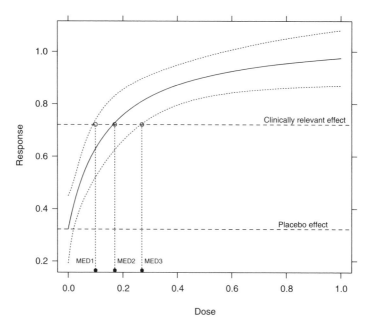

Figure 10.2. Estimated E_{max} model for the dose-finding example, with corresponding 60% confidence bands ($\gamma = 0.2$). Also shown are the estimated MES's using the formulas in Eq.(10.13)

selected, the dose level either equal to 0.17 or in close proximity to 0.17 would then be determined as the dose used for further drug development.

10.4   Model Uncertainty and Model Selection

In the previous sections we have described a variety of commonly used dose–response models and given some possibilities of deriving initial parameter estimates for constructing model contrasts. We have not yet discussed the problem of selecting a model for the final analysis. This is a particularly important issue in the regulated environment of pharmaceutical drug development, since it is required to prespecify completely the statistical analysis (and thus also the dose–response model used for the final analysis) prior to the start of a study.

The application of a model-based approach to analyze a given dose–response study may raise questions on the validity of the statistical results, since the true underlying dose–response relationship under investigation is typically unknown. This model uncertainty remains during the entire drug development until the late Phase III clinical trials. Thus, justification of a certain dose designated to be released on the market is based on the assumption of a particular dose–response model. Supporting statistical analyses are mainly conducted to obtain the best parameter estimates for a suitable description of the collected data. Even if the model specification is based on supporting information from prior trials, there is always a more or less remote possibility of model misspecification. Current statistical practice, however, mostly does not take this additional statistical uncertainty into account. Instead, current approaches believe on the truth of the underlying model and thus do not reflect the complete statistical decision process. This is of particular concern in standard confirmatory clinical trials, since in late drug development stages the statistical methods need to be defined up front, inherently including the definition of the unknown dose–response model.

In fact, model uncertainty is one of the major pitfalls when conducting statistical modeling. The intrinsic problem is the introduction of a new source of variability by selecting a particular model M (say) at any stage prior to the final analysis. Standard statistical analysis neglects this fact and reports the final outcomes without accounting for this extra-variability. It is common practice, for example, to compute the variance of a parameter estimate as $\text{var}(\hat{\mu})$ where in fact $\text{var}(\hat{\mu}|M)$ is the correct term. In addition, substantial bias in estimating the parameters of interest can be introduced due to the model selection process. Whereas, it is admittedly a more difficult task to compute unbiased estimates conditional on the selected model, ignoring completely the model uncertainty can lead to very undesirable effects (Chatfield, 1995; Draper, 1995; Hjorth, 1994).

A common approach in situations when one has to select the model that will ultimately be used to fit the data is to use information criteria based on a reasonable discrepancy measure to assess the lack of fit. Many model selection criteria are available and the discussion on the best method is still ongoing (Zucchini, 2000; Kadane and Lazar, 2004). A common approach is, for example, to consider the ratio R^2 of the sum of squares for regression to the total sum of squares. This number is reported by most software packages when performing a standard regression analysis. The problem with the R^2 is that the sum of squares for regression, and hence by construction R^2 itself, increases with the number of parameters and thus leads to over-fitting. If solely the (unadjusted) R^2 would be used, the selected model at the end would typically be among the most complex ones within the given set of candidate models. A variety of alternative measures have thus been proposed, which include a penalty term: as the model gets more complex, i.e., for larger number of parameters p, the penalty increases. The inclusion of a new variable is therefore only supported, if the amount of information gain (in form of a better prediction) is substantial as measured by the penalty correction. A well known information criterion is the penalized log-likelihood $\text{AIC} = -2\log(L) + 2p$ (Akaike, 1973), where L denotes the likelihood under the fitted model and p the number of corresponding parameters. A second information criterion of the same general form is the Bayesian information criterion $\text{BIC} = -2\log(L) + p\log(n)$ (Schwarz, 1978), which also depends on the sample size n. Although both methods are derived in completely different ways, the BIC differs from the AIC only in the second term, favoring simpler models than AIC as n increases.

Note that these and other information criteria are generally not suitable in dose–response analyses as they do not incorporate potential parameter constraints, such as the simple order restriction $\mu_1 \leq \ldots \leq \mu_k$. This observation parallels the results from the theory of order restricted inference that the maximum likelihood estimates for the mean level responses subject to a given order restriction are different from the unrestricted maximum likelihood estimates (Robertson et al., 1988). Anraku (1999) thus proposed to use an order restricted information criterion (ORIC) based on the isotonic regression theory. Simulation results suggest that the ORIC indeed behaves better than the AIC, in that it selects more often the correct target dose for varying model specifications and parameter configurations.

However, any measure of fit—either the AIC, ORIC or any other criterion—bears the inherent drawback of a missing error control. If we simply select the model corresponding to the best ORIC, say, we have no conclusion on the validity of our decision. In fact, once we have a candidate set of models, the application of the ORIC will always lead to the selection of one single model, irrespective of the goodness of fit given the observed data. Instead, model selection uncertainty should be incorporated into statistical inference in those cases, where the estimation process is sensitive to the ultimate model choice (Shen et al., 2004). In order to circumvent to a certain extent the problem of conditional inference on a selected model, weighting methods and computer-intensive simulation based inferences have been proposed.

We first consider the weighting methods, which incorporate rather than ignore model uncertainty by computing parameter estimates using a weighted average across the models. A straightforward solution in the line of the information criterion approaches above was introduced by Buckland, Burnham, and Augustin (1997). Let $\mathcal{M} = \{M_1, \ldots, M_L\}$ denote a set of L candidate models index by ℓ. Buckland et al. (1997) proposed to use the weighted estimate

$$\widehat{\mu} = \sum_\ell w_\ell \widehat{\mu}_\ell$$

where $\widehat{\mu}_\ell$ is the estimate of μ under model ℓ for given weights w_ℓ. The idea is, thus, to use estimates for the final data analysis which rely on the averaged estimates across all L models. Buckland et al. (1997) proposed the use of the weights

$$w_\ell = \frac{e^{-\frac{IC_\ell}{2}}}{\sum_{j=1}^{L} e^{-\frac{IC_j}{2}}}, \quad \ell = 1, \ldots, L \qquad (10.15)$$

which are defined in dependence of a common information criterion IC applied to each of the L models. Alternatively, Buckland et al. (1997) have proposed to set the weights w_ℓ as the proportions of bootstrap samples for which model M_ℓ was selected. Augustin et al., (2002) extended this resampling approach and proposed bootstrap aggregation methods instead. Note that although these approaches provide a simple and intuitive way to overcome some of the model uncertainty problems, one is still left with the open problem on how to ultimately choose the final model for further inferential problems. Similar in spirit, though based on a completely different theoretical reasoning, are Bayesian model averaging techniques. Having observed the data X, the posterior distributions $P(\mu|X, M_\ell)$ under each of the investigated models are weighted according to their posterior model probabilities $P(M_\ell|X)$, so that

$$P(\mu|X) = \sum_{\ell=1}^{L} P(\mu|X, M_\ell)P(M_\ell|X)$$

We refer to Hoeting et al., (1999) and Clyde and George (2004) for discussions of the related methods and several examples. Note that choosing the BIC for the calculation of the weights in Eq. (10.15) leads to results that are closely related to Bayesian model averaging (Augustin et al., 2002).

Cross-validation techniques are an example of computer-intensive simulation based approaches. A data set consisting of n observed data is split into two subsets. The first set of size n_1 is used for fitting the model (learning sample). The second set of size of size $n_2 = n - n_1$ is used for validating the fitted model, i.e., assessing its predictive ability (training sample). Clearly, using n_1 observations instead of the complete sample of size n may substantially reduce the performance of the fit. One possibility is to repeat the above procedure for all (or some) learning samples of size n_1 and to assess the average predicted ability. A common approach is thus to choose $n_2 = 1$ (leave-one-out method) and to repeat a large number of times the two steps (1) model fit based on the learning sample of size $n_1 = n - 1$ and (2) validation of the fitted model using the single remaining observation. Cross-validation then selects the model with the best predictive ability across the replications. We refer to Hjorth (1994) and Hastie et al., (2001) for further details on cross-validation and related techniques.

A different philosophy is to consider model selection as a multiple hypotheses testing problem, where the selection of a specific model is done while controlling the familywise error rate at a prespecified level α (Shimodaira, 1998; Junquera, et al., 2002). In this context, the FWER may be interpreted as $1 -$ Probability of Correct Model Selection. In addition, a reference set of good models is constructed rather than choosing a single model. Shimodaira (1998), for example, considered testing the set of hypotheses

$$H_\ell : \mathrm{E}(\mathrm{AIC}_{M_\ell}) \leq \min_{M_j \in \mathcal{M} \backslash M_\ell} \mathrm{E}(\mathrm{AIC}_{M_j})$$

$$\text{vs.} \quad K_\ell : \mathrm{E}(\mathrm{AIC}_{M_\ell}) > \min_{M_j \in \mathcal{M} \backslash M_\ell} \mathrm{E}(\mathrm{AIC}_{M_j})$$

where $\mathrm{E}(\mathrm{AIC}_{M_\ell})$ is the expected AIC value for model M_ℓ. The proposed multiple test procedure uses the standardized differences of any two AIC values within a variant of Gupta's subset selection procedure using bootstrap techniques to assess the joint distribution of the test statistics. A final reference set $\mathcal{T}$ of good models is obtained as

$$\mathcal{T} = \left\{ M_\ell \in \mathcal{M} : P_{M_\ell} \geq \alpha \right\},$$

where P_{M_ℓ} is the p-value associated with the ℓth model. By construction, if $P_{M_\ell} < \alpha$, it has been shown that the AIC value for the ℓth model M_ℓ is significantly larger than the minimum AIC of the remaining set $\mathcal{M} \setminus M_\ell$. Thus, the present approach includes all models at the beginning and only removes those models shown to behave inferior to the other models. This approach never leads $\mathcal{T} = \emptyset$ and may contain more than one model at the end.

10.5   Combining Modeling Techniques and Multiple Testing

10.5.1   Methodology

As seen in the previous sections, modeling techniques provide a flexible tool for describing functional dose–response relationships and subsequently selecting a suitable dose for the confirmatory Phase III studies. Typical model-based analyses, however, do not provide a rigid error control, as it is provided, for example, by multiple comparison procedures (Hochberg and Tamhane, 1987; Hsu, 1996). In this section, we consider a hybrid approach which provides the flexibility advantages of modeling based techniques within the framework of multiple comparisons (MCP-Mod, Bretz et al., 2005). We perform a detailed numerical simulation study to assess the operating characteristics of this approach.

The starting point of the MCP-Mod method is to recognize that the power of standard dose–response trend tests depends on the (unknown) dose–response relationship. Tukey et al. (1985) proposed the use of several transformations f of the single predictor variable $dose$ (i.e., of the dose levels d_i) and then to look at the minimum multiplicity adjusted P-value to decide for or against a significant trend. The P-values were obtained from the regression sum of squares based on the regression on the new set of carriers within a linearized model. In particular, Tukey et al. (1985) proposed the use of the following transformations at the initial step:

- arithmetic scaling: $f(d_i) = d_i$,
- ordinal scaling: $f(d_i) = i$,
- logarithmic scaling: $f(d_i) = \log(d_i)$,
- arithmetic-logarithmic scaling: $f(d_i) = d_i$, if $i = 1$, $f(d_i) = \log(d_i)$ otherwise.

The lowest P-value is then taken and—after an appropriate multiplicity adjustment—compared to the FWER α, see Tukey et al. (1985).

Bretz et al. (2005) formalized this approach and extended it in several ways. One starts with a candidate set of models $\mathcal{M}$. Each of the models $M_\ell \in \mathcal{M}$ is applied to the set of doses under investigation. Based on the resulting dose–response curves, optimum weights are calculated for the comparison of the different candidate models within a multiple hypotheses testing framework. Once the multiplicity adjusted P-values are obtained, different approaches of selecting the models and subsequent dose-finding steps are possible. In the following we describe the procedure in more detail before presenting the results of a simulation study.

Assume that a set $\mathcal{M}$ of parameterized candidate models is given together with initial parameter estimates as described in Section 10.3. The candidate set $\mathcal{M}$ may contain some of the models presented in Section 10.2 or any other models deemed to be suitable for the analysis. Applying these models to the doses $d_1, \ldots, d_k$ results in the means $\mu_\ell = (\mu_{\ell 1}, \ldots, \mu_{\ell k})$, which describe the dose–response of model ℓ at the given doses d_i. Each of these dose–response curves is tested by a single contrast test, which is defined as a standardized linear combination of the means. The choice of the weights (so called contrast coefficients) is free subject to the regularity condition that the weights sum up to zero. We refer to Abelson and Tukey (1963) for an early introduction of contrast tests in the context of dose–response analyses. Here, the associated coefficients are chosen such that they best reflect the assumed curves as characterized through μ_ℓ. A linear contrast test, for example, is defined such that the difference of any two adjacent contrast coefficients is a constant. Assuming that the standard linear model has been included in the candidate set $\mathcal{M}$, the linear contrast test is then a powerful test to detect the linear trend. Similarly, any dose–response relationship characterized through μ_ℓ can be tested equally powerfully by selecting an appropriate contrast test, whose coefficients are defined in dependence of the assumed μ_ℓ. Details on the computation of optimum contrast coefficients can be found in Bretz et al. (2005). Note that due to shift and scale invariance properties of contrast tests, it is sufficient to work with the standardized modeling functions f^0 to obtain the optimum contrast coefficients, as discussed in Section 10.2.

Every single contrast test thus translates into a decision procedure, whether a selected dose–response curve is significant given the observed data, while controlling the Type I error rate at level α. Under the assumptions stated in Eq. (10.1), the joint distribution of the contrast test statistics is seen to be multivariate t and available numerical integration routines can be used to compute the p-values and critical constants (Genz and Bretz, 2002). Those models that are associated with a significant contrast test result form a set of good models. This set may be regarded as a reference set of models, which includes the most significant model with the minimum p-value among all models initially considered in $\mathcal{M}$. While all models included in this reference set are statistically significant at the FWER α, the one with minimum p-value (or according to any other standard model selection criteria) may be regarded further for the dose selection step. Once a particular model has been selected, the final step is then to use this model to produce inferences on adequate doses, employing the methods described in Section 10.3. Note that in contrast to a direct application of a model based approach, these preliminary steps take care of possible model misspecifications and include the associated statistical uncertainty in a hypothesis testing environment. This approach therefore has the advantage of leading to a quantitative measure of reliability for selecting an adequate dose–response model. Basically, the multiple testing part is used mainly to establish PoA, while accounting for model uncertainty. In the second step, a single model from a suitable reference set of good models is selected, thus incorporating indirectly model uncertainty into the actual estimate of the MED. The simulation study of Section 10.5.3 shows that although one model is ultimately selected, the estimation bias is generally small, at least for $\widehat{MED}_2$ defined in Eq. (10.13).

As discussed in Section 10.3, the precision of the MED estimates can be assessed via bootstrap methods, either nonparametrically (by re-sampling with replacement subjects within each dose group), or parametrically (by re-sampling parameter vectors according to the asymptotic distribution of the estimated coefficients.) In the nonparametric case, the whole MCP-Mod procedure leading to the estimation of the MED should be repeated for each bootstrap sample, so as to incorporate the different sources of uncertainty involved in the MED estimation.

10.5.2   Proof-of-Activity Analysis in the Dose-Finding Example

We now re-analyze the data presented in Section 10.1 using the MCP-Mod approach outlined in Section 10.5.1. The set of candidate models includes $E_{\max}$, linear in log-dose, linear, exponential and quadratic (umbrella shape). Based on preliminary discussions, the logistic model is not included in this candidate set. Initial estimates for the different models are provided in Section 10.3. The test contrasts were obtained using the true parameter values for the corresponding standardized model, (e.g., $ED_{50} = 0.2$ for the $E_{\max}$ model). The resulting contrasts are presented in Table 10.3. There is considerable correlation between some of the test contrasts (e.g., linear and linear in log) indicating that it may be hard to discriminate between such models, as discussed later in Section 10.5.3.

Table 10.3. Test contrasts for models in candidate set, with corresponding pairwise correlations

Model	Contrast					Correlation with				
						linear-log	linear	exp	quad	logistic
$E_{\max}$	−0.643	−0.361	0.061	0.413	0.530	0.98	0.91	0.72	0.84	0.90
Linear-log	−0.539	−0.392	−0.083	0.373	0.640		0.98	0.84	0.75	0.96
Linear	−0.437	−0.378	−0.201	0.271	0.743			0.93	0.60	0.96
Exponential	−0.292	−0.286	−0.257	−0.039	0.875				0.26	0.81
Quadratic	−0.574	−0.364	0.155	0.713	0.070					0.72
Logistic	−0.396	−0.387	−0.308	0.496	0.595					

A summary of the multiple-comparison component of MCP-Mod, ordered by the magnitude of the observed t-values, is given in Table 10.4. The one-sided unadjusted (raw) p-values are presented and are accompanied with the corresponding adjusted one-sided p-values from the multivariate t-distribution. All contrast tests with an adjusted p-value less than 0.05 or equivalently with a t-value greater than 1.930 can be declared statistically significant having maintained the FWER at level 5%. Clearly all contrast tests are highly significant at the 5% level. In this example, the $E_{\max}$ model is the first model to be considered for the dose selection component of this analysis, see Section 10.3.

Table 10.4. Summary of contrast tests

Contrast	Estimate	t-value	Raw P-value	Adjusted P-value
$E_{\max}$	0.552	3.46	0.0004	0.0017
Linear-log	0.524	3.29	0.0007	0.0028
Quadratic	0.494	3.10	0.0013	0.0048
Linear	0.473	2.97	0.0019	0.0069
Exponential	0.353	2.22	0.0145	0.0448

10.5.3   Simulations

We now investigate, via simulation, the performance of the MCP-Mod dose finding methodology described in Section 10.5.1. Following the design of the case study of Section 10.1, we consider the comparison of the five dose levels $d = 0, 0.05, 0.2, 0.6$, and 1, with a single endpoint measured per patient. The outcome is assumed to be independently distributed as $\mathcal{N}(\mu\_d, \sigma^2)$. We set $\sigma = 0.65$, motivated by the residual standard deviation from the case study in Section 10.1. We restrict the simulations to balanced sample size allocations with $n = 10, 25, 50, 75, 100$ and 150 patients per dose group and no drop-outs. As in Section 10.1, a clinically relevant effect of $\Delta = 0.4$ was adopted in the dose selection algorithms. The confidence levels $(= 100(1 - 2\gamma)\%)$ used for these algorithms in the simulations were 50, 60, 70, 80, and 90% respectively. We generated a total of 10,000 simulation runs for each shape $\times$ sample-size combination.

Eight different shapes for the mean vector $\mu(d)$ were investigated in the simulations:

1. $E_{\max}$: $\mu(d) = 0.2 + 0.7d/(0.2 + d)$
2. linear in log-dose: $\mu(d) = 0.2 + 0.6 \log(5d + 1)/\log(6)$
3. linear: $\mu(d) = 0.2 + 0.6d$
4. exponential: $\mu(d) = 0.2 \exp[\log(4)d]$
5. quadratic: $\mu(d) = 0.2 + 2.0485d - 1.7485d^2$
6. logistic: $\mu(d) = 0.193 + 0.607/\{1 + \exp[10\log(3)(0.4 - d)]\}$,
7. double-logistic:

$$\mu(d) = \left\{0.198 + \frac{0.61}{1 + \exp[18(0.3 - d)]}\right\} I(d \leq 0.5)$$
$$+ \left\{0.499 + \frac{0.309}{1 + \exp[18(d - 0.7)]}\right\} I(d > 0.5)$$

8. convex: $\mu(d) = 0.2 + 0.6/\{1 + \exp[10(0.8 - d)]\}$.

Note that the shapes were selected such that the placebo response value at $d = 0$ is about 0.2. In addition, all shapes have a maximum response of about 0.8 within the dose range $[0, 1]$, such that the maximum dose effect is about 0.6. The dose–response profiles are shown in Fig. 10.3. Shapes 1 through 6 have been described in Section 10.2. They will also form the set of candidate models for the contrast tests. The last two shapes, 7 and 8, were included to evaluate the performance of

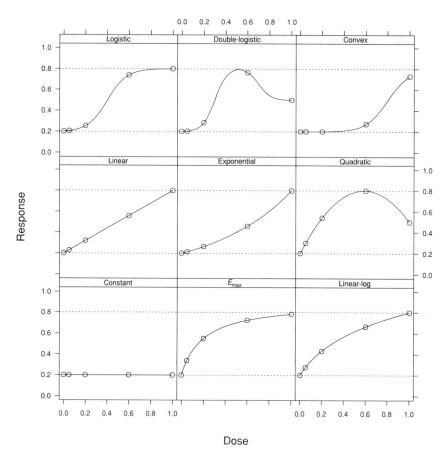

Figure 10.3. Dose–response shapes used in the simulation study with the response at the doses under investigation indicated by open dots.

the MCP-Mod method under model misspecification: they do not quite correspond to any of the model shapes in the candidate set, though can be approximated by some of the models in there.

The simulation power values to detect a significant dose–response relationship under the different shape scenarios are given in Table 10.5. Due to the small standard deviation, the power values are very close to 1 even for moderate to low sample sizes. It can be expected that increasing the variability reduces the power to detect a significant dose–response relationship (Bretz et al., 2005). Given the high power values, MCP-Mod will in most cases lead to at least one model associated with a significant contrast test in the following investigations.

The PoA power results also provide information about the ability of the contrast tests in the MCP-Mod method to discriminate between the models in the candidate set and thus to select the correct model for further inference. Table 10.6 gives the simulation probabilities of choosing the correct model for the six models in the

Table 10.5. PoA power values for MCP-Mod, under the model ×sample size combinations

n	E_{max}	Linear-log	Linear	Exponential	Quadratic	Logist	Double-logistic	Convex
				Data generating shape				
10	0.723	0.746	0.736	0.708	0.638	0.851	0.663	0.558
25	0.974	0.982	0.981	0.975	0.951	0.997	0.956	0.915
50	1.000	1.000	1.000	1.000	0.999	1.000	0.999	0.998
75	1.000	1.000	1.000	1.000	1.000	1.000	1.000	1.000
100	1.000	1.000	1.000	1.000	1.000	1.000	1.000	1.000
150	1.000	1.000	1.000	1.000	1.000	1.000	1.000	1.000

candidate set (e.g., the probability of the E_{max} model contrast yielding the largest t-statistic when in fact this is the correct model). The quadratic model has the highest discrimination power. This is because the quadratic shape is the most pronounced one and none of the other shapes is similar to it. Even for low sample sizes, the quadratic shape is correctly identified in about half of the cases. As expected, the linear and the log-linear shapes, being the two most similar to each other, have the lowest discrimination power and relatively high sample sizes are required to identify them.

In some cases, fitting the model with the minimum p-value does not work because of numerical instabilities. Such problems occur, for example, when the model to be fit contains many parameters in comparison to the number of doses, or when the doses are not spread evenly throughout the dose range under investigation. In our simulation study, this was particularly true for the logistic model, which involved the estimation of four parameters with the data being observed at five dose levels. In such instances, estimating the MED from the most promising model is not possible due to numerical convergence problems in fitting the model. To circumvent this problem in the simulations, we selected the second best model (assuming that it is significant at level α), fit it to the data and estimate the target dose if the fit was successful and otherwise continue with the next best model.

Table 10.7 gives the related simulation probabilities of using the correct model for the six models in the candidate set. Note that the probabilities in Table 10.7 are different from the ones presented in Table 10.6: the latter refers to the probabilities that the minimum p-value will correspond to the correct model, while the former gives the probabilities that the correct model will be used for dose estimation. The differences between the two tables result from the fact, mentioned above, that

Table 10.6. Probability of correctly identifying the response model

n	E_{max}	Linear-log	Linear	Exponential	Quadratic	Logistic
10	0.28	0.09	0.08	0.38	0.45	0.41
25	0.50	0.22	0.18	0.59	0.79	0.63
50	0.66	0.34	0.31	0.67	0.91	0.75
75	0.73	0.44	0.38	0.71	0.96	0.83
100	0.77	0.54	0.47	0.75	0.98	0.87
150	0.84	0.65	0.59	0.79	0.99	0.93

Table 10.7. Probability of using the correct dose–response model

n	E_{max}	Linear-log	Linear	Exponential	Quadratic	Logistic
10	0.38	0.19	0.19	0.56	0.73	0.08
25	0.51	0.29	0.25	0.63	0.84	0.15
50	0.66	0.38	0.36	0.68	0.92	0.27
75	0.73	0.47	0.42	0.71	0.96	0.37
100	0.77	0.56	0.50	0.76	0.98	0.44
150	0.84	0.66	0.60	0.79	0.99	0.55

it is not always possible to use the model with the minimum p-value for dose estimation, due to convergence problems. The probability of choosing the correct model is increased compared with that of selecting it based on the contrast tests for all models except for the logistic model. As indicated before, the logistic model ended up being used for dose selection considerably less frequently than it was initially selected by the contrast tests. An alternative approach would have been not to use the minimum p-value for the model selection process, but using other model selection criteria instead. Using the AIC, for example, could possibly ensure that the penalty term for the number of model parameters helps selecting models with a better numerically feasible fit to the data.

Two of the shapes used in the simulations, the double-logistic and the convex, do not correspond to any of the models included in the candidate set. It is interesting to consider which of the candidate models, if any, were chosen at the model selection step, when these shapes were used. The selection probabilities for the models in the candidate set for the double-logistic and convex shapes are presented in Tables 10.8 (contrast test) and 10.9 (dose selection). Similarly to Tables 10.6 and 10.7, these two tables convey information about two different selection probabilities— Table 10.8 refers to the probabilities that the minimum p-value will correspond to the different models in the candidate set, while Table 10.9 gives the probabilities that the different models are used for dose selection. As mentioned before,

Table 10.8. Selection probabilities for models in the candidate setbased on the contrast test.

Shape	n	None	E_{max}	Linear-log	Linear	Exponential	Quadratic	Logistic
Double-logistic	10	0.34	0.07	0.02	0.01	0.02	0.30	0.25
	25	0.04	0.06	0.02	0.01	0.00	0.47	0.41
	50	0.00	0.03	0.01	0.00	0.00	0.52	0.44
	75	0.00	0.02	0.00	0.00	0.00	0.52	0.46
	100	0.00	0.01	0.00	0.00	0.00	0.54	0.45
	150	0.00	0.01	0.00	0.00	0.00	0.54	0.45
Convex	10	0.45	0.03	0.02	0.03	0.41	0.00	0.05
	25	0.09	0.02	0.02	0.04	0.81	0.00	0.03
	50	0.00	0.00	0.00	0.02	0.96	0.00	0.01
	75	0.00	0.00	0.00	0.01	0.99	0.00	0.00
	100	0.00	0.00	0.00	0.00	1.00	0.00	0.00
	150	0.00	0.00	0.00	0.00	1.00	0.00	0.00

Table 10.9. Selection probabilities for models in the candidate set based on the dose-selection step

Shape	n	E_{max}	Linear-log	Linear	Exponential	Quadratic	Logistic
Double-logistic	10	0.11	0.15	0.10	0.03	0.57	0.03
	25	0.07	0.17	0.07	0.01	0.65	0.03
	50	0.04	0.18	0.03	0.00	0.72	0.04
	75	0.03	0.17	0.01	0.00	0.75	0.04
	100	0.02	0.15	0.00	0.00	0.79	0.04
	150	0.01	0.12	0.00	0.00	0.83	0.04
Convex	10	0.06	0.06	0.16	0.70	0.01	0.01
	25	0.02	0.02	0.07	0.88	0.00	0.01
	50	0.00	0.00	0.03	0.96	0.00	0.00
	75	0.00	0.00	0.01	0.99	0.00	0.00
	100	0.00	0.00	0.00	1.00	0.00	0.00
	150	0.00	0.00	0.00	1.00	0.00	0.00

the probabilities in the two tables differ because a model with minimum p-value may not be used for dose selection, due to convergence problems. It is clear from Table 10.8 that the double-logistic shape is approximated by either the quadratic or the logistic shape, while the convex shape is approximated by the exponential model. The discrimination among the different models increases with sample size, as expected, being quite small under the scenarios considered here, for sample sizes smaller than 50. The logistic model was frequently selected based on the contrast tests for the double-exponential shape, but was rarely the model actually used for dose selection, due to convergence problems.

Table 10.10 gives the target doses to achieve the desired clinically relevant effect of 0.4 (difference with respect to placebo) for the eight different shapes considered for dose selection. We now discuss the simulation results with respect to the dose-selection performance of the MED estimators, measured in terms of its proximity to and dispersion around the target dose (the doses producing an improvement of $\Delta = 0.4$ over placebo). Recall that the proposed MED estimates can be any dose within the dose range under investigation. Because the target doses differ with model, the performance of the estimator $\widehat{MED}_i$ is measured in terms of its relative deviation R_i from the target dose, where $R_i = 100(\widehat{MED}_i - MED)/MED$. The median and inter-quartile range (IQR) of R_i in the 10,000 simulated dose selections then characterize the relative bias and variability of $\widehat{MED}_i$. Due to the large number of combinations of sample sizes (n) and confidence levels ($1 - 2\gamma$) used in the simulations, only a subset of the scenarios are included here, namely $n = 25$, $n = 50$ and 150 and $\gamma = 0.1$ and 0.2 (corresponding to 80% and 60% level confidence intervals respectively). Table 10.11 gives the corresponding summary statistics for

Table 10.10. Target doses for clinically relevant effect of 0.4 under various simulations shapes

Shape	E_{max}	Linear-log	Linear	Exponential	Quadratic	Logistic	Double-logistic	Convex
Target dose	0.27	0.46	0.67	0.79	0.25	0.46	0.34	0.87

Table 10.11. Median relative bias and relative IQR of MED estimators under various models and scenarios

Model	n	γ	Median relative bias (%)			Relative IQR (%)		
			$\widehat{MED}_1$	$\widehat{MED}_2$	$\widehat{MED}_3$	$\widehat{MED}_1$	$\widehat{MED}_2$	$\widehat{MED}_3$
$E_{\max}$	25	0.10	−40.0	−2.5	31.2	86.2	116.2	120.0
		0.20	−28.8	−2.5	23.7	97.5	112.5	120.0
	50	0.10	−36.3	5.0	38.7	82.5	93.7	108.7
		0.20	−21.3	5.0	27.5	82.5	93.7	105.0
	150	0.10	−25.0	1.2	31.2	48.7	60.0	75.0
		0.20	−17.5	1.2	20.0	52.5	60.0	71.2
Linear in log-dose	25	0.10	−32.7	−4.4	19.5	69.5	76.0	84.7
		0.20	−24.0	−6.6	12.9	73.9	76.0	82.5
	50	0.10	−24.0	−0.1	23.8	56.5	63.0	71.7
		0.20	−17.5	−0.1	17.3	56.5	63.0	69.5
	150	0.10	−13.1	−0.1	17.3	28.2	36.9	43.4
		0.20	−8.8	−0.1	10.8	30.4	36.9	39.1
Linear	25	0.10	−29.5	−11.5	8.0	39.0	46.5	45.0
		0.20	−25.0	−11.5	2.0	42.0	46.5	46.5
	50	0.10	−22.0	−7.0	9.5	28.5	33.0	34.5
		0.20	−17.5	−7.0	5.0	30.0	33.0	34.5
	150	0.10	−11.5	−2.5	8.0	15.0	18.0	19.5
		0.20	−8.5	−2.5	5.0	16.5	18.0	18.0
Exponential	25	0.10	−27.2	−6.7	3.5	27.3	26.2	18.2
		0.20	−19.2	−6.7	1.3	26.2	26.2	20.5
	50	0.10	−17.0	−2.2	4.7	21.6	19.3	14.8
		0.20	−11.3	−2.2	2.4	21.6	19.3	17.1
	150	0.10	−6.7	0.1	4.7	12.5	11.4	10.2
		0.20	−4.4	0.1	3.5	12.5	11.4	10.2
Quadratic	25	0.10	−31.3	−7.1	21.2	28.3	44.4	56.5
		0.20	−23.3	−7.1	13.1	32.3	44.4	52.5
	50	0.10	−23.3	1.0	25.2	24.2	36.4	48.5
		0.20	−15.2	1.0	17.1	28.3	36.4	44.4
	150	0.10	−11.1	1.0	21.2	16.2	20.2	32.3
		0.20	−7.1	1.0	13.1	16.2	20.2	28.3
Logistic	25	0.10	−20.4	3.2	29.0	47.3	51.6	60.2
		0.20	−14.0	1.1	20.4	49.5	51.6	55.9
	50	0.10	−11.8	5.4	29.0	38.7	40.9	45.2
		0.20	−7.5	5.4	20.4	40.9	40.9	45.2
	150	0.10	−7.5	3.2	20.4	30.1	30.1	32.3
		0.20	−5.4	3.2	14.0	28.0	30.1	32.3
Double−logistic	25	0.10	−37.6	−10.9	12.9	44.6	68.3	71.3
		0.20	−28.7	−10.9	6.9	53.5	65.4	68.3
	50	0.10	−28.7	−4.9	18.8	44.6	59.4	65.4
		0.20	−19.8	−4.9	9.9	47.5	56.4	62.4
	150	0.10	−19.8	−4.9	12.9	23.8	32.7	41.6
		0.20	−16.8	−4.9	6.9	26.7	29.7	38.6
Convex	25	0.10	−21.0	−0.6	10.2	28.7	25.1	16.8
		0.20	−13.8	−0.6	7.8	26.3	25.1	20.4
	50	0.10	−9.0	5.4	12.6	20.4	18.0	10.8
		0.20	−4.2	5.4	10.2	19.2	18.0	14.4
	150	0.10	1.8	9.0	13.8	8.4	9.6	7.2
		0.20	4.2	9.0	11.4	9.6	9.6	7.2

t2 various models. It is seen that $\widehat{MED}_2$ tends to estimate the target dose with less bias than the alternative estimation methods. $\widehat{MED}_1$ tends to underestimate the target dose, while $\widehat{MED}_3$ tends to overestimate it. The precision of all three estimation methods depends on the sample sizes and on the underlying dose–response shape, though. With higher sample sizes, the precision of all three methods is considerably enhanced. Furthermore, the precision is considerably higher when the underlying dose–response shape is either a quadratic, convex or a exponential shape.

Similar results are observed for the other sample sizes and values of γ. We conclude that $\widehat{MED}_2$ seems preferable to the other methods. The dose-selection step offers additional and useful knowledge about the underlying dose–response profile that is not possible with traditional multiple comparison dose-selection methods. Greater precision in the estimation of the model would be obtained if more suitable designs were used.

10.6   Conclusions

In this chapter, we have described modeling methods for analyzing dose–response studies. We introduced the framework of modeling approaches with their advantages and disadvantages as compared to alternative analysis methods. We described some commonly used dose–response models, while discussing and interpreting their parameters together with strategies for obtaining initial estimates. We then presented methods to determine suitable dose levels to meet clinical effect requirements. Particular emphasis was laid on the inherent problems related to model uncertainty, such as increased variability and bias of the parameters estimates of interest.

In light of these results a hybrid strategy for analyzing dose finding studies was investigated in detail. The proposed methodology combines the advantages of multiple comparison and modeling approaches, consisting of a multi-stage procedure. In the first stage, multiple comparison methods are used to test for PoA and to identify statistically significant contrasts corresponding to a set of candidate models. Once the PoA is established in the first stage, standard model selection criteria are used to chose the best model, which is then used for dose-fining in subsequent stages. The advantage of this new approach, in comparison to more traditional multiple comparison dose finding methods, is its added flexibility in searching for and identifying an adequate dose for future drug development while alleviating the aforementioned model selection problems.

The emphasis of this chapter has been on the motivation and the methodological foundation of the MCP-Mod approach. We did not present or discuss in greater detail the implementation aspects of the methodology, due to space limitations. A separate manuscript dedicated to the practical aspects of utilizing MCP-Mod, including software for implementing the various steps of the methodology, is currently under preparation.

An important research topic that can significantly enhance the performance of the methods described here is the re-evaluation of study designs for dose finding studies which take modeling of the dose–response relationship into consideration. Traditionally, dose-finding designs were developed with multiple comparison methods in mind. From the point of view of modeling, it would be better to have more doses spread out in the range of possible doses. Of course this raises other important issues, like the feasibility of manufacturing such doses and managing a trial with a larger number of doses. Whether or not these may be practical restrictions will be study-dependent. However, the need to re-think traditional dose finding designs in light of the need to model the dose–response relationship is evident and certainly deserving more research.

References

Abelson, R.P., and Tukey, J.W. 1963. Efficient utilization of non-numerical information in quantitative analysis: General theory and the case of simple order. *The Annals of Mathematical Statistics* 34:1347–1369.

Akaike, H. 1973. "Information theory and an extension of the maximum likelihood principle" in *2nd International Symposium on Information Theory*, (B.N. Petrov and F. Csaki, editors) pp. 267–281, Budapest: Akademiai Kiado. Reprinted in *Breakthrough in Statistics 1*, (S. Kotz and N.L. Johnson editors) pp. 610–624. New York: Springer-Verlag

Anraku, K. 1999. An information criterion for parameters under a simple order restriction. *Biometrika*. 86:141–152.

Augustin, N.H., Sauerbrei, W., and Schumacher, M. 2002. *Incorporating model selection uncertainty into prognostic factor model predictions*. Technical report #76, Department of Biometry, University of Freiburg, Germany.

Bates, D.M., and Watts D.G. 1988. *Nonnlinear Regression Analysis and Its Applications*. New York: Willey.

Bretz, F., Pinheiro, J.C., and Branson, M. 2005. Combining multiple comparisons and modeling techniques in dose–response studies. *Biometrics*, 61:738–748.

Buckland, S.T., Burnham, K.P., and Augustin, N.H. 1997. Model selection: An integral part of inference. *Biometrics*, 53:603–618.

Chambers, J.M., and Hastie, T.J. 1992. Statistical Models in S. New York: Chapman & Hall.

Chatfield, C. 1995. Model uncertainty, data mining and statistical inference (with discussion). *Journal of the Royal Statistical Society* Series A, 158:419–466.

Clyde, M., and George, E.I. 2004. Model uncertainty. *Statistical Science*, 19:81–94.

Draper, D. 1995. Assessment and propagation of model uncertainty. *Journal of the Royal Statistical Society* Series B, 57:45–97.

Freund, R.J., and Littell, R.C. 2000. SAS System for Regression, 3rd ed. New York: BBU Press and Wiley.

Genz, A., and Bretz, F. 2002. Methods for the computation of multivariate t-probabilities. *Journal of Computational and Graphical Statistics* 11:950–971.

Hastie, T., Tibshirani, and Friedman, J. 2001. *The Elements of Statistical Learning*. New York: Springer-Verlag.

Hjorth, J.S.U. 1994. *Computer Intensive Statistical Methods – Validation, Model Selection and Bootstrap*. London: Chapman & Hall.

Hochberg, Y., and Tamhane, A.C. 1987. Multiple comparisons procedures. New York: Wiley.

Hoeting, J., Madigan, D., Raftery, A.E., and Volinsky, C.T. 1999. Bayesian model averaging. *Statistical Science*, 14:382–417.

Hsu, J.C. 1996. *Multiple Comparisons*. New York: Chapman and Hall.

ICH E4. 1994. *Dose–Response Information to Support Drug Registration.*

Junquera, J.P., Vázquez, E.G., and Riaño, P.L.G. 2002. Multiple comparison procedures applied to model selection. *Neurocomputing* 48:155–173.

Kadane, J.B., and Lazar, N.A. 2004. Methods and criteria for model selection. *Journal of the American Statistical Association* 99:279–290.

MacDougall, J. (2005) "Analysis of dose response studies - E_{max} model," in *Design and Analysis of Dose Response Clinical Trials*, (Ting, N editor). New York: Springer-Verlag.

Pinheiro, J.C., and Bates, D.M. 2000. *Mixed-Effects Models in S and S-PLUS*. New York Springer-Verlag.

Robertson, T., Wright, F.T., and Dykstra, R.L. 1988. *Order Restricted Statistical Inference*. New York: Wiley.

Ruberg S.J. 1995. Dose response studies I. Some design considerations. *Journal of Biopharmaceutical Statistics* 5(1):1–14.

Scheffé, H. 1953. A method for judging all contrasts in analysis of variance. *Biometrika* 40:87–104.

Schwarz, G. 1978. Estimating the dimension of a model. *The Annals of Statistics* 6:461–464.

Seber, G.A.F., and Wild, C.J. 1989. *Nonlinear Regression*. New York: Wiley.

Shen, X., Huang, H.-C., and Ye, J. 2004. Inference after model selection. *Journal of the American Statistical Association* 99:751–762.

Shimodaira, H. 1998. An application of multiple comparison techniques to model selection. *Annals of the Institute of Statistical Mathematics* 50:1–13.

Tamhane, A.C., Dunnett, C.W., and Hochberg, Y. 1996. Multiple test procedures for dose finding. *Biometrics*, 52:21–37.

Tukey, J.W., Ciminera, J.L., and Heyse, J.F. 1985. Testing the statistical certainty of a response to increasing doses of a drug. *Biometrics* 41:295–301.

Westfall, P.H., and Krishen, A. 2001. Optimally weighted, fixed sequence and gatekeeping multiple testing procedures. *Journal of Statistical Planning and Inference* 99:25–40.

Zucchini, W. 2000. An introduction to model selection. *Journal of Mathematical Psychology* 44:41–61.

11
Multiple Comparison Procedures in Dose Response Studies

AJIT C. TAMHANE AND BRENT R. LOGAN

11.1   Introduction

Dose–response studies are useful in Phase II and Phase III clinical trials to evaluate efficacy and toxicity of a drug in order to determine its effective and safe ranges. A zero dose is generally included as a control against which higher doses are compared. This naturally leads to multiple comparisons. The ordered nature of doses suggests the use of stepwise multiple test procedures. The purpose of this article is to give a brief overview of these procedures. In Section 11.2, we present step-down procedures for identifying the minimum effective dose (MinED). These procedures are applied to the problem of identifying the maximum safe dose (MaxSD) in Section 11.3. Examples are given in Section 11.4 followed by some extensions in Section 11.5. The paper concludes with a discussion in Section 11.6.

11.2   Identifying the Minimum Effective Dose (MinED)

11.2.1   Problem Formulation

Let $i = 0, 1, \ldots, k$ represent increasing dose levels, where 0 denotes the zero (control) dose. Assume that the efficacy measurements Y_{ij} ($1 \leq j \leq n_i$) on the ith dose are independent and normally distributed with mean μ_i and variance σ^2, denoted by $Y_{ij} \sim N(\mu_i, \sigma^2)$. We assume that a larger μ_i represents higher efficacy. Let $\overline{Y}_i \sim N(\mu_i, \sigma^2/n_i)$ be the sample mean and $S^2 \sim \sigma^2 \chi_\nu^2/\nu$ be the pooled sample variance based on $\nu = \sum_{i=0}^{k} n_i - (k+1)$ degrees of freedom (df).

It is common to use the mean efficacy of the zero dose as a benchmark for comparison purposes to decide if a particular dose is clinically effective. Two different measures are employed for this purpose. The first is the difference measure, $\delta_i = \mu_i - \mu_0$, with a specified additive threshold $\delta > 0$ that this difference must exceed in order for dose i to be deemed effective. The second is the ratio measure, $\lambda_i = \mu_i/\mu_0$, with a specified multiplicative threshold $\lambda > 1$ that this ratio must exceed in order for dose i to be deemed effective. Here we adopt the latter approach since it requires an investigator to specify the threshold in relative terms instead of absolute terms, which is often more difficult. Thus, e.g., if a 10% increase in the mean efficacy compared to the zero dose is regarded as clinically significant then $\lambda = 1.10$. However, it should be noted that the use of the multiplicative threshold assumes that $\mu_0 > 0$. If μ_0 is positive but close to zero, very large values of λ must be specified. Procedures using the additive threshold are briefly covered in Section 11.5.

The true MinED can be defined in two ways. A simple definition is

$$\text{MinED} = \min\{i : \mu_i > \lambda\mu_0\} \tag{11.1}$$

which is the lowest dose that is effective. For a stronger requirement on MinED the following definition is used:

$$\text{MinED} = \min\{i : \mu_j > \lambda\mu_0 \text{ for all } j \geq i\} \tag{11.2}$$

This is the lowest dose such that it and all higher doses are effective.

In some applications it is reasonable to assume that the dose–response curve satisfies a monotone property that if dose i is ineffective then all lower doses are also ineffective, and if dose i is effective then all higher doses are also effective. Formally,

$$\mu_i \leq \lambda\mu_0 \Rightarrow \mu_j \leq \lambda\mu_0 \quad \forall j < i \qquad \text{and}$$
$$\mu_i > \lambda\mu_0 \Rightarrow \mu_j > \lambda\mu_0 \quad \forall j > i \tag{11.3}$$

This will be referred to as the weak monotonicity assumption as opposed to the strong monotonicity assumption:

$$\mu_0 \leq \mu_1 \leq \cdots \leq \mu_k \tag{11.4}$$

If the dose–response relationship is weakly monotone, then the two definitions of MinED are equivalent.

We want to guarantee that the probability of any ineffective dose being declared effective is no more than a specified level α. Let $\widehat{\text{MinED}}$ denote the sample or estimated MinED. Under weak monotonicity, this requirement translates to

$$P(\widehat{\text{MinED}} < \text{MinED}) \leq \alpha \tag{11.5}$$

Our approach to identifying MinED will be via tests of the hypotheses

$$H_i : \mu_i \leq \lambda\mu_0 \ (1 \leq i \leq k) \tag{11.6}$$

against one-sided alternatives. If using definition (11.1), the estimated MinED is defined as

$$\widehat{\text{MinED}} = \min\{i : H_i \text{ is rejected }\} \tag{11.7}$$

If using definition (11.2), the estimated MinED is defined as

$$\widehat{\text{MinED}} = \min\{i : H_j \text{ is rejected for all } j \geq i\} \tag{11.8}$$

If a multiple test procedure controls the familywise error rate (FWE), defined as

$$\text{FWE} = P\{\text{Reject any true } H_i\} \tag{11.9}$$

strongly (for any combination of true and false H_i) at level α then the requirement in Eq. (11.5) is satisfied. However, note that if the dose response curve is not weakly monotone, then the interpretation of Eq. (11.5), and the associated FWE, as the probability of any ineffective dose being declared effective only holds for definition (11.1).

In the next two subsections we will consider two types of multiple test procedures. The SD1PC procedure estimates the MinED according to definition (11.1). The SD2PC procedure estimates the MinED according to definition (11.2). When it is reasonable to assume monotonicity, the two definitions are equivalent and either SD1PC or SD2PC may be used.

11.2.2   Review of Multiple Test Procedures

Various procedures based on different contrasts of the dose means have been proposed in the literature (Ruberg, 1989, Tamhane et al., 1996, Dunnett and Tamhane, 1998). Here we will only consider step-down procedures based on pairwise contrasts because (1) as shown by Bauer (1997), only pairwise contrasts yield procedures that control the FWE even when the dose response is not monotone, (2) they are simple to use, and (3) they can be easily extended to nonnormal data by using appropriate two-sample statistics.

The traditional method for deriving step-down multiple test procedures is based on the closure principle due to Marcus et al., (1976). More recently, Hsu and Berger (1999) and Finner and Strassburger (2002) have proposed the partitioning principle to derive more powerful test procedures. We now explain these principles and the resulting test procedures.

11.2.2.1   Closure Principle: SD1PC Procedure

The closure principle requires a closed family of hypotheses. If we define the hypotheses $H_i' = \bigcap_{j=1}^{i} H_j$ meaning all doses at or below dose i are ineffective, then $\{H_i' \ (1 \leq i \leq k)\}$ is a closed family. (Note that this does not require the monotonicity assumption.) The closure principle tests each hypothesis H_i', if it is not already accepted, at level α. If H_i' is not rejected then the closure principle accepts all H_j' that are implied by H_i' without further tests. The representation $H_i' = \bigcap_{j=1}^{i} H_j$ shows that all H_j' for $j < i$ are implied by H_i'. This leads to a step-down test procedure in which H_k' is tested first. If H_k' is not rejected then all hypotheses are accepted and no dose is declared effective. Otherwise H_{k-1}' is tested next and the testing sequence continues. If H_i' is the last rejected hypothesis then $\widehat{\text{MinED}} = i$.

For the normal data assumed here, define the pairwise t-statistic corresponding to hypothesis H_i as

$$T_i = \frac{\overline{Y}_i - \lambda \overline{Y}_0}{S\sqrt{\lambda^2/n_0 + 1/n_i}} \qquad (1 \leq i \leq k). \qquad (11.10)$$

Then using the union-intersection (UI) method of Roy (1953), the statistic for testing H_i' is $T_{i,\max} = \max_{1 \leq j \leq i} T_j$. Under H_i' (assuming the least favorable configuration $\mu_j = \lambda \mu_0 \ \forall \ j \leq i$, which maximizes the FWE), the joint distribution of $T_1, T_2, \ldots, T_i$ is an i-variate t-distribution with ν df and correlation matrix $R_i = \{\rho_{j\ell}\}$, which has a product correlation structure, $\rho_{j\ell} = \tau_j \tau_\ell$, with

$$\tau_j = \frac{\lambda}{\sqrt{\lambda^2 + r_j}} \quad \text{and} \quad r_j = \frac{n_0}{n_j} \quad (1 \leq j \leq k) \qquad (11.11)$$

If $n_1 = n_2 = \cdots = n_k = n$ and $r = n_0/n$ then $\rho_{j\ell} \equiv \rho = \lambda^2/(\lambda^2 + r)$. Let $t_{i,\nu,R_i}^{(\alpha)}$ denote the upper α equicoordinate critical point of this i-variate t-distribution. Then the closed procedure rejects H_i' at level α iff $H_k', \ldots, H_{i+1}'$ have been rejected and

$$T_{i,\max} > t_{i,\nu,R_i}^{(\alpha)}$$

This is referred to as the SD1PC procedure. Note that the critical constants used in SD1PC are different if smaller μ_i's represent higher efficacies with the threshold $\lambda < 1$. This is so because the $\rho_{j\ell}$ are not invariant to the transformation $\lambda \leftarrow 1/\lambda$ or $\lambda \leftarrow \lambda - 1$. Also, as pointed out earlier, the SD1PC procedure is appropriate for definition (11.1) of the MinED in the sense that it will control the error rate in Eq. (11.5) for this definition, but it can also be used for definition (11.2) under the assumption of monotonicity, in which case $H_i' = H_i = \bigcap_{j=1}^{i} H_j$.

11.2.2.2   Partitioning Principle: SD2PC Procedure

The partitioning principle reformulates the hypotheses (11.6) so that they are disjoint. There are different ways to accomplish this. One way is to write the hypotheses as

$$H_i^* : \mu_i \leq \lambda \mu_0, \ \mu_j > \lambda \mu_0 \quad \forall \ j > i \ (1 \leq i \leq k) \qquad (11.12)$$

For the sake of completeness, add the hypothesis $H_0^* : \mu_j > \lambda \mu_0 \ \forall \ j$, which need not be tested. This partitioning is appropriate when efficacy is expected to increase with dose. Note that the hypotheses H_i^* are disjoint with their union being the whole parameter space, and the true parameter configuration belongs to exactly one of the H_i^*. Therefore, no multiplicity adjustment is needed to perform the tests and each H_i^* can be tested at level α independently of the others. Final inferences drawn must be logically consistent with the H_i^* that are not rejected. This procedure controls the error rate in Eq. (11.5) corresponding to the more stringent definition (11.2) of the MinED.

Note that the above formulation of the hypotheses implies that doses must be tested in a step-down manner in the order $H_k^*, H_{k-1}^*, \ldots$, stopping as soon as any hypothesis is accepted. For example, suppose $k = 5$, and all five hypotheses are tested, but only H_5^*, H_4^* and H_2^* are rejected. Then we can only conclude that doses 5 and 4 are effective, but not dose 2. Thus, we get $\widehat{\text{MinED}} = 4$ and so testing can be stopped once H_3^* is accepted.

The main difficulty in applying the partitioning principle is that it is not easy to derive tests of the hypotheses H_i^*. However, by noting that H_i^* is a subset of H_i, we see that an α-level test of H_i provides a conservative α-level test of H_i^*. This leads to a step-down test procedure on the family $\{H_i \ (1 \leq i \leq k)\}$. Therefore, for testing H_i, we use the ordinary Student's t-test, which rejects H_i (assuming that $H_k, \ldots, H_{i+1}$ have been rejected) if $T_i > t_{\nu,\alpha}$, where $t_{\nu,\alpha}$ is the upper α critical point of the univariate Student's t-distribution with ν df. The resulting step-down procedure is referred to as the SD2PC procedure.

Although we have derived the SD2PC procedure by using the partitioning principle, it can also be derived by noting that the a priori ordering of the hypotheses results in their nesting: $H_k \subseteq H_{k-1} \subseteq \cdots \subseteq H_1$. This approach is employed by Maurer et al. (1995) to show that SD2PC controls the FWE strongly.

Finally we note that both SD1PC and SD2PC are pre-determined testing procedures since they both test the hypotheses $H_k, H_{k-1}, \ldots$ in a pre-determined order not in a sample-determined order (see Chapter 12).

11.2.3   Simultaneous Confidence Intervals

Bretz et al. (2003) proposed stepwise confidence intervals for the ratios $\lambda_i = \mu_i/\mu_0$ based on Fieller's (1954) method. Consider the r.v.

$$T_i = \frac{\overline{Y}_i - \lambda_i \overline{Y}_0}{S\sqrt{\lambda_i^2/n_0 + 1/n_i}}$$

which is t-distributed with ν df. By solving the inequality $T_i \leq t_{\nu,\alpha}$, which is an event of probability $1 - \alpha$, we get the following $100(1 - \alpha)\%$ lower confidence bound on λ_i:

$$\lambda_i \geq L_i = \frac{\overline{Y}_0 \overline{Y}_i - \sqrt{a_0 \overline{Y}_i^2 + a_i \overline{Y}_0^2 - a_0 a_i}}{\overline{Y}_0^2 - a_0}$$

where $a_i = t_{\nu,\alpha}^2 S^2/n_i$ $(0 \leq i \leq k)$.

For identifying the MinED Bretz et al. (2003) embedded these marginal $100(1 - \alpha)\%$ confidence intervals into the following step-down procedure, which does not require any multiplicity adjustment according to the results of Hsu and Berger (1999).

STEP 1: If $L_k \leq \lambda$ then conclude that $\lambda_k \geq L_k$, all doses are ineffective and stop. Otherwise conclude that $\lambda_k > \lambda$ (dose k is effective) and go to Step 2.

STEP i: If $L_{k-i+1} \leq \lambda$ then conclude that $\lambda_{k-i+1} \geq L_{k-i+1}$, doses $1, \ldots, k - i + 1$ are ineffective and stop. Otherwise conclude that $\lambda_{k-i+1} > \lambda$ (dose $k - i + 1$ is effective) and go to Step $i + 1$.

STEP $k + 1$: Conclude that $\min_{1 \leq i \leq k} \lambda_i \geq \min_{1 \leq i \leq k} L_i$.

This test procedure is equivalent to the SD2PC procedure because it is derived from it. However, additionally, it yields lower confidence bounds on the λ_i's for all doses found effective and the first dose found ineffective.

11.3   Identifying the Maximum Safe Dose (MaxSD)

All of the preceding discussion extends naturally to the problem of identifying the MaxSD in toxicity studies with a few minor changes as we note below. In order to keep the forms of the hypotheses (11.6) and the test statistics in Eq. (11.10) the same, and also to conform with the past literature, we will assume that lower μ_i implies a more toxic (less safe) dose. Toxicity generally increases with dose level and the zero dose has the least toxicity. Therefore the μ_i's are generally decreasing and the threshold $\lambda < 1$. Thus, dose i with $\mu_i > \lambda\mu_0$ is regarded as safe, while dose i with $\mu_i \leq \lambda\mu_0$ is regarded as unsafe. For example, $\lambda = 0.90$ means that a 10% decrease in safety level (increase in toxicity) is regarded as clinically unsafe.

The maximum safe dose (MaxSD) for specified $\lambda < 1$ is defined as

$$\text{MaxSD} = \max\{i : \mu_j > \lambda\mu_0 \; \forall \; j \leq i\}$$

Analogous to the discussion of the MinED, there could be two definitions of the MaxSD. However, we assume monotonicity of the toxicity response so that the definitions are identical. The hypotheses are the same as in Eq. (11.6) (where now H_i states that the ith dose is unsafe). If

$$\widehat{\text{MaxSD}} = \max\{i : H_j \text{ is rejected } \forall \; j \leq i\}$$

denotes the estimated MaxSD then we want to guarantee that

$$P(\widehat{\text{MaxSD}} > \text{MaxSD}) \leq \alpha \tag{11.13}$$

Since the goal is now to find the MaxSD, both SD1PC and SD2PC start by testing H_1 and proceed to testing H_2 if H_1 is rejected (dose 1 is declared safe) and so on. If H_1 is not rejected then all H_i are accepted without further tests and all doses are declared unsafe, i.e., there is no MaxSD. SD1PC rejects H_i using the representation $H_i = \bigcap_{j=i}^{k} H_j$ if

$$T_{i,\max} = \max_{i \leq j \leq k} T_j > t_{\ell,\nu,R_\ell}^{(\alpha)}$$

where $\ell = k - i + 1$ and $R_\ell = \{\rho_{ij}\}$, while SD2PC rejects H_i if $T_i > t_{\nu,\alpha}$. For details see Tamhane et al.

11.4   Examples

Example 1 (Identifying the MinED): Tamhane and Logan (2002) cite an example of a Phase II randomized, double-blind, placebo-controlled parallel group clinical trial of a new drug for the treatment of arthritis of the knee using four increasing doses (labeled 1 to 4). While they consider both efficacy and safety outcomes in that study, here we focus only on the efficacy data. A total of 370 patients were randomized to the five treatment groups. The efficacy variable is the pooled WOMAC (Western Ontario and McMaster Universities osteoarthritis index) score, a composite score computed from assessments of pain (5 items), stiffness (2 items), and physical function (17 items). The composite score is normalized to a scale of 0–10. An increase in WOMAC from the baseline indicates an improvement in disease condition. We will consider a 30% improvement in WOMAC scores over the baseline mean compared to that for the zero dose group a clinically significant improvement, so that $\lambda = 1.3$.

The summary data are given in Table 11.1. Normal plots were found to be satisfactory, and the Bartlett and Levene tests for homogeneity of variances yielded nonsignificant results. The sample sizes are approximately equal so that $r_i \approx r = 1$ and $\rho_{ij} \approx \rho = 1.30^2/(1.30^2 + 1) = 0.628$. The pooled estimate of the standard deviation is 1.962 with $\nu = 365$ df. The t-statistics computed using Eq. (11.10) are given in Table 11.2.

Table 11.1. Summary statistics for changes from baseline in WOMAC score

	Dose level				
	0	1	2	3	4
Mean	1.437	2.196	2.459	2.771	2.493
SD	1.924	2.253	1.744	1.965	1.893
n	76	73	73	75	73

Table 11.2. t-Statistics and unadjusted p-values for WOMAC scores

	Comparison			
	1 vs. 0	2 vs. 0	3 vs. 0	4 vs. 0
T_i	0.881	1.588	2.439	1.680
p_i	0.189	0.056	0.007	0.047

The SD1PC procedure begins by comparing $T_{4,\max} = 2.439$ with the critical value $t_{4,365,0.628}^{(.05)} = 2.123$. Since $2.439 > 2.123$, we step down to compare dose 3 with the control. In fact, we can take a shortcut and step down to compare dose 2 with the control, since $T_{4,\max} = T_3 = 2.439$ and the multivariate T-critical values decrease with dimension implying rejection of H_3. So, next we compare $T_{2,\max} = 1.588$ with the critical value $t_{2,365,0.628}^{(.05)} = 1.900$. Since $1.588 < 1.900$, we accept hypothesis H_2 and by implication hypothesis H_1, leading to the conclusion that MinED = 3.

The SD2PC procedure begins by comparing $T_4 = 1.680$ with the critical value $t_{365,.05} = 1.649$. Both T_4 and $T_3 = 2.439$ exceed 1.649, so we reject H_4 and H_3.

Next $T_2 = 1.588 < 1.649$, so we stop and accept H_2 and hence H_1 by implication, leading to the same conclusion that $\widehat{\text{MinED}} = 3$.

To compute stepwise 95% confidence intervals using the Bretz et al. method we first compute

$$L_1 = 1.136, \ L_2 = 1.288, \ L_3 = 1.468, \ L_4 = 1.308$$

Since L_4 and L_3 are both greater than $\lambda = 1.30$ we conclude that both doses 4 and 3 are effective. But $L_2 < \lambda = 1.30$, and so we stop and conclude that dose 2 is ineffective and $\lambda_2 \geq 1.288$. Obviously, we get the same conclusion as SD2PC, but additionally we get confidence bounds on λ_4, λ_3 and λ_2.

Example 2 (Identifying the MaxSD): Tamhane et al. (2001) cite an aquatic toxicology study in which daphnids, or water fleas (*Daphnia magna*), were exposed over 21 days to a potentially toxic compound. Daphnids of the same age and genetic stock were randomly assigned to a water control, a solvent control, or one of six concentrations of a pesticide. The safety endpoint of interest was the growth, as measured by the lengths of the daphnids after 21 days of continuous exposure. Because there was no significant difference between the two control groups, they were combined for subsequent analysis. Six nominal concentrations of the pesticide were tested: $0.3125, 6.25, 12.5, 25, 50$, and 100 ppm. Forty daphnids were randomly assigned to each group, but because some died during the course of the experiment they were not evaluable. Also, because of excessive mortality in the 100 ppm dose group, it was omitted from subsequent analysis. This follows the recommendation of Capizzi et al. (1985) for a two-stage approach, in which survival is studied in the first stage, and sublethal effects (such as growth) are compared among those doses which do not significantly affect survival. In the toxicology community, opinions about what constitutes a biologically significant effect have ranged from 5 to 25% adverse effect. If we take an average of this range, i.e., 15% reduction in length or $\lambda = 0.85$ as biologically unsafe, then we would like to know which dose is the MaxSD for this value of λ.

The summary statistics are given in Table 11.3. Normal plots were found to be satisfactory, and the Levene test for homogeneity of variances was nonsignificant. The pooled estimate of the standard deviation is 0.1735 with $v = 254$ df. Additional analyses of variance were performed on the data as discussed in Tamhane et al. (2002), but we do not elaborate on them here. The sample sizes in the nonzero dose groups were all approximately equal, so that $r_i \approx r = 80/36 = 2.222$ and $\rho_{ij} \approx \rho = 0.85^2/(0.85^2 + 2.222) = 0.245$. The t-statistics computed using Eq. (11.10) are given in Table 11.4.

Table 11.3. Summary statistics for daphnid length data

	Dose level					
	0	1	2	3	4	5
Mean	4.0003	3.9908	3.8108	3.6306	3.4600	3.2106
SD	0.1496	0.2110	0.1504	0.1961	0.1726	0.1829
n	80	38	39	35	35	33

Table 11.4. t-Statistics and unadjusted p-values
for daphnid length data

	Comparison				
	1 vs. 0	2 vs. 0	3 vs. 0	4 vs. 0	5 vs. 0
T_i	18.082	12.692	6.838	1.774	−5.505
p_i	0.000	0.000	0.000	0.038	1.000

For the SD1PC procedure, the critical values are $t_{5,254,0.245}^{(.05)} = 2.307, t_{4,254,0.245}^{(.05)} = 2.224, t_{3,254,0.245}^{(.05)} = 2.114, t_{2,254,0.245}^{(.05)} = 1.952$, and $t_{1,254,0.245}^{(.05)} = 1.652$. The SD1PC procedure proceeds by comparing the statistics $T_{i,\max}$ to the critical values in sequence, starting with $T_{1,\max} = 18.082$. These are rejected in sequence until we come to $T_{4,\max} = 1.774$, which is less than 1.952. Therefore, we conclude that $\widehat{\text{MaxSD}} = 3$.

The SD2PC procedure proceeds by comparing each t-statistic with the critical value $t_{254,.05} = 1.652$, starting with dose 1. H_4 is the last hypothesis rejected, since $T_4 = 1.774 > 1.652$ and $T_5 = -5.505 < 1.652$. Therefore, we stop and accept H_5, leading to the conclusion that $\widehat{\text{MaxSD}} = 4$. Note that SD2PC found dose 4 to be safe, whereas SD1PC did not.

11.5 Extensions

Several extensions of the basic methods described above have been studied in the literature. We briefly summarize a few below.

1. Multiple test procedures based on general contrasts are given in Ruberg (1989), Tamhane et al. (1996), Dunnett and Tamhane (1998), and Tamhane et al. (2001). The first three papers use the difference measure approach. Specifically, when using the difference measure approach for the MinED problem, a general contrast for testing $H_i : \mu_i \leq \mu_0 + \delta$ is given by

$$C_i = c_{i0}(\overline{Y}_0 + \delta) + c_{i1}\overline{Y}_1 + \cdots + c_{ik}\overline{Y}_k \quad (1 \leq i \leq k)$$

where the contrast coefficients c_{ij} sum to zero. The corresponding test statistic is

$$T_i = \frac{C_i}{\text{s.e.}(C_i)} = \frac{C_i}{S\sqrt{\sum_{j=0}^{I} c_{ij}^2/n_j}} \quad (1 \leq i \leq k)$$

The T_i have a multivariate t-distribution with correlations that depend on the c_{ij} and the n_i. If the dose response shape is known a priori then the c_{ij} can be chosen to mimic its shape, e.g., if the shape is roughly linear then one can use linear contrasts in which the c_{ij} form an arithmetic progression. However, often such knowledge is lacking. Previous simulation studies have shown that the procedures based on Helmert contrasts, in which $c_{ij} = -1$, for $j = 0, 1, \ldots, i-1$, $c_{ii} = i$ and $c_{ij} = 0$ for $j > i$, perform better than those based on other contrasts when the minimum effective dose is at the high end or when the dose response shape is convex, and do not perform too badly in other cases. Another advantage of Helmert contrasts is that for a balanced design ($n_0 = n_1 = \cdots = n_k$) they are uncorrelated, i.e., $\rho_{ij} = 0$. Effectively, the ith Helmert contrast compares the ith dose level mean with the average of all the lower dose level means (including the zero dose).

Other trend tests are available as well for testing the hypotheses at each stage of the step-down procedure. Abelson and Tukey (1963) propose a contrast test which minimizes the maximum power loss over the alternative hypothesis space. Stewart and Ruberg (2000) propose using the maximum of several well-defined contrast tests to improve the robustness of the trend test to different dose–response shapes. Tests could alternatively be based on isotonic regression (Robertson et al. 1988; Williams 1971, 1972).

2. The problem of identifying the MinED and MaxSD simultaneously is considered in Tamhane and Logan (2002); see also Bauer et al. (2001). The therapeutic window is defined as the interval [MinED, MaxSD] if this interval is nonempty. This interval is estimated by [$\widehat{\text{MinED}}$, $\widehat{\text{MaxSD}}$] subject to the requirement that the probability that [$\widehat{\text{MinED}}$, $\widehat{\text{MaxSD}}$] contains any ineffective or unsafe doses is less than or equal to a prespecified level α, i.e.,

$$P\left\{\widehat{\text{MinED}} < \text{MinED or } \widehat{\text{MaxSD}} > \text{MaxSD}\right\} \le \alpha$$

Tamhane and Logan (2002) investigated several strategies, including α-splitting, where the MinED is identified with Type I error α_E and the MaxSD is identified with Type I error α_S so that $\alpha_E + \alpha_S = \alpha$. They also proposed more efficient bootstrap procedures which take into account the correlation between efficacy and safety variables.

3. In many applications the assumption of homoscedasticity of variances is not satisfied. In Tamhane and Logan (2004), we give extensions of the procedures discussed here as well as those based on Helmert contrasts when the dose response data are heteroscedastic.

4. Nonparametric extensions of the step-down procedures for identifying the MinED are given by Chen (1999), Sidik and Morris (1999), Chen and Jan (2002), and Jan and Shieh (2004).

11.6   Discussion

In this section, we compare the methodology proposed in this paper with that currently practiced by the U.S. Food and Drug Administration (FDA). For simplicity assume a single dose or drug. Then the FDA's criterion for efficacy consists of the proof of statistical significance and of clinical significance. Denoting the means for the control and the drug by μ_0 and μ_1, respectively, the statistical significance criterion is met if $H_0 : \mu_1 \le \mu_0$ is rejected in favor of the one-sided alternative $H_1 : \mu_1 > \mu_0$ at the α-level (usually 2.5%). For clinical significance, if the ratio measure is adopted then it is required that $\widehat{\mu}_1/\widehat{\mu}_0 > \lambda$, where $\lambda > 1$ is a specified threshold. Thus it is required that the $100(1 - \alpha)\%$ confidence interval for μ_1/μ_0 lie above 1, but only the point estimate of μ_1/μ_0 lie above the threshold λ. On the other hand, our approach tests $H_0 : \mu_1 \leq \lambda\mu_0$ vs. $H_1 : \mu_1 > \lambda\mu_0$ and thus requires that the $100(1 - \alpha)\%$ confidence interval for μ_1/μ_0 lie above λ, which is a stricter requirement. The two approaches are equivalent if $\lambda = 1$. We recommend that the stricter requirement with $\lambda > 1$ be adopted since requiring that the point estimate $\widehat{\mu}_1/\widehat{\mu}_0 > \lambda$ does not guarantee that the true ratio $\mu_1/\mu_0 > \lambda$ with $100(1 - \alpha)\%$ confidence. Similar discussion applies if the difference measure is used. In either case, another practical problem is how to specify the threshold.

Acknowledgments

The authors are grateful to two referees and Dr. Naitee Ting for their comments and suggestions which significantly improved the paper.

References

Abelson, R. P., and Tukey, J. W. 1963. Efficient utilization of non-numerical information in quantitative analysis: general theory and the case of simple order. *Annals of Mathematical Statistics* 34:1347–1369.

Bauer, P. 1997. A note on multiple testing procedures for dose finding. *Biometrics* 53:1125–1128.

Bauer, P., Brannath, W., and Posch, M. 2001. Multiple testing for identifying effective and safe treatments. *Biometrical Journal* 43:605–616.

Bretz, F., Hothorn, L. A., and Hsu, J. C. 2003. Identifying effective and/or safe doses by stepwise confidence intervals for ratios. *Statistics in Medicine* 22:847–858.

Capizzi, T., Oppenheimer, L., Mehta, H., and Naimie, H. 1985. Statistical considerations in the evaluation of chronic toxicity studies. *Environmental Science and Technology* 19:35–43.

Chen, Y. I. 1999. Nonparametric identification of the minimum effective dose. *Biometrics* 55:126–130.

Chen, Y. I., and Jan, S-L 2002. Nonparametric identification of the minimum effective dose for randomized block designs. *Communications in Statistics* Ser. B 31:301–312.

Dunnett, C. W., and Tamhane, A. C. 1998. Some new multiple test procedures for dose finding. *Journal of Biopharmaceutical Statistics* 8:353–366.

Fieller, E. C. 1954. Some problems in interval estimation. *Journal of the Royal Statistical Society* Ser. B 16:175–185.

Finner, H., and Strassburger, K. 2002. The partitioning principle: A powerful tool in multiple decision theory. *Annals of Statistics* 30:1194–1213.

Hsu, J. C., and Berger, R. L. 1999. Stepwise confidence intervals without multiplicity adjustment for dose response and toxicity studies. *Journal of the American Statistical Association* 94:468–482.

Jan, S-L. and Shieh, G. 2004. Multiple test procedures for dose finding. *Communications in Statistics* Ser. B 34:1021–1037.

Marcus, R., Peritz, E., and Gabriel, K. R. 1976. On closed testing procedures with special reference to ordered analysis of variance. *Biometrika* 63:655–660.

Maurer, W., Hothorn, L. A., and Lehmacher, W. 1995. "Multiple comparisons in drug clinical trials and preclinical assays: A-priori ordered hypotheses," in *Testing Principles in Clinical and Preclinical Trials (J. Vollmar, editor)* Stuttgart, Gustav Fischer Verlag, pp. 3–18.

Robertson, T., Wright, F. T., and Dykstra, R. L. 1988. *Order Restricted Statistical Inference.* New York Wiley.

Roy, S. N. 1953. On a heuristic method of test construction and its use in multivariate analysis. *Annals of Mathematical Statistics* 24:220–238.

Ruberg, S. J. 1989. Contrasts for identifying the minimum effective dose. *Journal of the American Statistical Association* 84:816–822.

Sidik, K., and Morris, R. W. 1999. Nonparametric step-down test procedures for finding the minimum effective dose. *Journal of Biopharmaceutical Statistics* 9:217–240.

Stewart, W. H., and Ruberg, S. J. 2000. Detecting dose response with contrasts. *Statistics in Medicine* 19:913–921.

Tamhane, A. C., Dunnett, C. W., Green, J. W., and Wetherington, J. F. 2001. Multiple test procedures for identifying the maximum safe dose. *Journal of the American Statistical Association* 96:835–843.

Tamhane, A. C., Hochberg, Y., and Dunnett, C. W. 1996. Multiple test procedures for dose finding. *Biometrics* 52:21–37.

Tamhane, A. C., and Logan, B. R. 2002. Multiple test procedures for identifying the minimum effective and maximum safe doses of a drug. *Journal of the American Statistical Association* 97:293–301.

Tamhane, A. C., and Logan, B. R. 2004. Finding the maximum safe dose for heteroscedastic data. *Journal of Biopharmaceutical Statistics* 14:843–856.

Williams, D. A. 1971. A test for differences between treatment means when several dose levels are compared with a zero dose level. *Biometrics* 27:103–117.

Williams, D. A. 1972. The comparison of several dose levels with a zero dose control. *Biometrics* 28:519–531.

12
Partitioning Tests in Dose–Response Studies with Binary Outcomes

XIANG LING, JASON HSU, AND NAITEE TING

12.1 Motivation

As discussed in Chapter 1, the main purpose of Phase II studies is dose finding and most of these studies are designed to help estimate the dose–response relationships. On the other hand, Phase III studies are designed to confirm findings from early phases, and results from Phase III studies are used for submission to regulatory agencies for drug approval. Hence, Phase III studies are designed for decision making. In terms of hypotheses testing, ways of controlling the family-wise error rate (FWER) strongly should be well specified prior to unmasking the study data. In many cases, these prespecification need to be clearly communicated with regulatory agencies for mutual agreement.

Although a wide range of different doses may have been studied at Phase II, it is still of interest to test a few doses in Phase III. There are many reasons for doing this—one reason could be that one or a few of the target doses may not have been studied in Phase II, another reason could be that the target dose was not exposed long enough in Phase II. Therefore, it is common to see that several doses are studied at Phase III. In situations where Phase III studies include multiple doses against a control, the null and alternative hypotheses need to be clearly stated, and procedures of multiple comparisons need to be specified prior to unmasking the study data. In many Phase III studies, the control group is a known active treatment; however, placebo is still commonly used in Phase III.

This chapter introduces the partitioning tests (Stefansson, et al., 1988; Hsu and Berger, 1999; Finner and Strassburger, 2002) as a method to construct multiple comparison procedures for binary outcomes. Three types of partitioning tests are introduced in this chapter: Section 12.3.1 covers the predetermined step-down method, Section 12.3.2 discusses the sample-determined step-down method, and Section 12.3.3 discusses the sample-determined step-up method. Suppose a given Phase III trial was designed with a low dose, a high dose of the test drug, plus a placebo control. Then the objective is to show that either the low dose, or the high dose, or possibly both doses are clinically meaningfully better than placebo. Therefore, two null hypotheses—H_{0H}: high dose is no better than placebo, and

H_{0L}: low dose is no better than placebo—may be of interest. Partitioning testing is a general principle which is useful in conducting multiple comparisons. There are various ways of implementing these tests. Our focus in this chapter is to apply partitioning tests in Phase III dose response settings where the primary efficacy variable of interest is a binary variable.

Binary variables are frequently used in clinical trials. For example, at the end of a study, each patient is classified as a responder or a nonresponder to the study treatment. A typical primary efficacy analysis is to compare the numbers and proportions of responders between treatment groups. The responder variable is a binary variable. In some other cases the primary efficacy variable may be a time-to-event variable and, hence, the primary efficacy analysis would be a survival analysis. If, however, the interest is in the number of such events observed at a particular time point during this study, then the outcome variable is a binary variable (number of events observed from each treatment group up to that time point). Although Chapter 13 discusses the analysis of dose–response studies with binary endpoints from a traditional tests of equalities point of view, this chapter concentrates on formulating the dose–response problem to to illuminate the partitioning principle that cleaves through single-step and stepwise methods. Some connection between partition testing and closed testing can be seen in Chapter 11.

For hypothesis testing of binary variables, two approaches are introduced in this chapter: large sample approximation tests and small sample exact tests. The large sample tests are derived using the normal approximation to the binary distribution (Chuang-Stein and Tong, 1995). The small sample exact tests are derived using the multivariate hypergeometric distribution.

Section 12.2 provides a review, Section 12.3 derives the partitioning test with binary outcome, an example is given in Section 12.4 and Section 12.5 concludes this chapter.

12.2   Comparing Two Success Probabilities in a Single Hypothesis

In this section, we briefly review the tests for comparing two unknown success probabilities, p_0 and p_1. Let us first consider testing the null hypothesis of equality

$$H_0: \ p_0 = p_1 \tag{12.1}$$

There are exact tests and large sample approximate tests available for testing this simple null hypothesis. Let n_0 and n_1 represent the sample sizes in the two groups. Let X_0 and X_1 be the numbers of successes and x_0 and x_1 be the observed numbers of successes in each group. Then $X_0 \sim \text{Binomial}(n_0, p_0)$ and $X_1 \sim \text{Binomial}(n_1, p_1)$.

For large sample sizes n_0 and n_1, we can use normal approximation. The estimators of p_0 and p_1, $\hat{p}_0 = x_0/n_0$ and $\hat{p}_1 = x_1/n_1$, are approximately normally distributed, based on the central limit theorem. Hence $\hat{p}_0 - \hat{p}_1$ follows a normal distribution. Under the null hypothesis, we can use the pooled standard error for $\hat{p}_0$ and $\hat{p}_1$, so

$$
SE(\hat{p}_0 - \hat{p}_1) = \sqrt{\hat{p}(1-\hat{p})\left(\frac{1}{n_0} + \frac{1}{n_1}\right)} \tag{12.2}
$$

where $\hat{p} = (x_0 + x_1)/(n_0 + n_1)$. As $\hat{p}$ converges in probability to the common success rate, by Slutsky's theorem, the test statistic

$$
\frac{\hat{p}_0 - \hat{p}_1}{SE(\hat{p}_0 - \hat{p}_1)}
$$

has asymptotically a standard normal distribution under H_0.

If the sample sizes n_0 and n_1 are small, we must use exact tests instead of approximate procedures. Let x be the total observed number of successes from both groups. Fisher (1934) introduced a conditional test using the fact that under the null hypothesis the variable X_1 given n_0, n_1, x, follows a hypergeometric distribution. That is,

$$
Pr(X_1 = x_1 | n_0, n_1, x) = \frac{\binom{n_1}{x_1}\binom{n_0}{x-x_1}}{\binom{n_1+n_0}{x}} \tag{12.3}
$$

where $\max(0, x - n_0) \leq x_1 \leq \min(x, n_1)$.

Once we have the distribution (asymptotic distribution or conditional distribution) of the test statistics, it is trivial to test the simple hypothesis in Eq. (12.1).

Now let us consider comparing two success probabilities in a composite hypothesis. Suppose the null hypothesis of interest is

$$
H_{01} : p_1 \leq p_0 + \delta \tag{12.4}
$$

where δ is a prefixed constant. For a large sample test, since we cannot use the pooled variance under this null hypothesis, the test statistic is

$$
Z_1 = \frac{\hat{p}_1 - \hat{p}_0 - \delta}{SE^*(\hat{p}_1 - \hat{p}_0)} \tag{12.5}
$$

where

$$
SE^*(\hat{p}_1 - \hat{p}_0) = \sqrt{\frac{\hat{p}_1(1-\hat{p}_1)}{n_1} + \frac{\hat{p}_0(1-\hat{p}_0)}{n_0}}
$$

The null hypothesis is rejected if the test statistic is larger than the $(1-\alpha)$ quantile of the standard normal distribution.

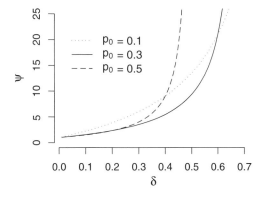

Figure 12.1. The relationship between δ and ψ for a few values of p_0.

As for a small-sample exact test, it can be shown that

$$\Pr(X_1 = x_1 | n_0, n_1, x) = \frac{\binom{n_1}{x_1}\binom{n_0}{x-x_1}\psi^{x_1}}{\sum_{j=L}^{U}\binom{n_1}{j}\binom{n_0}{x-j}\psi^j} \tag{12.6}$$

for L$\leq x_1 \leq$U, where $\psi = \frac{p_1}{1-p_1} / \frac{p_0}{1-p_0}$ is the odds ratio, L= max$(0, x - n_0)$, and U= min(n_1, x). A difference on the linear scale, i.e., δ, is now replaced by a nonlinear odds ratio ψ. Figure 12.1 shows the relationship between δ and ψ for a few values of p_0. Notice that $p_1 \leq p_0$ is equivalent to $\psi \leq 1$, and the distribution reduces to Eq. (12.3) when $p_1 = p_0$, or, $\psi = 1$.

It can also be shown that for $\psi > 0$, the distribution in Eq. (12.6) has monotone likelihood ratio in X_1. That is, for

$$\psi' > \psi, h(x_1) = \Pr_{\psi_1}(X_1 = x_1|n_0, n_1, x)/\Pr_\psi(X_1 = x_1|n_0, n_1, x) \propto (\psi'/\psi)^{x_1}$$

is non-decreasing in X_1. Therefore, the Type I error probability is maximized when $\psi = \frac{p_0+\delta}{1-p_0-\delta} / \frac{p_0}{1-p_0}$, or equivalently $p_1 = p_0 + \delta$. That is,

$$\Pr_{p_1 < p_0+\delta}(X_1 \geq m) \leq \Pr_{p_1=p_0+\delta}(X_1 \geq m)$$

for any m. When $\delta = 0$, the rejection region for the null hypothesis Eq. (12.4) is $X_1 \geq m_0$, where m_0 is the smallest integer such that $\Pr_{\psi=1}(X_1 \geq m_0) \leq \alpha$. For $\delta \neq 0$, ψ depends on the unknown parameter p_0 under null hypothesis. Thus the null hypothesis in Eq. (12.4) with $\delta \neq 0$ can not be tested using Fisher's exact test. We assume $\delta = 0$ for Fisher's exact test for the rest of the paper.

Although a null hypothesis of non-zero location shift cannot be tested using Fisher's exact test, the hypothesis of $\psi \leq \theta$ can be tested for any $\theta > 0$. The rejection region for $\psi \leq \theta$ is $X_1 \geq m_0'$, where m_0' is smallest integer such that $\Pr_{\psi=\theta}(X_1 \geq m_0') \leq \alpha$. The problem of comparing two success probabilities can be either in terms of the difference of the two probabilities or the odds ratio, but they are generally not the same unless $\delta = 0$ and $\theta = 1$. Next, we will discuss several methods for multiple comparisons of success probabilities.

12.3   Comparison of Success Probabilities in Dose–Response Studies

In dose–response studies, there are usually multiple composite null hypotheses of interest. Let the notation be the same as before, with the subscript denoting the dose group. For example, let p_i, $i = 0, 1, 2, \ldots, k$ denote the success probabilities of the placebo, the lowest dose, the second lowest dose, ..., and the highest dose respectively. Suppose a dose i is considered effective if $p_i > p_0 + \delta$, $i = 1, \ldots, k$, where δ is a pre-specified non-negative quantity that reflects practical significance. Then, the null hypotheses are:

$$H_{0i} : p_i \leq p_0 + \delta, \quad i = 1, \ldots, k \tag{12.7}$$

12.3.1   Predetermined Step-Down Method

The partitioning principle partitions the entire parameter space into disjoint null hypotheses, hence testing each at level α without multiplicity adjustment controls the familywise error rate (FWER) strongly (the probability of at least one wrong rejection).

Suppose our expectation is that the sample will show increasing efficacy with increasing dose. Then a set of partitioning hypotheses could be

$$H_{0k}^* : p_k \leq p_0 + \delta$$
$$H_{0(k-1)}^* : p_{k-1} \leq p_0 + \delta < p_k$$
$$\vdots$$
$$H_{0i}^* : p_i \leq p_0 + \delta < p_j \quad \text{for all } j, \ i < j \leq k \tag{12.8}$$
$$\vdots$$
$$H_{01}^* : p_1 \leq p_0 + \delta < p_j \quad \text{for all } j, \ 1 < j \leq k$$

In words, the null hypotheses are:

$$H_{0k}^* : \text{Dose } k \text{ is ineffective}$$
$$H_{0(k-1)}^* : \text{Dose } k \text{ is effective but dose } k - 1 \text{ is ineffective}$$
$$\vdots$$
$$H_{0i}^* : \text{Doses } i + 1, \ldots, k \text{ are effective but dose } i \text{ is ineffective}$$
$$\vdots$$
$$H_{01}^* : \text{Doses } 2, \ldots, k \text{ are effective but dose } 1 \text{ is ineffective.}$$

The partitioned parameter space is plotted in Figure 12.2 (left) for $k = 2$. We can see that if H_{0k}^* fails to be rejected, then none of the doses can be inferred to be effective, regardless of the results from testing the remaining hypotheses. Similarly, if H_{0i}^* fails to be rejected, then dose 1 to dose $i - 1$ cannot be inferred to

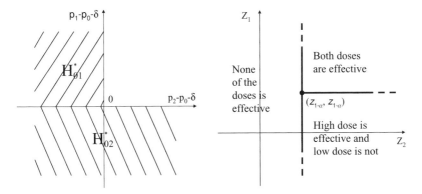

Figure 12.2. The partitioned parameter space (left) and inferences (right) of a pre-determined step-down procedure for comparing two doses with a placebo.

be effective. Therefore, by this formulation of null hypotheses, we can test those null hypotheses in a step-down fashion with H_{0k}^* tested first, then $H_{0(k-1)}^*$, and so on. We stop the procedure once a null hypothesis fails to be rejected. If H_{0k}^* fails to be rejected, then the remaining null hypotheses are not tested, and none of the doses can be inferred to be effective. For any integer $i \geq 1$, if H_{0j}^*, $j = i, \ldots, k$, are all rejected, then the logical inference is doses $i, \ldots, k$ are all efficacious. The dose levels inferred to be efficacious are naturally contiguous. By testing the dose levels expected to show more efficacy in the sample first, the method also takes advantage of the expected response shape, if it turns out to be true.

In practice, the null hypotheses typically tested (in Hsu and Berger (1999) for example)

$$H_{0k} : p_k \leq p_0 + \delta$$
$$H_{0(k-1)} : p_{k-1} \leq p_0 + \delta$$
$$\vdots$$
$$H_{0i} : p_i \leq p_0 + \delta \qquad\qquad (12.9)$$
$$\vdots$$
$$H_{01} : p_1 \leq p_0 + \delta$$

Since each H_{0i}^* implies H_{0i}, a level-α test for H_{0i} is automatically a level-α test for H_{0i}^*. Therefore, any family of level-α tests for Eq. (12.9) controls the FWER of Eq. (12.8) strongly. Thus, one can apply the large sample test/exact test for Eq.(12.4) to each of H_{0i}, $i = k, \ldots, 1$. Let z_{1-a} denote the $100(1 - a)\%$ percentage of the standard normal distribution. The right plot in Figure 12.2 shows the inferences of a predetermined step-down procedure for comparing two doses with a placebo.

Inference resulting from the predetermined step-down method is valid (in terms of FWER) without any prior assumption on the shape of the response curve. That is, it does not require a predetermined ordering of p_i. If, however, the expected response curve turns out be be not true, and the dose levels giving the higher sample responses are not the ones tested early in the steps, the predetermined stepwise method has weak power. When the shape of the sample response curve can not be reasonably anticipated, the sample-determined step-down method can be used.

12.3.2   Sample-Determined Step-Down Method

Consider the set of partitioning hypotheses:

$$H_{0I}^* : \text{Doses } i \ (i \in I) \text{ are not effective but doses } j \ (j \notin I) \text{ are effective}$$
(12.10)

for all $I \subseteq \{1, \ldots, k\}$. The partitioned parameter space for $k = 2$ is illustrated in the left plot of Figure 12.3. Similarly, a level-α test for H_{0I}, Doses i ($i \in I$) are not effective, is a level-α test for H_{0I}^*. As there are 2^k potential null hypotheses, applying a multiple comparison method to each of the H_{0I} would be computationally inefficient especially when k is large. Sample-determined step-down procedure is a computational shortcut to partition testing, reducing the number of tests to be performed to at most k. Specifically, if dose i_0 appears to be most significantly better than placebo among the doses whose indices are in the set I and the rejection of H_{0I} guarantees the rejection of all null hypotheses $H_{0I'}$, $i_0 \in I' \subset I$, then a shortcut can be taken by skipping testing $H_{0I'}$.

The idea of the sample-determined step-down procedure is to decide first whether there is sufficient evidence to infer that the dose that appears to be most significantly better than the control is indeed efficacious while guarding against the possibility that all k doses are actually worse than the control. If the answer is "yes", then at the next step one decides if the next dose that is most significantly better than the control is indeed efficacious while guarding against the possibility that all the remaining $k - 1$ doses are actually worse than the control, and so on (Naik, 1975; Marcus, et al., 1976; Stefansson, et al., 1988). A method of this form is called a step-down test because it steps down from the most statistically significant to the least statistically significant.

Let M_i, $i = 1, \ldots, k$, denote the test statistics for each treatment-control comparison. For large sample tests $M_i = Z_i$ (defined in Eq.(12.5) with subscript 1 replaced by i), and $M_i = X_i$ for Fisher's small sample tests. Let $[1], [2], \ldots, [k]$ denote the random indices such that $M_{[1]}, M_{[2]}, \ldots, M_{[k]}$ are the 'p-ordered' statistics of M_i, meaning that when applying a test to each of H_{0i}, $i = 1, \ldots, k$, $M_{[1]}$ is the M_i with the largest p-value, $M_{[2]}$ is the M_i with the second largest p-value, and so on. For large sample tests and Fisher's small sample tests with equal sample sizes for dose groups, the 'p-ordered' statistics are the usual order statistics of M_i, and

$$M_{[1]} \leq M_{[2]} \leq \ldots \leq M_{[k]}$$
(12.11)

For Fisher's small sample test with unequal sample sizes, the test statistics X_i follow different hypergeometric distributions. Therefore, the 'p-ordered' statistics are in general different from the usual order statistics and Eq.(12.11) does not hold.

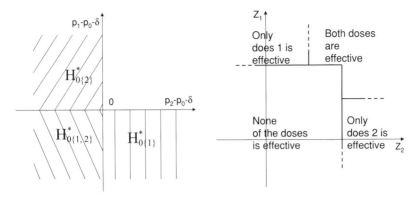

Figure 12.3. The partitioned parameter space (left) and inferences (right) of a sample-determined step-down procedure for comparing two doses with a placebo.

For instance, X_i could be large because of large n_i and/or large p_i, and $M_{[k]}$ may not be the largest X_i.

Let m_I, $I \subseteq \{1, \ldots, k\}$, denote suitable critical values for use in the procedure given below. The sample-determined step-down method proceeds as follows.

Step 1

Is $M_{[k]} > m_{\{[1],\ldots,[k]\}}$?
Yes, infer $p_{[k]} > p_0 + \delta$ and go to step 2;
No, stop.

Step 2

Is $M_{[k-1]} > m_{\{[1],\ldots,[k-1]\}}$?
Yes, infer $p_{[k-1]} > p_0 + \delta$ and go to step 3;
No, stop.

Step 3

Is $M_{[k-2]} > m_{\{[1],\ldots,[k-2]\}}$?
Yes, infer $p_{[k-2]} > p_0 + \delta$ and go to step 4;
No, stop.

$\vdots$

Step k

Is $M_{[1]} > m_{\{[1]\}}$?
Yes, infer $p_{[i]} > p_0 + \delta$ for $i \leq k$ and stop;
No, stop.

The right plot in Figure 12.3 shows the inferences of a sample-determined step-down procedure for comparing two doses with a placebo.

One should be aware that such shortcut may not be valid under some conditions. Hsu (1996) provides an example (pp. 136–137) of an erroneous shortcutting computer implementation of such a statistical method, demonstrating with data explicitly why shortcuts cannot be taken. The key condition needed to effect a shortcut is roughly that the rejection of a more restrictive hypothesis implies the rejection of certain less restrictive null hypotheses. Thus, if one starts by testing more restrictive null hypotheses and then skips the testing of less restrictive hypotheses as such implications allow, then the resulting shortcut version of a closed/partition test is a step-down test. One condition that guarantees that a step-down method strongly controls the familywise error rate is the subset pivotality condition given on page 42 of Westfall and Young (1993). Alternativly, we give a precise set of sufficient conditions for such shortcutting to be valid as follows.

S1: Tests for all hypotheses are based on statistics M_i, $i = 1, \ldots, k$, whose values do not vary with H_{0I};

S2: The level-α test for H_{0I} is to reject H_{0I} if the test statistic with the smallest p-value among M_i, $i \in I$, is more extreme than a suitable critical value;

S3: Critical value for H_{0I} is no smaller than that for $H_{0I'}$ if $I' \subset I$.

One should verify that either conditions S1–S3 are satisfied, or subset pivotality is satisfied, before implementing a stepdown test, for otherwise the stepdown test may not control the familywise error rate strongly.

There are several multiple comparison methods for binary outcomes (Piegorsch 1991). We can apply different comparison methods in the step-down procedure.

12.3.2.1 Sample-Determined Step-Down Procedure Using a Method for Comparisons With a Control

It is ideal to apply a method for multiple comparisons with a control, like Dunnett's method, to each H_{0I} (Stefansson, et al., 1988; Chapter 3 of Hsu, 1996). Dunnett's method is for situations where a common unknown variance for all groups is assumed. In the case of binary outcomes, the variances are related to the means and cannot be assumed to be equal. Therefore, Dunnett's method is not directly applicable. In the following, we develop a procedure for multiple comparisons with a control for binary response variable.

Let us first consider large sample tests. Let d_k be the first step critical value such that

$$\Pr(W_i \leq d_k, \ i = 1, \ldots, k) \tag{12.12}$$

is approximately $1 - \alpha$ for large sample sizes, where

$$W_i = \frac{\hat{p}_i - \hat{p}_0 - (p_i - p_0)}{\sqrt{\hat{p}_i(1 - \hat{p}_i)/n_i + \hat{p}_0(1 - \hat{p}_0)/n_0}} \tag{12.13}$$

Define the vectors $P = (p_0, \ldots, p_k)'$ and $\hat{P} = (\hat{p}_0, \ldots, \hat{p}_k)'$, where $\hat{p}_i = x_i/n_i$ as before. By the multivariate central limit theorem, $\hat{P}$ is asymptotically normally distributed with mean P and a diagonal variance covariance matrix $\Sigma = \{\sigma_{ii} = p_i(1 - p_i)/n_i\}$. After transforming, standardizing and replacing p_i with their consistent estimators $\hat{p}_i$, we have a vector of W_i being asymptotic multivariate normal with zero means, unit variances, and covariances

$$\frac{\hat{p}_0(1 - \hat{p}_0)/n_0}{\sqrt{\hat{p}_i(1 - \hat{p}_i)/n_i + \hat{p}_0(1 - \hat{p}_0)/n_0}\sqrt{\hat{p}_j(1 - \hat{p}_j)/n_j + \hat{p}_0(1 - \hat{p}_0)/n_0}}, \quad i \neq j$$

(12.14)

Denote the cumulative distribution function (cdf) of this k-dimensional multivariate normal distribution as F, then Eq. (12.12) is just $F(d_k, d_k, \ldots, d_k)$. Therefore, critical value d_k, for which the probability of Eq. (12.12) is approximately equal to the desired confidence level $1 - \alpha$, can be determined using a computer program for multivariate normal distribution such that $F(d_k, d_k, \ldots, d_k) = 1 - \alpha$. More simply, the critical value in step 1, $m_{\{[1],\ldots,[k]\}}$, is d_k, the $(1-\alpha)$ quantile of $W_{[k]}$, where $W_{[1]} \leq W_{[2]} \leq \ldots \leq W_{[k]}$. Similarly, the critical value in step 2, $m_{\{[1],\ldots,[k-1]\}} = d_{k-1}$, the $(1-\alpha)$ quantile of $W_{[k-1]}$, such that $F_{k-1}(d_{k-1}, \ldots, d_{k-1}) = 1 - \alpha$, where F_{k-1} is the $(k-1)$-dimensional $c.d.f.$ for the same multivariate normal density without elements corresponding to $W_{[k]}$. The critical value in step 3, $m_{\{[1],\ldots,[k-2]\}}$, is d_{k-2}, which is the $(1-\alpha)$ quantile of $W_{[k-2]}$, and so on. Since $W_{[1]} \leq W_{[2]} \leq \ldots \leq W_{[k]}$ and d_i is the $1 - \alpha$ quantiles of $W_{[i]}, i = 1, \ldots, k$, we have $d_1 \leq d_2 \leq \ldots \leq d_k$.

For the small-sample exact test, the joint probability of X_i, $i \in I$, $I \subseteq \{1, \ldots, k\}$, given the total number of successes from all groups in I plus the placebo group, denoted as x_{I_0} where $I_0 = I \cup \{0\}$, is a (non-central) multivariate hypergeometric distribution:

$$\Pr(X_i = x_i, \ i \in I | n_0, n_i, x_{I_0}) \propto \binom{n_0}{x_0} \prod_{i \in I} \binom{n_i}{x_i} \psi_i^{x_i}$$

where $\psi_i = \frac{p_i}{1 - p_i} / \frac{p_0}{1 - p_0}$. Therefore, the small-sample test procedure involves a multivariate hypergeometric distribution. For instance, assume equal sample sizes for the dose groups: $n_1 = n_2 = \ldots = n_k$, and let $\psi = (\psi_1, \ldots, \psi_k)'$. The null hypotheses in Eq. (12.9) are equivalent to $\psi \leq \mathbf{1}$, that is, $\psi_i \leq 1$ for all i, and $\Pr_{\psi \leq 1}(X_i \geq m, \ i = 1, \ldots, k)$ is increasing in ψ. Hence, the critical value of Fisher's small sample test in step 1 is $m_{\{1,\ldots,k\}} = d'$ where d' is the smallest integer such that $\Pr_{\psi=1}(X_i \geq d', \ i = 1, \ldots, k | n_0, n_i, x_{I_0}) \leq \alpha$. In general, the critical values m_I are the smallest integers such that $\Pr_{\psi=1}(X_i \geq m_I, \ i \in I | n_0, n_i, x_{I_0}) \leq \alpha$. Routines for calculating the probabilities of multivariate hypergeometric distributions are not available in major statistical packages. For small sample sizes, it is more convenient to use a step-down procedure based on the Bonferroni method.

12.3.2.2   Sample-Determined Step-Down Method Using Bonferroni Method—Holm's Step-Down Procedure

Holm's (1979) step-down method uses the Bonferroni method to test each H_{0I}. For a large sample test, Bonferroni method is used to guarantee that Eq. (12.12) is at least $1 - \alpha$. The critical value for step 1 is $z_{1-\alpha/k}$, the critical value for step 2 is $m_{\{[1],...,[k-1]\}} = z_{1-\alpha/(k-1)}$, and so on. That is, the critical value for step i is $z_{1-\alpha/(k-i+1)}$. For a small-sample exact test, the critical value for step i, $m_{\{[1],...,[k-i+1]\}}$, is the smallest integer d'' such that $\Pr(Y \geq d'') \leq \alpha/(k-i+1)$, where Y follows a hypergeometric distribution $H(n_0, n_{[k-i+1]}, x_{[k-i+1]} + x_0)$, where $n_{[k-i+1]}$ and $x_{[k-i+1]}$ are the sample size and the number of observed successes in the dose group corresponding to $X_{[k-i+1]}$, the $(k - i + 1)th$ largest p-ordered test statistic. Note that the critical values of Bonferroni method are conservative compared to those of the method for comparisons with a control.

Since $m_J < m_{\{1,...,k\}}$ for $J \subset \{1, \ldots, k\}$ in the step-down testing and $m_{\{1,...,k\}}$ is the critical value for non-stepwise tests, given the same data set and error rate, this sample-determined step-down procedure with a multiple comparison method applied to the partitioned hypotheses will infer the same or more doses to be efficacious compared to a non-stepwise procedure with the same multiple comparison method.

12.3.3   Hochberg's Step-up Procedure

This is also a sample-determined stepwise procedure, similar to that in Section 12.3.2. While Holm's step-down testing is a shortcut version of the partition testing based on Bonferroni methods, Huang and Hsu (2005) show that Hochberg's step-up testing is also a special case, or shortcut version, of a partition testing based on Simes' test. Although more powerful than Bonferroni method/Holm's procedure, Simes' test/Hochberg's procedure control the Type I error rate/familywise error rate at α only when the test statistics are independent (Simes, 1986). Sarkar (1998) proves that Simes' test controls the probability of a Type I error at or below α when the test statistics have joint null distributions with multivariate totally positive of order two (MTP$_2$, implying that the test statistics are positively dependent) with common marginals. Conservativeness of Simes' test for some other positively dependent multivariate distributions is proved or supported by simulation results and anti-conservativeness of Simes's test for negatively associated test statistics is observed (Sarkar and Chang, 1997, Sarkar, 1998).

Since the correlations of the large sample test statistics as in Eq. (12.14) are positive, it is reasonable to use Hochberg's step-up procedure. Here, we show that the correlation matrix of the test statistics has 1-factor structure (Hsu, 1996) and is MTP$_2$. By definition, a correlation matrix of the distribution has 1-factor structure if and only if the correlation matrix can be written in the form of $\lambda\lambda' + \Omega$, where Ω is a diagonal matrix and λ is a column vector. In our case,

$$\lambda_i = \sqrt{\frac{\hat{p}_0(1 - \hat{p}_0)}{n_0}} \Bigg/ \left(\frac{\hat{p}_0(1 - \hat{p}_0)}{n_0} + \frac{\hat{p}_i(1 - \hat{p}_i)}{n_i}\right), \quad i = 1, \ldots, k \qquad (12.15)$$

and Ω has elements $1 - \lambda_i^2$. By theorem A.5.1 of Srivastava (2002), the inverse of the correlation matrix is

$$\Omega^{-1} - \Omega^{-1}\lambda(1 + \lambda'\Omega^{-1}\lambda)^{-1}\lambda'\Omega^{-1},$$

which has all off diagonal elements non-positive. Then, asymptomatically, the test statistics have MTP$_2$, by Fact 1.3. of Karlin and Rinott (1980). This justifies the use of Hochberg's procedure.

The idea of a step-up multiple comparison method is to decide, at step 1, whether there is sufficient evidence to infer that the dose that appears to be least significantly better than the control is indeed better. If the answer is "yes," then we infer all the doses to be better than the placebo and stop. If the answer is "no," then at step 2, one uses a larger critical value to decide whether the dose that appears to be the next least significantly better than the placebo is indeed better, and so on. The critical values for large sample testing, $z_{1-\alpha}$, are the $1 - \alpha$ quantiles of a standard normal distribution. Define the critical values for a small sample test, $d^*_{1-\alpha}$, as the smallest integer such that $\Pr(Y \geq d^*_{1-\alpha}) \leq \alpha$, where Y follows hypergeometric distribution H($n_0, n_{[i]}, x_{[i]} + x_0$), where $n_{[i]}$, $x_{[i]}$ are the sample size and the number of observed successes in the dose group corresponding to the test statistic in each step. The Hochberg's (1988) step-up method proceeds as follows, with $M_{[i]}$ being the p-ordered' statistics.

Step 1
Is $M_{[1]} > z_{1-\alpha}$ or $d^*_{1-\alpha}$?
Yes, infer $p_{[i]} > p_0 + \delta$ for $i = 1, ..., k$ and stop;
No, go to step 2.

Step 2
Is $M_{[2]} > z_{1-\alpha/2}$ or $d^*_{1-\alpha/2}$?
Yes, infer $p_{[i]} > p_0 + \delta$ for $i = 2, ..., k$ and stop;
No, go to step 3.

⋮

Step k
Is $M_{[k]} > z_{1-\alpha/k}$ or $d^*_{1-\alpha/k}$?
Yes, infer $p_{[k]} > p_0 + \delta$ and stop;
No, stop.

12.4   An Example Using Partitioning Based Stepwise Methods

A dose–response trial study with four active doses of an experimental compound versus a placebo was reported by Stewart and Ruberg (2000). The experiment was planned to study the effectiveness of the drug of different doses in preventing nausea and vomiting for patients undergoing surgery. The response variable was "complete response", that is, no emetic episodes over a 24-hour observation period. The data are as follows.

Dose	Placebo	12.5 mg	25 mg	50 mg	100 mg
Number of responders	102	123	111	119	121
N	208	206	203	205	208
% responders	49%	60%	55%	58%	58%

The sample sizes are large enough for the asymptotic normality assumption of the large sample test. The large sample test statistics for dose groups 12.5, 25, 50, and 100 mg versus the placebo are 2.19, 1.15, 1.84 and 1.88 mg respectively. Let the familywise error rate be controlled strongly at $\alpha = 0.05$.

Let us first use the predetermined step-down method to test from high dose to low dose. For large sample tests, the critical value for large sample test for each step is $z_{0.95} = 1.64$. Hence, the predetermined step-down method infers the 100 and 50 mg doses to be efficacious. For small sample exact tests, the procedure leads to the same conclusion.

For the sample-determined step-down procedure using the method for comparisons with a control, the critical values for large sample tests can be calculated using the R package *mvtnorm*, which calculates the probability for a multivariate normal distribution with any specified mean vector and variance-covariance matrix. The R package *mvtnorm* is described in Hothorn, et al. (2001), which is available at http://cran.r-mirror.de/doc/Rnews/Rnews 2001- 2.pdf. The ProbMC function in SAS can also be used since the correlation matrix here has 1-factor structure.

The syntax of the ProbMC function in SAS is

```
probmc(distribution, q, prob, df, nparms<, parameters>)
```

In our case distribution = "dunnett1," which refers to the one-sided Dunnett; the quantile, q, is what we want to compute and is not specified; prob is the cumulative probability, which is 1-alpha; the degrees of freedom, df, is missing here, which is interpreted as an infinite value. In step 1, using $\boldsymbol{\lambda} = (\lambda_1, \lambda_2, \lambda_3, \lambda_4)'$ for the parameters of the ProbMC function,

```
data binary_Dunnett;
    array drug{5}$;
    array count{5};
    array mu{5};
    array temp{5};
    array lambda{4};
    array q{2};

    /* input the table */
    do i = 1 to 5;
        input drug{i} count{i} mu{i};
    end;
```

```
    /* input alpha */
input alpha;
    /* compute the lambdas    */
do i = 1 to 5;
    temp {i} = (mu{i}/count{i})*(1-mu{i}/count{i})/count{i};
end;
do i = 1 to 4;
    lambda{i} = sqrt(temp {1}/(temp{i+1} + temp{1}));
end;

    /* run the one-sided Dunnett's test */
q{1} = probmc("dunnett1",.,1-alpha,.,4, of lambda1-lambda4);
put q{1} e18.13;
datalines;
P 208 102
A 206 123
B 203 111
C 205 119
D 208 121
0.05
;
```

This gives us the critical value of 2.16, which is smaller than the largest test statistic. Thus, dose 12.5 mg is declared efficacious. In step 2, we delete λ_1 which corresponds to the largest test statistic and use $\boldsymbol{\lambda} = (\lambda_2, \lambda_3, \lambda_4)'$:

```
q{2} = probmc("dunnett1", ., 1-alpha, ., 3, of lambda2-lambda4);
```

The resulting critical value for step 2 is 2.06, larger than the second largest test statistic, hence dose 100 mg is declared not efficacious. Therefore, only dose 12.5 mg, which has the largest response rate, is inferred to be efficacious.

For Holm's step-down procedure with large sample tests, the critical value for step 1 is $z_{1-0.05/4} = 2.24$, which is bigger than the largest test statistic. Therefore, none of the doses is inferred to be efficacious, which shows the conservativeness of Bonferroni method compared with the method for comparisons with a control. For Hochberg's step-up method with large sample tests, the critical values from Step 1 to 4 are is 1.64, 1.96, 2.13 and 2.24, which are bigger than the corresponding ordered test statistics. Hence, none of the doses is inferred to be efficacious. However, both Holm's and Hochberg's stepwise procedures with small sample tests infer dose 12.5 mg is effective.

12.5   Conclusion and Discussion

In dose–response studies, when the purpose is to test for one or a few doses that are more efficacious than placebo, the principle of partitioning provides a powerful testing procedure for constructing multiple tests which control the FWER strongly.

In this chapter, two partitioning test procedures for binary responses are introduced. One is a predetermined step-down method and the other is a sample determined step-down method. Choice of the appropriate procedure depends on the anticipated dose response relationship. If it is anticipated that the relationship is monotonic, then the pre-determined step-down method is recommended because it is more powerful.

The general use of multiple comparison adjustment in dose response studies is introduced in Chapter 11. In that chapter, additional statistical concerns and methods are discussed in further detail. Binary data is a type of categorical data. Chapter 13 has more discussion about handling categorical data in dose response studies.

References

Chuang-Stein, C., Tong, D.M. 1995. Multiple comparison procedures for comparing several treatments with a control based on binary data. *Statistics in Medicine* 14:2509–2522.

Finner, H., and Strassburger, K. (2002) The partitioning principle: A powerful tool in multiple decision theory. *The Annals of Statistics* 30:1194–1213.

Fisher, R.A. 1934. *Statistical Methods for Research Workers*, 5th ed. Edinburgh: Oliver & Boyd.

Hochberg, Y. 1988. A sharper Bonferroni procedure for multiple tests of significance. *Biometrika* 75:800–802.

Holm, S. 1979. A simple sequentially rejective multiple test procedure. *Scandanavian Journal of Statistics* 6:65–70.

Hothorn, T., Bretz, F., and Genz, A. 2001. On multivariate t and Gauss probabilities in R. *R News* 1:27–28.

Hsu, J.C. 1996. *Multiple Comparisons: Theory and Methods*. London: Chapman & Hall.

Hsu, J.C., and Berger, R.L. 1999. Stepwise confidence intervals without multiplicity adjustment for dose response and toxicity studies. *Journal of the American Statistical Association* 94:468–482.

Huang, Y., and Hsu J.C. 2005. Hochberg's step-up testing: A special case of Partition testing. *Technical Report 756*, The Ohio State University.

Karlin, S., and Rinott, Y. 1981. Total positivity properties of absolute value multinormal variables with applications to confidence interval estimates and related probabilistic inequalities. *The Annals of Statistics* 9:1035–1049.

Marcus, R., Perits, E., and Gabriel, K.R. 1976. On closed testing procedures with special reference to ordered analysis of variance. *Biometrika* 63:655–660.

Naik, U. D. 1975. Some selection rules for comparing p processes with a standard. Communication in Statistics 4:519–535.

Piegorsch, W. W. 1991. Multiple comparisons for analyzing dichotomous response. *Biometrics* 47:45–52.

Sarkar, S. 1998. Probability inequalities for ordered MTP$_2$ random variables: A proof of the Simes conjecture. *The annals of Statistics* 26:494–504.

Sarkar, S., and Chang, C.K. 1997. Simes' method for multiple hypothesis testing with positively dependent test statistics. *Journal of the American Statistical Association* 92:1601–1608.

Simes R. J. 1986. An improved Bonferroni procedure for multiple tests of significance *Biometrika* 73:751–754.

Srivastava M. S. 2002. Methods of multivariate statistics. New York: Wiley

Stefansson, G., Kim, W., and Hsu, J.C. 1988. "On confidence sets in multiple comparisons," in *Statistical Decision Theory and Related Topics IV* (Gupta, S. S. and Berger, J. O., editors) vol. 2, pp. 89–104. New York: Springer-Verlag.

Stewart, W., and Ruberg S. (2000) Detecting dose response with contrasts. *Statistics in Medicine* 19:913–921.

Westfall P.H., Young S.S. (1993) *Resampling-based Multiple Testing*. New York: Wiley.

13
Analysis of Dose–Response Relationship Based on Categorical Outcomes

CHRISTY CHUANG-STEIN and ZHENGQING LI

13.1 Introduction

In an eloquent article prepared in defense of the dichotomy, Lewis (2004) wrote that one of the most important ways in which we learned to understand the world was to describe complicated phenomena using simple categories. Thus, it is hardly surprising that medical researchers often seek to categorize data in their attempt to make sense of unfamiliar measurement scales and treatment effects of uncertain implication. For this reason, threshold values based on continuous measurements are frequently used to help guide the decision to initiate medical interventions. Examples include a diastolic blood pressure greater than 90, a fasting cholesterol level higher than 200, and a CD4 count lower than 200. Normal ranges were constructed to screen subjects for possible lab abnormalities. Even though this black-and-white dichotomy appears to be crude in many situations, its simplicity helps human minds make decisions, decisions that are often binary in nature.

As we became more sophisticated in our views of the world, so did our descriptions of the surroundings. Being normal or abnormal alone is no longer enough. We want to know the extent of abnormality to decide if immediate actions are necessary. Experiencing pain alone is not enough to decide if pain relief medications are necessary. Similarly, recovery from a major trauma can mean recovery with major disability, with minor disability, or essentially with no noticeable disability. The human minds realized that creating a finer grid between the two extremes of black and white could help us make better decisions on many occasions.

Over the past 30 years, researchers have been busy developing scales to subdivide the space between the black and white extremes. The proliferation of scales is most prevalent in the area of outcome research where scales are used to record a patient's and the treating physician's global assessments of the clinical symptoms associated with the underlying disorders. Scales are also used to record the extent of relief patients receive from the medications. These activities have led to the collection of categorical data in many clinical trials.

In this chapter, we will focus on analyzing dose–response relationship when the primary endpoint is either ordinal or binary. We will treat the ordinal case first in Section 13.2 and regard the binary case as a special case of the former. The binary case will be covered in Section 13.3. In Section 13.4, we will discuss multiple comparisons procedures that are applicable to categorical data when multiplicity adjustment is considered necessary because of the confirmatory nature of the trial. Readers are referred to Chapter 12 for a more general discussion on multiple comparisons. We will comment briefly in Section 13.5 the use of a titration design to explore the dose–response relationship with a binary outcome. In addition, we will discuss in that section issues related to sample size. Finally, we encourage our readers to use simulations to help evaluate the planned study at the design stage.

In this chapter, we provide numerical examples along with methodology. This is a deliberate effort to emphasize the applied nature of this chapter. To help implement the methodology, we include in the Appendix simple SAS codes that could be used to produce most of the results in Sections 13.2 and 13.3.

This chapter draws heavily from a review article by Chuang-Stein and Agresti (1997) on testing a monotone dose–response relationship with ordinal response data. Readers who wish to learn more about the technical details of the methodologies are encouraged to read the original publication.

13.2   When the Response is Ordinal

Consider the data in Table 13.1 where five ordered categories ranging from "death" to "good recovery" were used to describe the clinical outcome of patients who suffered from subarachnoid hemorrhage. The five outcome categories make up the Glasgow Outcome Scale (GOS). Three doses of an investigational drug (low, medium, and high) and a vehicle infusion (placebo) were included in the trial. For this type of data, one can either model the probability of an ordinal response as a function of the dose or conduct hypothesis testing to test for a dose–response relationship. In this section, we will briefly describe the modeling approach first followed by procedures that focus on hypothesis testing.

13.2.1   Modeling Dose–Response

Let p_{ij} be the probability that a subject in the ith dose group ($i = 1, 2, 3, 4$) will have a response in the jth ($j = 1, 2, \ldots, 5$) category. For each dose group, p_{ij}'s

Table 13.1. Responses measured on the Glasgow Outcome Scale from a trial comparing three doses of a new investigational treatment with a control (Chuang-Stein and Agresti, 1997)

Treatment group		Glasgow Outcome Scale				
	Death	Vegetative state	Major disability	Minor disability	Good recovery	Total
Placebo	59	25	46	48	32	210
Low dose	48	21	44	47	30	190
Medium dose	44	14	54	64	31	207
High dose	43	4	49	58	41	195

satisfy $\Sigma_j p_{ij} = 1$. We will use Y_{ij} to denote the number of subjects in the ith dose group whose responses are in the jth category. We assume that within each dose group $\{Y_{ij}, j = 1, \ldots, 5\}$ follows a multinomial distribution $(n_i; \{p_{ij}\})$ where $n_i = \Sigma_j Y_{ij}$. Here, we are treating $\{n_i\}$ as fixed constants since most trials have a target figure for $\{n_i\}$. Furthermore, we assume in this chapter that the response categories are arranged in such a way that higher response categories correspond to a more desirable outcome. The dose groups are arranged in an ascending order. If there is a placebo group, the placebo group will be the first dose group.

There are many ways to take advantage of the ordinal nature of the response when modeling the dose response relationship. The most popular one is probably the one using logits of the cumulative probabilities defined as (McCullagh, 1980)

$$\ln\left(\frac{\sum_{l=1}^{j} p_{il}}{\sum_{l=j+1}^{5} p_{il}}\right) = \alpha_j - \beta_i \qquad (13.1)$$

In Eq. (13.1), "ln" represents the natural logarithm and $i = 1,2,3,4$ and $j = 1,2,3,4$. In Eq. (13.1), the parameters $\{\alpha_j\}$ associated with the response categories do not depend on the dose group. As a result, if one looks at the ratio of the cumulative odds between two dose groups, the ratio is constant across response categories. For this reason, model (13.1) is called the proportional odds model. The appropriateness of the proportional odds assumption can be checked by the likelihood ratio statistic obtained by comparing the proportional odds model to the saturated model.

One can further simplify model (13.1) by fitting β_i as a function of the dose as in Eq. (13.2) or the dose on the logarithmic scale if there is reason to believe that the treatment effect is a monotone function of the dose.

$$\ln\left(\frac{\sum_{l=1}^{j} p_{il}}{\sum_{l=j+1}^{5} p_{il}}\right) = \alpha_j - \beta\, d_i \qquad (13.2)$$

Parameters in Eqs. (13.1) and (13.2) could be estimated by the maximum likelihood method. The procedure PROC LOGISTIC in SAS® can be employed to estimate the parameters. Testing the equality of the $\{\beta_i\}$ in Eq. (13.1) and $\beta = 0$ in Eq. (13.2) can be done using the likelihood ratio test. In either case, the likelihood ratio statistic has an asymptotic χ^2 distribution with degrees of freedom determined by the difference in the number of parameters included in the two models under comparison. For example, the likelihood ratio statistic for testing $\beta = 0$ in Eq. (13.2) has an asymptotic χ^2 distribution with 1 degree of freedom under the null hypothesis.

When employing model (13.2), one is typically interested in testing $\beta = 0$ against $\beta > 0$ so that rejecting $\beta = 0$ will infer that higher doses tend to produce more favorable response. Despite this, we will report two-sided p-values when testing the significance of the slope parameter to reflect the current regulatory requirement on reporting two-sided p-values even if the interest is clearly one-sided. Unless mentioned otherwise in this chapter, one-sided p-values can be obtained by halving the two-sided p-values.

By setting $\beta_1 = 0$ in model (13.1), we obtained the maximum likelihood estimates for β_2 to β_4 from PROC LOGISTIC as $\hat{\beta}_2 = 0.118$ (SE$=0.178$), $\hat{\beta}_3 = 0.317$ (SE $= 0.175$), and $\hat{\beta}_4 = 0.521$ (SE $= 0.178$). Since the β's estimates increase with the dose, model (13.1) suggests that the cumulative odds for the lower response categories are a decreasing function of the dose. The likelihood ratio test for the goodness-of-fit of model (13.2) relative to model (13.1), obtained as the difference of -2 log-likelihood values between the two models, results in a likelihood ratio statistic of 0.13 with 2 degrees of freedom. The low value of the likelihood ratio statistic (therefore a high p-value) strongly suggests that the simpler model in (13.2) is appropriate for the data when compared to the model in (13.1).

The maximum likelihood estimate for β in (13.2) is $\hat{\beta} = 0.175$ (SE $= 0.056$). For Table 13.1, this means that as we move from one dose to the next higher dose, the odds of obtaining a more desirable outcome against a less desirable one is increased by 19% ($e^{0.175} = 1.19$). The Wald test for $\beta = 0$ produces a χ^2 statistic of 9.709 with 1 degree of freedom. This statistic is highly significant ($p = 0.002$ for a two-sided test), suggesting a monotone dose–response relationship on the cumulative odds scale.

Other choices to take advantage of the ordered categories include the adjacent-categories logit model that looks at the odds of being in two adjacent categories, i.e., $\ln(p_{ij}/p_{i,j+1})$, and the continuation-ratio logit model. The latter looks at $\ln(p_{ij}/\sum_{l=j+1}^{5} p_{il})$, the logarithmic odds of being in one category versus the categories above. While these other logit models are all reasonable models for ordinal response, the cumulative odds logit model is a natural extension of the binary response case because the former becomes the regular logit model when one chooses to collapse the ordinal response categories into two categories.

All the logit models can be further extended to include stratifying factors. Assuming that there are S strata defined by patient's characteristics at baseline, a straightforward extension of model (13.1) is model (13.3) in which the terms β_h^S, $h = 1, \ldots, H$, represent the stratum effect and β_i^D represent the dose effect. There is no treatment by stratum interaction in model (13.3). Furthermore, the proportional odds assumption now applies not only to dose groups but also to subgroups defined by the strata as well as those jointly defined by the dose and the stratum. PROC LOGISTIC can be used to estimate the model parameters and to test various hypotheses concerning β_i^D

$$\ln\left(\frac{\sum_{l=1}^{j} p_{ihl}}{\sum_{l=j+1}^{5} p_{ihl}}\right) = \alpha_j - \beta_h^S - \beta_i^D \tag{13.3}$$

13.2.2   Testing for a Monotone Dose–Response Relationship

A frequently asked question in dose–response studies is whether a monotone relationship exists between dose and the response. Section 13.2.1 discussed how the question on monotonicity could be addressed under a modeling approach. Following the discussion in Section 13.2.1, monotonicity can be interpreted as a more favorable response with a higher dose. Since a more favorable outcome implies a smaller probability for the lower end of the response scale, the question on monotonicity can translate to a comparison on the cumulative probabilities. In other words, monotonicity can be evaluated by checking if $\sum_{l=1}^{j} p_{il}$ is a nonincreasing function of the dose $\{d_i, i = 1, 2, 3, 4\}$ for all $j = 1, \ldots, 4$. The latter implies testing a null hypothesis of equal distributions against a monotone stochastic ordering among the four dose groups as described below:

$$H_0: \ p_{1j} = p_{2j} = p_{3j} = p_{4j}, \quad j = 1, \ldots, 4$$

$$H_A: \ \sum_{l=1}^{j} p_{1l} \geq \sum_{l=1}^{j} p_{2l} \geq \sum_{l=1}^{j} p_{3l} \geq \sum_{l=1}^{j} p_{4l}, \quad j = 1, \ldots, 4$$

Strict inequality holds for at least one j for one of the three inequalities included in the alternative hypothesis above. The subscript j above goes from 1 to 4 since $\sum_{l=1}^{5} p_{il} = 1$ for all i.

It should be pointed out that testing H_0 versus H_A as formulated above forces one to make a choice between a flat dose–response and a monotone one. Even though monotone dose–response is very common, other types of dose–response relationships are also possible. If there are reasons to anticipate beforehand that the dose–response relationship is substantially different from monotone, testing H_0 versus H_A as shown above will not be appropriate.

13.2.2.1   Tests Based on Association Measures

Since the response categories are ordinal, one can treat the response scale as quantitative and assign scores to the categories. One can also assign numerical values to the dose groups. With the assigned scores, one can use correlation-type association measures to tease out the linear component of the dose–response relationship and construct a χ^2 statistic with 1 degree of freedom to test for the significance of the correlation.

The most commonly used scores for the response categories are the equally spaced ones. When the desirability of moving from one category to the next depends strongly on the categories involved, other scores might be more appropriate. For example, it might be more appropriate to assign scores $\{0, 1, 2, 4, 8\}$ than $\{1, 2, 3, 4, 5\}$ to the response categories in Table 13.1. From our experience, conclusions are generally robust to the scores assigned to the response categories unless the data are highly imbalanced with many more observations falling in some categories than others. Because of this potential issue, it is often prudent to check the robustness of the conclusion by using several sets of scores.

For the dose group, one can use equally spaced scores, the actual doses, or the logarithmic doses to represent the treatment groups. Since trials typically randomize patients to the treatment groups, treatment groups are represented either similarly or according to a prespecified ratio. As a result, the above three choices of the numerical scores for the dose groups usually lead to similar conclusions on the existence of a linear relationship between the dose and the response.

One approach that does not require assigning scores is to use ranks of the observations. All observations in the same response category will have the same rank r_j defined in Eq. (13.4). These ranks $\{r_j\}$ are called the midranks. Midranks are nothing but the averages of all ranks that would have been assigned to the observations in the same response category if we rank observations from the entire trial

$$r_j = y_{+1} + y_{+2} + \cdots + \frac{y_{+j}}{2} \tag{13.4}$$

In Eq. (13.4), $y_{+l} = \sum_{i=1}^{4} y_{il}$ is the total number of subjects with a response in the lth category.

The use of midranks seems appealing because one does not need to assign any scores. On the other hand, midranks cannot address the unequal spacing of the response categories from the clinical perspective. In addition, when one particular response category has very few observations, this response category will have a midrank similar to the preceding one. The latter might not be desirable if the two categories represent very different outcomes with drastically different medical implications.

Using PROC FREQ (CMH1 option) with scores $\{1, 2, 3, 4\}$ for the four dose groups and $\{1, 2, 3, 4, 5\}$ for the five response categories, we obtained a χ^2 test statistic of 9.61 with 1 degree of freedom. Under the null hypothesis of a zero correlation, this statistic produced a two-sided p-value of 0.002. Using $\{1, 2, 3, 4\}$ for doses and midranks for the response categories yielded a χ^2 statistic of 9.42 with a two-sided p-value of 0.002. Finally, using $\{1, 2, 3, 4\}$ for the dose groups and $\{0, 1, 2, 4, 8\}$ for the response categories produced a χ^2 statistic of 7.39 with a two-sided p-value of 0.007. In this case, the three sets of response scores produced similar results, all confirming a higher chance for a more favorable outcome with higher doses.

13.2.2.2   Tests Treating the Response as Continuous

Another application of assigning scores to the ordered categories is to treat the data as if they come from continuous distributions and apply standard normal theory methods to the data. The latter include approaches such as the analysis of variance and regression-type of analysis. There is evidence that treating ordinal data as continuous can provide a useful approximation as long as the number of categories is at least five (Heeren and D'Agostino, 1987). Under this approach, all methods developed for continuous data can be applied here. Interested readers are referred to other chapters in this book for a detailed account of the methods for continuous data.

One can, however, take into account the nonconstant response variance by explicitly incorporating the multinomial distribution structure when estimating the mean response for each dose group. Assuming that scores $\{s_j\}$ are assigned to the five response categories, the mean response score for the ith dose group, denoted by m_i, is defined by

$$m_i = \frac{\sum_{j=1}^{5} s_j \times p_{ij}}{\sum_{j=1}^{5} s_j}$$

Under the above definition, m_i can be thought of as a weighted average of $\{p_{ij}\}$ within each dose.

Grizzle et al. (1969) proposed to model $\{m_i\}$ as a function of the dose as in Eq. (13.5). The $\{m_i\}$ can be estimated by replacing p_{ij} with the observed proportions. Using multinomial distributions, one can calculate the variance of the estimated mean response for each group. The inverse of the variances can then be used as the weights when estimating the regression coefficients in Eq. (13.5) using the least-squares methods,

$$m_i = a + b \times (\text{dose}_i) \tag{13.5}$$

SAS® procedure PROC CATMOD with weight option can be used to estimate the parameters a and b in Eq. (13.5). Testing a monotone dose–response relationship (i.e., $b = 0$) can be accomplished using a χ^2 test statistic. Using $\{1, 2, 3, 4\}$ for the dose groups and $\{1, 2, 3, 4, 5\}$ for the response categories, PROC CATMOD produced a χ^2 statistic of 9.58 with a two-sided p-value of 0.002. Using the same dose scores but $\{0, 1, 2, 4, 8\}$ as the scores for the response categories produced a χ^2 statistic of 7.08. The latter has a two-sided p-value of 0.008.

Applying weighted least squares method to the mean response model in Eq. (13.5), we conclude that there is a monotone relationship between the mean response and the dose. As the dose increases, the mean response increases accordingly.

13.2.2.3   Jonckheere–Terpstra Test

Assume d_i and $d_{i'}$ are two doses such that $d_{i'} > d_i$. Consider the Wilcoxon-Mann-Whitney (WMW) statistic for testing equal distributions in response to these two doses against a stochastic ordering with response to dose $d_{i'}$ being stochastically greater than that to dose d_i. Let $\{r_{(i,i')j}\}$ represent the midranks constructed from dose groups d_i and $d_{i'}$ only, i.e.,

$$r_{(i,i')j} = (y_{i1} + y_{i'1}) + (y_{i2} + y_{i'2}) + \cdots + \frac{(y_{ij} + y_{i'j})}{2}$$

The WMW statistic for comparing groups i and i' can be constructed as

$$WMW_{i,i'} = \sum_{j=1}^{5} r_{(i, \, i')j} y_{i'j} - \frac{n_{i'}(n_{i'} + 1)}{2}$$

If there is a stochastic ordering between the response distributions to doses d_i and $d_{i'}$, we would expect the observed rank sum for dose $d_{i'}$ to be greater than the rank sum expected for that group if there is no difference between the two groups. In other words, we would expect $WMW_{i,i'}$ to be generally positive under the alternative hypothesis of a stochastic ordering between d_i and $d_{i'}$.

For four dose groups, there are six pairs of dose groups and six WMW statistics to compare the response distributions within each pair. Constructing WMW in such a way that the WMW statistic always looks at the difference between the expected and observed rank sums of the higher dose groups, we can express the

Jonckheere–Terpstra (Jonckheere, 1954; Terpstra, 1952) statistic (*JT*-statistic for short) as below

$$JT = \sum_{i'=2}^{4} \sum_{i=1}^{i'-1} WMW_{i,i'}$$

For large samples, the standardized value

$$z = \frac{JT - E(JT)}{\sqrt{var(JT)}}$$

provides a test statistic that has a standard normal distribution under the null hypothesis of equal response distributions across dose groups. Both SAS (PROC FREQ) and the StatXact (1995) software could conduct this test. For the data in Table 13.1, the standardized *JT*-statistic is 3.10, producing a two-sided *p*-value of 0.002. The conclusion from the *JT*-test is similar to that obtained from other approaches.

13.2.2.4   Summary

If the number of categories is at least five and the sample size is reasonable, the simplest approach is to treat the response as if it is continuous. This approach is particularly relevant if one intends to look at the change in the response at a follow-up visit from that at the baseline. In this case, change from baseline can be constructed using the scores assigned to the ordinal categories. This approach could be extended to include baseline covariates using an analysis of covariance model.

On the other hand, if there is much uncertainty in assigning scores to the categories or if the primary interest is in estimating the probability of a response in a particular category, modeling approach becomes a natural choice. Modeling approach is especially useful for dose-finding studies at the early stage of drug development when there is very little information on the dose response relationship. In this case, modeling allows us to borrow information from adjacent doses to study the effect of any particular dose.

13.3   When the Response is Binary

Binary endpoints are very popular in clinical trials. Frequently, "success" and "failure" are used to describe the outcome of a treatment. Even if the endpoint is continuous, there is an increasing tendency to define criteria and classify subjects as a "responder" or a "nonresponder". For example, patients in antidepressants trials are frequently referred to as a responder if they experience a 50% reduction in the HAM-D score from their baseline values. The American College of Rheumatology (ACR) proposed to use ACR20 as the basis to determine if the treatment is a success or not for an individual. ACR20 is defined as

- $\geq$ 20% improvement in tender joint count
- $\geq$ 20% improvement in swollen joint count
- $\geq$ 20% improvement in at least three of the following five assessment

- Patient pain assessment
- Patient global assessment
- Physician global assessment
- Patient self-assessed disability
- Acute phase reactant

The above definition combines multiple endpoints into a single dichotomous endpoint. By setting a criterion to classify treatment outcome, the medical community implicitly provides a target for treatment success. The popularity of responder analysis arises from the above desire even though dichotomization can lead to the loss of information (Senn, 2003).

There are situations when binary response makes sense. Examples include "alive" or "dead" for patients in salvage trials with end stage cancer. In anti-infective trials, it is natural to consider if an individual is cured of the underlying infection, both clinically and microbiologically. There are many situations where dichotomizing subject's response in a manner that makes clinical sense is not a trivial matter. This is especially so when the response is measured using an instrument. Does a 50% improvement in the HAM-D scale from the baseline in depressed patients translate to clinically meaningful improvement? Is the rule we use to dichotomize patients sensitive to drug effect? All these are important questions when determining the responder definition.

We will assume that a binary endpoint is appropriately defined and the objective is to explore the relationship between the likelihood of the desirable outcome and the dose. Using Table 13.1 as an example, we will assume that it is reasonable to collapse the three categories of death, vegetative state, and major disability into one category and combining minor disability and good recovery into another. The first (combined) category is deemed undesirable while the second (combined) category is the desirable one. Following our previous notations, we will label the two response categories as $j = 1$ and 2. The four dose groups will be labeled as $i = 1, 2, 3, 4$, respectively. Response categories after combination are given in Table 13.2.

The binary case can be considered as a special case of the ordinal response discussed in Section 13.2. For example, the logit model in (13.6) is subsumed in the proportional odds logit model described in (13.1). Similarly, the logit model

Table 13.2. Collapsing the first three response categories and the last two response categories in Table 13.1 to form a binary response consisting of "undesirable" and "desirable" categories

Treatment group	Outcome		Total
	Undesirable	Desirable	
Placebo	130	80	210
Low dose	113	77	190
Medium dose	112	95	207
High dose	96	99	195

in (13.7) is subsumed in the proportional odds logit model in (13.2).

$$\ln\left(\frac{p_{i2}}{p_{i1}}\right) = \alpha - \beta_i \qquad (13.6)$$

$$\ln\left(\frac{p_{i2}}{p_{i1}}\right) = \alpha - \beta \, d_i \qquad (13.7)$$

Because of the relationship between the above and their counterparts for the ordinal response, estimation and testing related to models (13.6) and (13.7) can be conducted similar to those for models (13.1) and (13.2). Setting $\beta_1 = 0$, the maximum likelihood estimates for $\{\beta_i\}$ in (13.6) are $\hat{\beta}_2 = 0.102$ (SE $= 0.205$), $\hat{\beta}_3 = 0.321$ (SE $= 0.199$), and $\hat{\beta}_4 = 0.516$ (SE $= 0.202$). Maximum likelihood estimate for β in Eq. (13.7) is $\hat{\beta} = 0.176$ (SE $= 0.064$). The Wald test for $\beta = 0$ produced a two-sided p-value of 0.006.

As for approaches that assign scores to response categories, one can easily show that with only two response categories, one will reach identical conclusions regardless of the scores assigned. Since there are only two response categories for a binary outcome, the approach of treating the data as if they are from continuous distributions (Section 13.2.2.2) is generally not encouraged. On the other hand, the mean response model with parameters estimated using the weighted least-squares method is still appropriate. In the latter case, one can choose $(0, 1)$ scores so that the mean response is actually the probability of the desirable response. The mean response model in (13.5) now reduces to

$$p_{i2} = a + b \times (\text{dose})_i \qquad (13.8)$$

In general, fitting model (13.8) could be a challenge if one wants to incorporate the constraint that $\{p_{i2}, i = 1, 2, 3, 4\}$ are between 0 and 1. For Table 13.2, with numerical scores $\{1, 2, 3, 4\}$ for the doses, the weighted least-squares estimates for a and b are 0.331 and 0.043 with standard errors of 0.042 and 0.016, respectively. These estimates produced weighted least-squares estimates of 0.374, 0.417, 0.460, and 0.503 for $\{p_{i2}, i = 1, 2, 3, 4\}$.

For the binary case, the association-based approach is closely related to the Cochran-Armitage (1955) test that is designed to detect a linear trend in the response probabilities with dose. Mancuso et al. (2001) proposed to use isotonic regression to increase the power of common trend tests in situations where a monotone dose response relationship is imposed. They developed the isotonic versions of the Cochran-Armitage type trend tests and used bootstrap method to find the empirical distributions of the test statistics. Using simulations, they demonstrated that the order-restricted Cochran-Armitage type trend tests could increase the power of the regular Cochran-Armitage trend test. When using $\{1, 2, 3, 4\}$ as the scores for doses, the Cochran-Armitage test for detecting a linear trend in $\{p_{i2}\}$ produced a χ^2 statistic of 7.65 with a two-sided p-value of 0.006.

For the data in Table 13.1 and the collapsed data in Table 13.2, all approaches confirm a monotone dose–response relationship. As the dose increases, so is the probability for a more favorable outcome. Since the binary case is a simplified case of the ordinal data, we will not devote more attention to this special case.

13.4   Multiple Comparisons

Dose–response studies can be conducted at different stages of a drug development program. They can be the studies to establish proof of concept or to establish a dose to bring into the confirmatory phase. Because the objectives of dose–response studies at various development phases are different, the analytic approaches to handling the data should vary accordingly. For dose response studies to establish proof of concept, the focus is to see if the response varies with the dose to suggest any drug activity. Therefore, the analysis will focus on estimation. This also applies to many Phase IIb studies that are designed to correctly identify the dose(s) with adequate treatment benefit. In this case, studying the trend and identifying doses by the observed mean responses will be key since the studies might not be sufficiently powered to detect a clinically meaningful difference between doses. There are also situations where studies are powered to differentiate between pairs of groups, but not powered to do so with adjustment for multiple comparisons. In any cases, the analysis should be conducted to specifically address their objectives.

When multiple doses are included in a confirmatory trial and the goal is to test the efficacy of each dose against the control (often a placebo), statistical analyses should be adjusted for multiple comparisons. The latter will be the focus of this section. Unlike the previous two sections where hypothesis testing, when employed, is to check for a monotone dose–response relationship, a monotone dose response is not necessarily the basis for hypothesis testing in this section. Instead, definitively differentiating between treatment groups (especially doses of an investigational medication from the control) will be the primary objective.

The primary objective of a multiple testing procedure is to control the overall probability of erroneously rejecting at least one null hypothesis irrespective of which and how many of the null hypotheses of interest are in fact true. Many multiple testing procedures have been proposed in the literature. In general, they fall in two classes. The first class includes procedures that are developed specifically for continuous data such as the Dunnett's method (1965) and the procedure by William (1971). The second class includes procedures that are "distributional free" in the sense that their implementation does not depend on any particular distributional assumption. Most of the procedures in this class are derived from the closed testing procedure proposed by Marcus et al. (1976) and work directly with the p-values produced from individual tests. As such, procedures in the second class are readily applicable to categorical data.

We will assume in this section that the objective of pairwise comparisons is to unequivocally identify doses that have significantly different effect from the control. For data in Tables 13.1 and 13.2, this means comparing low, medium, and high doses against the placebo. Except for the Dunnett's procedure described in Section 13.4.5, we will focus on approaches that compare p-values to adjusted significance levels with adjustments determined by the multiple testing procedures. We will look at four most commonly used procedures.

When the proportional odds model (13.1) is employed to analyze the ordinal response data such as in Table 13.1 with the convention of $\beta_1 = 0$, comparing each dose group to the placebo is equivalent to testing if $\beta_i = 0$ for $i = 2, 3, 4$. Dividing β_i estimate by its asymptotic standard error, we obtained z-statistics of 0.663, 1.811, and 2.937 for testing $\beta_2 = 0$, $\beta_3 = 0$, and $\beta_4 = 0$, respectively. The two-sided p-values associated with these three z-statistics under their respective null hypotheses are 0.507, 0.070, and 0.003.

We can also obtain p-values for comparing each dose to the placebo by assigning scores to the ordinal categories and treating the data as if they are continuous. When doing this, multiple comparison procedures developed for normal distribution could be applied. Alternatively, one can apply the Wilcoxon-Mann-Whitney test to compare each dose group to the placebo. Similarly, one can either use the modeling approach or compare two proportions directly for the binary case. For Sections 13.4.1 through 13.4.4, we will assume that p-values corresponding to the hypotheses of interest have been produced. We will assume throughout Section 13.4 that the overall Type I error rate is to be controlled at the 5% level.

We would like to point out that multiplicity adjustment for model-based approaches with large sample sizes may be done using parametric re-sampling techniques. Macros for doing these are provided in Westfall et al. (1999) and an example for binary outcome is given in Chapter 12 of that book. For the rest of this chapter, large sample asymptotic normal approximations are used to derive the significance levels.

13.4.1   Bonferroni Adjustment

Under this approach, we will compare each p-value to 0.0167 (=0.05/3) since we will make three comparisons. Because of its simplicity, Bonferroni adjustment is often used despite its conservativeness. Taking the three p-values cited above, i.e., 0.507, 0.070 and 0.003, only 0.003 is smaller than 0.0167. Thus, applying the Bonferroni procedure, one could only conclude that the high dose produced a significantly better result than the placebo.

13.4.2   Bonferroni–Holm Procedure

This procedure calls for ordering the p-values from the smallest to the largest. In our case, this lead to the order of 0.003 (high dose), 0.070 (medium dose), and 0.507 (low dose). If the smallest p-value is smaller than 0.0167 (=0.05/3), we will move to the next smallest p-value; otherwise we will stop and conclude that no dose group is significantly different from the placebo. In our case, 0.003 is less than 0.0167, so we continue to 0.070, the next smallest p-value. We will compare 0.070 to 0.025 (0.05/2). Since 0.070 is greater than 0.025, we will stop the comparison and conclude that only the high dose produced results that are significantly different from the placebo. Should the second smallest p-value be smaller than 0.025, we would proceed to the next p-value in the ordered sequence. In other words, we continue the process with a significance level that is 0.05 divided by the number of hypotheses remaining to be tested at each stage unless the p-value under comparison exceeds the current significance level. When this occurs, we will conclude significance for all comparisons before the present one.

13.4.3   Hochberg Procedure

This procedure is among the most popular multiple comparison procedures by pharmaceutical statisticians. Instead of ordering the p-values from the smallest to the largest, this procedure orders the p-values from the largest to the smallest. In our example, the ordered p-values are 0.507 (low dose), 0.070 (medium dose), and 0.003 (high dose). The largest p-value will be compared to 0.05. If it is smaller than 0.05, we will stop the testing and conclude significance for all comparisons; otherwise we will move to the second highest p-value. In our case, the largest p-value, i.e., 0.507 is greater than 0.05, so we will continue. The second largest p-value will be compared to 0.025 (=0.05/2). If it is smaller than 0.025, we will stop and conclude significance for this comparison and all subsequent ones that produced p-values smaller than the current one. Since 0.07 is greater than 0.025, we will continue. The smallest p-value in our example will be compared to 0.0167 (0.05/3). Since 0.003 is smaller than 0.0167, we will conclude a significant difference between the high dose and the placebo. Under the Hochberg procedure, the process starts with the largest p-value and the significance level decreases as we proceed. The significance level for the kth step is given by $0.05/k$. Unlike the Holm procedure, the Hochberg procedure continues the testing until we reach a statistical significance, otherwise it will conclude that none of the doses is statistically different from the placebo.

13.4.4   Gate-Keeping Procedure

This procedure is also known as predetermined step-down or the hierarchy procedure (Bauer and Budde, 1994; Bauer et al., 1998). In short, this procedure follows a prespecified sequence. Testing will be conducted at the 0.05 level at each stage and it will continue as long as the p-value is significant at the 0.05 level. Testing will stop at the first instance when a p-value is above 0.05.

   This procedure is used very frequently when there is a prior belief of a monotone dose–response relationship and therefore it is logical to start with the highest dose first. This procedure is especially helpful when looking for the minimum effective dose (Tamhane et al., 1996). To look for a minimum effective dose under the strong belief of a monotone dose–response relationship, one can start by comparing the highest dose with the control and working our way down the doses. The minimum effective dose is often defined as the smallest dose for which the null hypothesis of no effect is rejected. Another appealing feature is that all comparisons are conducted at the level of 0.05. Despite its appeal and ease to implement, if the prior belief turns out to be false and the dose–response relationship turns out to be umbrella-shaped, the predetermined step-down procedure can miss the opportunity to identify effective doses.

In our example, if we choose (high, medium, low) as the testing sequence based on biologic considerations, we will reach the same conclusion as the previous procedures. That is, the high dose is the only one demonstrating a statistically different effect from the placebo.

13.4.5 A Special Application of Dunnett's Procedure for Binary Response

Chuang-Stein and Tong (1995) examined three approaches for comparing several treatments with a control using a binary outcome. The first approach relies on the asymptotic theory applied to the Freeman and Tukey (1950) transformation of the observed proportions. The second finds an acceptance region based on the binomial distributions estimated under the joint null hypotheses. The third approach applies Dunnett's procedure to the binary data. The authors found that for sample sizes typical of the confirmatory trials, applying Dunnett's critical values to the z-statistics obtained from comparing proportions results in an actual overall Type I error rate generally at the desirable level.

For the data in Table 13.2, the z-statistics for comparing each dose against the placebo are 0.497 for the low dose, 1.618 for the medium dose, and 2.585 for the high dose. Dunnett's critical value for three comparisons and a sample sizes greater than 160 per group is 2.212 (Hsu, 1996, Table E.3). Compared to 2.212, only the comparison between the high dose and the placebo reached statistical significance at the 0.05 level.

Occasionally, one might want to compare among doses that have been established to be efficacious. Our recommendation is to make these comparisons without worrying about multiplicity adjustment. This is because the latter are secondary to the primary objective of identifying efficacious doses.

Ruberg (1995a,b) noted that dose–response studies routinely ask four questions. They are (1) Is there any evidence of a drug effect? (2) Which doses exhibit a response different from the control group? (3) What is the nature of the dose–response relationship? (4) Which is the optimal dose? One can discuss the first three questions either in the context of safety (Hothorn and Hauschke, 2000) or efficacy data. The prevailing practice is to focus on safety and efficacy data separately without making a conscious effort to integrate them. Compared to the first three, the last question can only be answered when safety and efficacy are considered jointly. The latter is outside the scope of this chapter.

13.5 Discussion

Ordinal data occur frequently in real life. Likert scale is frequently used to record a subject's response to a question or to an external intervention. Because of the way the scale is constructed, it is intuitive to use scores such as $\{-2, -1, 0, 1, 2\}$ for the five-category scale and $\{-3, -2, -1, 0, 1, 2, 3\}$ for the seven-category scale. Other examples of ordinal response come from using instruments to record outcome reported by both patients and their treating physicians. Many instruments contain questions that are ordinal in nature. Even though the score summed over the various questions is often the primary point of interest, analysis of specific questions leads to the analysis of ordinal data.

In this chapter, we discussed both the modeling and the testing approaches. In our opinion, modeling approach, for all its advantages, is underutilized. Modeling approach can handle covariates and predict the chance for achieving certain response for a given dose as well as the uncertainty associated with the prediction. In addition, a fitted model can be used to estimate the dose within the dosing range that has a desirable probability to produce certain response. By plotting the observed logit against the dose (or ln dose), one can get some indication whether the assumption of a monotone dose–response relationship is likely to be supported by the data or not. For example, if there is a downward trend in response when the dose moves toward the high end, one might want to consider including a quadratic term in dose (or ln dose) to describe the umbrella-like relationship. In addition to modeling, distribution-free tests for umbrella alternatives were studied by Chen and Wolfe (1990).

To be useful, models typically come with accompanying assumptions to aid interpretation. The proportional odds logit models require constant odds ratios among dose groups on the cumulative probability scale. Models such as those in (13.2) and (13.7) describe a linear dose effect. Some researchers (e.g., Mantel, 1963) considered such requirements appropriate as long as the required conditions constitute a major component of the phenomenon under examination. For example, the linear models as in (13.2) and (13.7) are reasonable as long as the linearity assumption holds for the underlying dose–response relationship. In using a linear model, we are able to construct a powerful test for a hypothesis that suggests a monotone dose–response relationship. In most cases, the linearity assumption and the proportional odds assumption can be checked via the goodness-of-fit based on the likelihood ratio tests.

Calculating sample size for binary outcome when comparing each dose group against the control is straightforward. If multiplicity adjustment is needed, a conservative approach is to use the Bonferroni significance level as the Type I error in the calculation. Sample size calculated in this way will be adequate when other more efficient multiple comparison procedures are used in the analysis. If the number of categories associated with an ordinal response is at least five and the analysis calls for treating the data as continuous, the calculation of the sample size can proceed as for the continuous case. A detailed discussion on sample sizes needed for dose response studies is provided in Chapter 14 of this book.

Sample size calculation for the modeling approach is more complicated. Whitehead (1993) discussed the case of comparing two groups based on the proportional odds logit model. Suppose we want an 80% power in a two-sided 5% test for detecting a size of β_0 in a model like (13.2). Assuming a randomization ratio of A to 1 to the two groups and $\{\overline{p}_j, j = 1, \ldots, J\}$ the anticipated marginal proportions of the response categories, Whitehead showed that the total required sample size is

$$N = \frac{3(A+1)^2(z_{0.975} + z_{0.80})^2}{A\beta_0^2\left(1 - \sum_j \overline{p}_j^3\right)}$$

where z_c above represents the $100 \times c\%$ percentile of the standard normal distribution. A lower bound for N can be obtained by substituting $1/J$ for $\overline{p}_j$ in the above formula. Whitehead showed that the required sample size did not differ much from this lower bound unless a single dominant response category occurred. It can be easily seen that equal allocation, i.e., $A = 1$, produces the smallest sample size.

Using Whitehead formula, Chuang-Stein and Agresti (1997) discussed the effect of the choice of the number of response categories on the sample size. In particular, they discussed the sample size required for J categories $N(J)$ and that required for two categories $N(2)$ for the case of equal marginal response probabilities. The ratio of $N(J)$ to $N(2)$ is

$$\frac{N(J)}{N(2)} = \frac{0.75}{1 - J^{-2}}$$

For $J = 5$, the above ratio is about 78%, suggesting a substantial loss of information when collapsing five response categories into two. This observation is consistent with our earlier comments on the loss of information when dichotomizing a nonbinary response. Even though Whitehead's original discussion was applied to two-arm trials, the discussion is relevant to dose–response studies when the primary focus is to compare each dose group against, for example, the placebo.

For dose–response studies conducted at the earlier development phase, the objective might not be to statistically differentiate between doses, but to correctly identify doses that have better efficacy. For example, when studying a new antibiotic at the Phase II stage, the primary objective of a dose–response trial is often to pick a dose to bring to the confirmatory phase. Such a trial might contain only doses of the new antibiotic. The major consideration for sample size decision is to make sure that we have enough patients at each dose so that the probability of correctly identifying the dose with the best efficacy using the observed success rate is at a desirably high level. For example, we might want to have an 80% chance that the observed success rates will correctly reflect the ordering in the true response rates when the underlying true rates are 60% and 50%, respectively. If this is the objective, then we will need approximately 35 patients per dose group. On the other hand, if one wants to differentiate between these two doses with an 80% power using a hypothesis testing procedure at a two-sided 5% significance level, one will need 408 patients per dose group. The latter is excessive for a Phase II antibiotic trial, especially when in vitro testing and animal model have already confirmed the antibacterial activity of the compound under investigation. Some design considerations for dose–response studies can be found in Wong and Lachenbruch (1998).

The analysis approaches discussed in this chapter are applicable to a parallel design under which subjects are randomized to receive one of the treatments (doses) under comparison. In some therapeutic areas, early phase dose–response studies are done using a titration design. Under a titration design, subjects typically start with the lowest dose and have their doses titrated upwards until treatment intolerance or the obtainment of a response. The exploration of a dose–response relationship with a binary outcome in a titration study requires special care because of the selective nature of the titration scheme. For more details on the analysis of such studies, the readers are referred to Chuang (1987).

There is a great flexibility in analyzing dose–response studies when the endpoint is measured on an ordinal scale. Since most of the discussion in this chapter is for the average situation, one might want to consider evaluating the use of a general-purpose approach for a particular situation more thoroughly. To this end, we would like to encourage our readers to diligently use simulations to evaluate various design options. The latter includes the sample size. For example, one can simulate studies under various conditions to see if the planned size provides adequate power to address the research objectives. In addition to sample size, how missing data are handled (e.g., the baseline response category carried forward, the worse response category experienced by the individual, or the worst response category) could have a significant impact on power. Furthermore, most multiple comparison procedures, when applied to categorical data, rely on the asymptotic behaviors of the underlying test statistics. Whether the asymptotic approximation is adequate for a particular application needs to be assessed for the planned sample size, the response profiles, the dropout patterns, as well as the choices of the analytical approaches (modeling vs. comparing proportions directly). With the convenience of modern computing power, it is highly desirable to take advantage of these tools so we have a good understanding of the operating characteristics of the procedures chosen before we initiate a clinical trial.

References

Agresti, A. 2000. *Categorical Data Analysis*, 2nd ed. New York: Wiley.

Armitage, P. 1955. Tests for linear trends in proportions. *Biometrics* 11:375–386.

Bauer, P., and Budde, M. 1994. Multiple testing for detecting efficient dose steps. *Biometrical Journal* 36:3–15.

Bauer, P., Rohmel, J., Maurer, W., and Hothorn, L. 1998. Testing strategies in multi-dose experiments including active control. *Statistics in Medicine* 17:2133–2146.

Chen, Y.I., and Wolfe, D.A. 1990. A study of distribution-free tests for umbrella alternatives. *Biometrical Journal* 32:47–57.

Chuang, C. 1987. The analysis of a titration study. *Statistics in Medicine* 6:583–590.

Chuang-Stein, C., and Tong, D.M. 1995. Multiple comparison procedures for comparing several treatments with a control based on binary data. *Statistics in Medicine* 14:2509–2522.

Chuang-Stein, C., and Agresti, A. 1997. A review of tests for detecting a monotone dose–response relationship with ordinal response data. *Statistics in Medicine* 16:2599–2618.

Dunnett, C.W. 1965. A multiple comparisons procedure for comparing several treatments with a control. *Journal of the American Statistical Association* 60:573–583.

Freeman, M.F., and Tukey, J.W. 1950. Transformations related to the angular and the square root. *Annals of Mathematical Statistics* 21:607–611.

Grizzle, J.E., Starmer, C.F. and Koch, G.G. (1969) Analysis of categorical data by linear models. *Biometrics* 25, 489–504.

Heeren, T., and D'Agostino, R. 1987. Robustness of the two independent sample *t*-test when applied to ordinal scale data. *Statistics in Medicine* 6:79–90.

Hothorn, L.A., and Hauschke, D. 2000. Identifying the maximum safe dose: A multiple testing approach. *Journal of Biopharmaceutical Statistics* 10:15–30.

Hsu, J.C. 1996. *Multiple Comparisons—Theory and Methods*. London, UK: Chapman & Hall.

Jonckheere, A.R. 1954. A distribution-free K sample test against ordered alternatives. *Biometrika* 41:133–145.

Lewis, J.A. 2004. In defence of the dichotomy. *Pharmaceutical Statistics* 3:77–79.

Mancuso, J.Y., Ahn, H. and Chen, J.J. (2001) Order-restricted dose-related trend tests. Statistics in Medicine 20, 2305–2318.

Mantel, N. 1963. Chi-square tests with one degree of freedom: extensions of the Mantel-Haenszel procedure. *Journal of the American Statistical Association* 58:690–700.

Marcus, R., Peritz, E., and Gabriel, K.R. 1976. On closed testing procedures with special reference to ordered analysis of variance. *Biometrika* 63:655–660.

McCullagh, P. 1980. Regression model for ordinal data (with discussion). *Journal of the Royal Statistical Society Series B* 42:109–142.

Ruberg, S.J. 1995. Dose-response studies I: Some design considerations. *Journal of Biopharmaceutical Statistics* 5:1–14.

Ruberg, S.J. 1995. Dose-response studies II: Analysis and interpretation. *Journal of Biopharmaceutical Statistics* 5:15–42.

SAS, version 9.0. 2003. Cary, NC: SAS Institute Inc.

Senn, S. 2003. Disappointing dichotomies. *Pharmaceutical Statistics* 2:239–240.

StatXact 1995. *StatXact3 for Windows: Statistical Software for Exact Nonparametric Inference, User Manual*. Cytel Software.

Tamhane, A.C., Hochberg, Y., and Dunnett, C.W. 1996. Multiple test procedures for dose finding. *Biometrics* 52:21–37.

Terpstra, T.J. 1952. The asymptotic normality and consistency of Kendall's test against trend, when ties are present in one ranking. *Indigationes Mathematicae* 14:327–333.

Westfall, P.H., Tobias, R.D., Rom, D., Wolfinger, R.D., and Hochberg, Y. 1999. *Multiple Comparisons and Multiple Tests Using the SAS System*. Cary, North Carolina: SAS Institute Inc.

Whitehead, J. 1993. Sample size calculations for ordered categorical data. Statistics in Medicine 12, 2257–2271.

William, D.A. 1971. A test for difference between treatment means when several dose levels are compared with a zero dose control. *Biometrics* 27:103–117.

Wong, W.K., and Lachenbruch, P.A. 1998. Designing studies for dose response. *Statistics in Medicine* 15:343–359.

Appendix: SAS Code for Performing Various Analyses

SAS code for performing various analyses with data in Table 13.1

```
data one;
input dose outcome count @ @;
group = 1;
cards;
1 1 59 1 2 25 1 3 46 1 4 48 1 5 32
2 1 48 2 2 21 2 3 44 2 4 47 2 5 30
3 1 44 3 2 14 3 3 54 3 4 64 3 5 31
4 1 43 4 2  4 4 3 49 4 4 58 4 5 41
proc freq data=one; *CMH test with scores entered in the data;
weight count;
tables group*dose*outcome/cmh1;
run;

proc freq data=one; *CMH test with mid-rank scores;
weight count;
tables group*dose*outcome/cmh1 scores=ridit;
run;

proc catmod data=one order=data; *mean response model;
weight count;
population dose;
response 1 2 3 4 5; direct dose; *use scores (1,2,3,4,5);
model outcome=dose;
run;

proc logistic data=one; *proportional odds model (ML);
freq count;
model outcome=dose;
run;

proc catmod data=one; *proportional odds model (WLS);
weight count;
response clogits;
direct dose;
model outcome=_response_ dose;
run;

proc catmod data= one; *adjacent cat. Logit model (WLS);
weight count;
response alogits;
direct dose;
```

```
model outcome=_response_ dose;
run;
```

SAS code for performing various analyses after classifying data in Table 13.2

```
data two;
input dose outcome count;
cards;
1 0 130
1 1 80
2 0 113
2 1 77
3 0 112
3 1 95
4 0 96
4 1 99
proc logistic data=two; *treating dose levels as a continuous variable;
freq count;
model outcome=dose;
run;

data three;
set two; *create dummy variables for dose levels;
if dose=2 then idose2=1; *placebo group is treated as a reference level;
else idose2=0;
if dose=3 then idose3=1;
else idose3=0;
if dose=4 then idose4=1;
else idose4=0;
run;

proc logistic data=three; *treating dose levels as nominal categories;
freq count;
model outcome=idose2 idose3 idose4;
run;

proc freq data=two; *Cochran-Armitage trend test;
weight count;
tables dose*outcome/trend;
run;
```

14
Power and Sample Size for Dose Response Studies

MARK CHANG AND SHEIN-CHUNG CHOW

14.1 Introduction

In this chapter, we will study sample size issues in dose–response trials. As indicated in 21 CFR 312.21, Phase I clinical investigation provides an initial introduction of an investigational new drug in humans. The primary objectives are to (1) determine the metabolism and pharmacological activities of the drug, the side effects associated with increasing dose and early evidence in effectiveness and (2) obtain sufficient information regarding the drug's pharmacokinetics and pharmacological effects to permit the design of well-controlled and scientifically valid Phase II clinical studies. Thus, Phase I clinical investigation includes studies of drug metabolism, bioavailibility, dose ranging, and multiple dose. For dose-escalation studies, clinical researchers usually start with low dose which is unlikely to present any harmful effects to subjects. Then, several cohorts of subjects are treated at progressively higher doses until a predetermined level of drug-related toxicity is reached. The level of drug-related toxicity is usually referred to as dose-limiting toxicity (DLT). In practice, since the test drug for progressive disease such as oncology is usually toxic and only a small number of patients are allowed for the study due to ethical consideration, the efficiency of the design is not only measured by its power but also the number of DLTs and accuracy for determination of maximum tolerated dose (MTD). In Phase II, dose–response studies are focused on the efficacy. Four questions are often of interest (Ruberg, 1995a, b): (1) Is there any evidence of the drug effect? (2) What doses exhibit a response different from the control response? (3) What is the nature of the dose–response? (4) What is the optimal dose? The first question is often essential and most hypothesis test methods try to answer this question; The second question can usually be addressed by Williams' test for minimum effective dose. The third question can be addressed by model-based approaches, either of frequentist or Bayesian type. The last question is multiple dimensional involving at least efficacy and safety components. We will limit our discussion on the sample size calculations for answering the first three questions. Specifically, in next section, some general concepts regarding sample size calculation are briefly reviewed. Section 14.3 provides a formula for sample size calculation for various study endpoints under multiple-arm response trials, including Williams' test for minimum effective dose for normal response, Cocharan-Armitage trend test for binary response, and a newly derived contrasts test for survival endpoint. Sample size estimation and related operating characteristics of Phase I dose escalation designs are discussed in Section 4. A brief concluding remark is given in the last section.

14.2   General Approach to Power Calculation

When testing a null hypothesis $H_0 : \varepsilon \leq 0$ against an alternative hypothesis $H_a : \varepsilon > 0$, where ε is the treatment effect (difference in response), the Type I error rate function is defined as

$$\alpha(\varepsilon) = \Pr\{\text{reject } H_0 \text{ when } H_0 \text{ is true}\}.$$

Similarly, the type-II error rate function β is defined as

$$\beta(\varepsilon) = \Pr\{\text{fail to reject } H_0 \text{ when } H_a \text{ is true}\}.$$

For hypothesis testing, we need to know the distribution of the test statistic T, $\Phi_0(T)$, under H_0. For sample size calculation, we need to know its distribution under a particular H_a. To control the overall Type-I error rate at level α under any point of the H_0 domain, the condition $\alpha(\varepsilon) \leq \alpha^*$ for all $\varepsilon \leq 0$ must be satisfied, where α^* is a threshold which is usually larger than 0.05 unless it is a Phase III trial. If $\alpha(\varepsilon)$ is monotonic function of ε, then the maximum Type-I error occurs when $\varepsilon = 0$ and test statistic should be derived under this condition. For example, for the null hypothesis $H_0 : \mu_2 - \mu_1 \leq 0$, where μ_1 and μ_2 are the means of the two treatment group, the maximum Type-I error occurs on the boundary of H_0 when $\mu_2 - \mu_1 = 0$. Thus, $\Phi_0(T)$ is the cumulative distribution function (CDF) of the test statistic on the boundary of this null hypothesis domain.

The power of the test statistic T under a particular H_a can be expressed as follows:

$$Power = \Pr(T \geq \Phi_o^{-1}(1 - \alpha; n)|H_a) = 1 - \Phi_a(\Phi_o^{-1}(1 - \alpha; n); n) \qquad (14.1)$$

where Φ_a is CDF under the alternative hypothesis H_a. Figure 1 is an illustration of the power function of α and the sample size n. Note that Φ_o and Φ_a are often CDF for normal distribution. In this situation, we can derive an sample size formula as follows:

$$n = \frac{(z_{1-a}\hat{\sigma}_0 + z_{1-\beta}\hat{\sigma}_a)^2}{\varepsilon^2} \qquad (14.2)$$

where ε is treatment difference. If homogeneous variances hold among treatment groups, i.e., $\sigma_0^2 = \sigma_a^2 = \sigma^2$, then the sample size is simply given by

$$n = \frac{(z_{1-a} + z_{1-\beta})^2\sigma^2}{\varepsilon^2} \qquad (14.3)$$

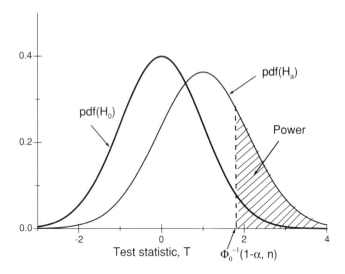

Figure 14.1. Power as a function of α and n.

Table 14.1. Sample sizes for different types of endpoints

Endpoint	Sample size	variance
One mean	$n = \dfrac{(z_{1-a} + z_{1-\beta})^2\sigma^2}{\varepsilon^2}$	
Two means	$n_1 = \dfrac{(z_{1-a} + z_{1-\beta})^2\sigma^2}{(1 + 1/r)^{-1}\varepsilon^2}$	
One proportion	$n = \dfrac{(z_{1-a} + z_{1-\beta})^2\sigma^2}{\varepsilon^2}$	$\sigma^2 = p(1 - p)$
Two proportions	$n_1 = \dfrac{(z_{1-a} + z_{1-\beta})^2\sigma^2}{(1 + 1/r)^{-1}\varepsilon^2}$	$\sigma^2 = \bar{p}(1 - \bar{p});$ $\bar{p} = \dfrac{n_1 p_1 + n_2 p_2}{n_1 + n_2}.$
One survival curve	$n = \dfrac{(z_{1-a} + z_{1-\beta})^2\sigma^2}{\varepsilon^2}$	$\sigma^2 = \lambda_0^2\left(1 - \dfrac{e^{\lambda_0 T_0} - 1}{T_0\lambda_0 e^{\lambda_0 T_s}}\right)^{-1}$
Two survival curves	$n_1 = \dfrac{(z_{1-a} + z_{1-\beta})^2\sigma^2}{(1 + 1/r)^{-1}\varepsilon^2}$	$\sigma^2 = \dfrac{r\sigma_1^2 + \sigma_2^2}{1 + r},$ $\sigma_i^2 = \lambda_i^2\left(1 - \dfrac{e^{\lambda_i T_0} - 1}{T_0\lambda_i e^{\lambda_i T_s}}\right)^{-1}$

Note: $r = \dfrac{n_2}{n_1}$. λ_0 = expected hazard rate, T_0 = uniform patient accrual time and T_s = trial duration.
Log rank-test is used for comparison of the two survival curves.

Based on Eq. (14.1), sample sizes for comparing means, proportions and survival endpoints with one or two groups can all be easily derived, which are summarized in Table 14.1 (see also, Chow et al., 2003).

Note that the selection of Type-I error rate α and Type-II error rate β should be based on study objectives that may vary from phase to phase of clinical trials.

It depends efficacy, safety, and other aspects of the trial. From safety perspective, the number of patients should be gradually increased from early phases to later phases due to potential toxicity of the test drug. From efficacy point of view, for early phases, we are more concerned about missing good candidates and less concerned about false positive rate. In this case, a larger α is recommended. For later phase, a small α may be considered to meet regulatory requirements. In practice, it is suggested that the benefit-risk ratio should be taken into consideration when performing sample size calculation. In such case, Bayesian decision theory is a useful tool.

14.3   Multiple-Arm Dose Response Trial

To characterize the response curve, multiple groups at different dose levels including a control group are usually studied. Such a multiple-arm trial is informative for the drug candidates with a wide therapeutic window. Whether a model-based or a nonparametric approach is adopted, any prior information about dose–response curve such as linear or monotonic is helpful. This prior information not only allows user to decide a more powerful test statistic (e.g., linear contrasts of the means), but also to perform power analysis under an appropriate model. In what follows, we will consider sample size calculation in multiple-arm dose response trials with various study endpoints.

A linear contrast test is commonly used in dose–response studies. For a one-sided hypothesis testing problem

$$H_o: L(\mathbf{u}) = \sum_{i=0}^{k} c_i u_i \leq 0; \text{ vs. } H_a: L(\mathbf{u}) = \sum_{i=0}^{k} c_i u_i = \varepsilon > 0$$

where u_i can be the mean, proportion, or ranking score, ε a constant, and the contrast coefficients c_i satisfy the equality $\sum_{i=0}^{k} c_i = 0$.

The pivotal statistic (when H_a is true) and test statistic (when H_o is true) can be expressed as

$$T = \frac{L(\hat{\mathbf{u}}|H)}{\sqrt{var(L(\hat{\mathbf{u}})|H_o)}}, \quad H \in H_o \cup H_a$$

where $\hat{\mathbf{u}}$ is an unbiased estimator of $\mathbf{u}$.

Let

$$\varepsilon = E(L(\hat{\mathbf{u}})|H_a), \quad v_o^2 = var(L(\hat{\mathbf{u}})|H_o), \text{ and } v_a^2 = var(L(\hat{\mathbf{u}})|H_a).$$

We then have the large sample test statistic

$$T(H_o) = \frac{L(\hat{\mathbf{u}})|H_o}{v_o} \sim N(0, 1)$$

and

$$T(H_a) = \frac{L(\hat{u})}{v_o} \sim N\left(\frac{\varepsilon}{v_o}, \frac{v_a^2}{v_o^2}\right)$$

where

$$\begin{cases} v_o^2 = var(L(\hat{u})|H_o) = \sum_{i=0}^k c_i^2 var(\hat{u}_i|H_o) = \sigma_o^2 \sum_{i=0}^k \frac{c_i^2}{n_i} \\ v_a^2 = var(L(\hat{u})|H_a) = \sum_{i=0}^k c_i^2 var(\hat{u}_i|H_a) = \sum_{i=0}^k \frac{c_i^2 \sigma_i^2}{n_i} \end{cases}$$

That is,

$$\begin{cases} v_o^2 = \frac{\sigma_o^2}{n} \sum_{i=0}^k \frac{c_i^2}{f_i} \\ v_a^2 = \frac{1}{n} \sum_{i=0}^k \frac{c_i^2 \sigma_i^2}{f_i} \end{cases}$$

where the size fraction $f_i = \frac{n_i}{n}$ with $n = \sum_{i=0}^k n_i$, σ_o^2 and σ_i^2 are the variances of the response under H_0 and H_a, respectively.

14.3.1   Normal Response

Let μ_i be the population mean for group i. The null hypothesis of no treatment effect can be written as follows:

$$H_0 : \mu_0 = \mu_1 = ... = \mu_k \tag{14.4}$$

or

$$H_0 : L(\mu) = \sum_{i=0}^k c_i \mu_i = 0 \tag{14.5}$$

where contrasts satisfy the condition that $\sum_{i=0}^k c_i = 0$.

Note that if H_0 in Eq. (14.5) is rejected for some $\{c_i\}$ satisfying $\sum_{i=0}^k c_i = 0$, then H_0 in Eq. (14.4) is also rejected. We are particularly interested in the following alternative hypothesis:

$$H_a : L(\mu) = \sum_{i=0}^k c_i \mu_i = \varepsilon \tag{14.6}$$

Under the alternative hypothesis in Eq. (14.6) and the condition of homogeneous variance, the sample size can be obtained as

$$n = \left[\frac{(z_{1-\alpha} + z_{1-\beta})\sigma}{\varepsilon}\right]^2 \sum_{i=0}^k \frac{c_i^2}{f_i}$$

where f_i is the sample size fraction for the ith group and the population parameter σ, for the purpose of sample size calculation, can be estimated using the pooled standard deviation if prior data are available.

Example   In a Phase II asthma study, a design with 4 dose groups (0, 20, 40, and 60 mg) of the test drug is proposed. The primary efficacy endpoint is percent change from baseline in FEV1. Based on limited information from previous studies, it is assumed that 5%, 12%, 14%, and 16% improvement over baseline for the control group, 20, 40, and 60 mg groups, respectively, and a homogeneous standard deviation of 22% for the FEV1 change from baseline. Therefore, we propose the following contrast which is consistent with the assumed dose–response shape: $c_1 = -6$, $c_2 = 1$, $c_3 = 2$, $c_4 = 3$ such that $\sum c_i = 0$. Thus, we have $\varepsilon = \sum_{i=0}^{k} c_i \bar{\mu}_i = 58\%$, where $\bar{\mu}_i$ is the observed FEV1 improvement in the ith group.

Using a balanced design ($f_i = 1/4$) with one-sided $\alpha = 0.05$ (Since this is Phase II, we do not have to use $\alpha = 0.025$), the sample size required to detect the difference of $\varepsilon = 0.58$ with 80% power is given by

$$
n = \left[\frac{(z_{1-\alpha} + z_{1-\beta})\sigma}{\varepsilon} \right]^2 \sum_{i=0}^{k} \frac{c_i^2}{f_i}
$$

$$
= \left[\frac{(1.645 + 0.842)(0.22)}{0.58} \right]^2 4((-6)^2 + 1^2 + 2^2 + 3^2) = 178
$$

Thus, a total sample size of 178 (45 per group) is required.

To study how the different combinations of response shapes and contrasts may affect the sample size and power, we consider the following five different shapes (Table 14.2).

Sample sizes required for different combinations of responses and contrasts are presented in Table 14.3. It can be seen that when response and contrasts have the same shapes, a minimum sample size is required. If an inappropriate contrast set is used, the sample size could be 30 times larger than the optimal design.

Table 14.2. Response and contrast shapes

Shape	μ_0	μ_1	μ_2	μ_3	c_0	c_1	c_2	c_3
Linear	0.1	0.3	0.5	0.7	−3.00	−1.00	1.00	3.00
Step	0.1	0.4	0.4	0.7	−3.00	0.00	0.00	3.00
Umbrella	0.1	0.4	0.7	0.5	−3.25	−0.25	2.75	0.75
Convex	0.1	0.1	0.1	0.6	−1.25	−1.25	−1.25	3.75
Concave	0.1	0.6	0.6	0.6	−3.75	1.25	1.25	1.25

Table 14.3. Sample size per group for various contrasts

Response	Linear	Step	Contrast Umbrella	Convex	Concave
Linear	31	35	52	52	52
Step	39	35	81	52	52
Umbrella	55	74	33	825	44
Convex	55	50	825	33	297
Concave	55	50	44	297	33

Note: $\sigma = 1$, one-sided $\alpha = 0.05$

14.3.1.1   Williams test for minimum effective dose (MED)

Under the assumption of monotonicity in dose response, Williams (1971, 1972) proposed a test to determine the lowest dose level at which there is evidence for a difference from control. Williams considered the following alternative hypothesis:

$$H_a : \mu_0 = \mu_1 = \ldots = \mu_{i-1} < \mu_i \leq \mu_{i+1} \leq \ldots \leq \mu_k$$

and proposed the following test statistic:

$$T_i = \frac{\hat{\mu}_i - \bar{Y}_0}{\hat{\sigma} \sqrt{\frac{1}{n_i} + \frac{1}{n_0}}}$$

where $\hat{\sigma}^2$ is an unbiased estimate of σ^2, which is independent of $\bar{Y}_i$, the mean response of the n_i patient in the ith group, and is distributed as $\sigma^2 \chi_v^2 / v$ and $\hat{\mu}_i$ is the maximum likelihood estimate of μ_i which is given by

$$\hat{\mu}_i = \max_{1 \leq u \leq i} \min_{i \leq v \leq k} \left\{ \frac{\sum_{j=u}^{v} n_j \bar{Y}_j}{\sum_{j=u}^{v} n_j} \right\}$$

When $n_i = n$ for $i = 0, 1, \ldots, k$, this test statistic can be simplified as

$$T_i = \frac{\hat{\mu}_i - \bar{Y}_0}{\hat{\sigma} \sqrt{2/n}}$$

We then reject the null hypothesis of no treatment difference and conclude that the ith dose level is the minimum effective dose if

$$T_j > t_j(\alpha) \quad \text{for all } j \geq i$$

where $t_j(\alpha)$ is the upper αth percentile of the distribution of T_j. The critical values of $t_j(\alpha)$ are given in the Table 12.11 of Chow et al., (2003).

Since the power function of the above test is rather complicated, as an alternative, Chow et al., (2003) considered the following approximation to obtain the required sample size per dose group:

$$\text{power} = \Pr \{\text{reject } H_0 | \mu_i \geq \mu_0 + \Delta \text{ for some i}\}$$

$$> \Pr \left\{\text{reject } H_0 | \mu_0 = \mu_1 = \ldots = \mu_{k-1}, \mu_k = \mu_0 + \Delta\right\}$$

$$\geq \Pr \left\{ \frac{\bar{Y}_k - \bar{Y}_0}{\sigma \sqrt{2/n}} > t_k(\alpha) | \mu_k = \mu_0 + \Delta \right\}$$

$$= 1 - \Phi \left(t_k(\alpha) - \frac{\Delta}{\sigma \sqrt{2/n}} \right)$$

where Δ the clinically meaningful minimal difference. To have a power of $1 - \beta$, required sample size per group can be obtained by solving

$$\beta = \Phi\left(t_k(\alpha) + \frac{\Delta}{\sigma\sqrt{2/n}}\right)$$

$$n = \frac{2\sigma^2\left[t_k(\alpha) + z_\beta\right]^2}{\Delta^2} \tag{14.7}$$

It should be noted that this approach is conservative.

Example   We consider the previous example of asthma trial. For power $= 80\%$, $\sigma = 0.22$, one-sided $\alpha = 0.05$ (Note that there is no two-sided William's test.), Since the critical value $t_k(\alpha)$ is dependent on the degree of freedom ν that is related to sample size n which is unknown. Iterations are usually needed. However, for the current case we know that $\nu > 120$ or ∞, which leads to $t_3(0.05) = 1.75$. Assume that 11% improvement in FEV1 over placebo is the minimum effect that is both clinically and commercially meaningful. Thus, the sample size for this study is given by

$$n = \frac{2(0.22)^2(1.75 + 0.8415)}{0.11^2} = 53 \text{ per group}$$

Note that this sample size formulation has a minimum difference from that based the two sample t-test with the maximum treatment difference as the treatment difference. For the current example, $n = 54$ from the two sample t-test.

14.3.2   Binary Response

Binary response is a commonly used endpoint in clinical trials. Denote p_i the proportion of response in the ith group. Suppose we are interested in testing the following null hypothesis

$$H_0 : p_0 = p_1 = \ldots = p_k \tag{14.8}$$

against the following alternative hypothesis

$$H_a : L(\mathbf{p}) = \sum_{i=0}^{k} c_i p_i = \varepsilon \tag{14.9}$$

where c_i are the contrasts satisfying $\sum_{i=1}^{k} c_i = 0$.

Similarly, by applying the linear contrast approach, the sample size can be obtained as

$$N \geq \left[\frac{z_{1-\alpha}\sqrt{\sum_{i=0}^{k} \frac{c_i^2}{f_i}\bar{p}(1-\bar{p})} + z_{1-\beta}\sqrt{\sum_{i=0}^{k} \frac{c_i^2}{f_i}p_i(1-p_i)}}{\varepsilon}\right]^2 \tag{14.10}$$

where $\bar{p} = \sum_{i=0}^{k} f_i p_i$.

The effects of different contrasts on sample size are summarized in Table 14.4.

As it can be seen from Table 14.4, an appropriate selection of contrasts yields a minimum sample size required for achieving the desired power.

Table 14.4. Total sample size comparisons for binary data

			Contrast		
Response	Linear	Step	Umbrella	Convex	Concave
Linear	26	28	44	48	44
Step	28	28	68	48	40
Umbrella	48	68	28	792	36
Convex	28	36	476	24	176
Concave	36	44	38	288	28

Note: One-sided $\alpha = 0.05$, $\sigma_o^2 = \bar{p}(1 - \bar{p})$.

Other commonly used methods include Cochran–Armitage test (Cochran, 1954, and Amitage, 1955) and Nam's test (Nam, 1987) for monotonic trend. These methods can be reviewed as regression based approaches. Therefore, using these methods, the rejection of the null hypothesis implies the dose–response has an *overall* monotonic "trend" in the regression sense. However the global monotonic trend is not a proof of monotonicity among all dose levels.

14.3.2.1   Nam's formula for Cochran-Armitage test

Let x_i be the k mutually independent binomial variates representing the number of responses among n_i subjects at dose level d_i for $i = 0, 1, \ldots, k - 1$. Define average response rate $\hat{p} = \frac{1}{N} \sum_i x_i$, $N = \sum_i n_i$, $\hat{q} = 1 - \hat{p}$, and $\bar{d} = \frac{1}{N} \sum n_i d_i$. $U = \sum_i x_i (d_i - \bar{d})$.

Assume that the probability of response follows a linear trend in logistic scale

$$p_i = \frac{e^{\gamma + \lambda d_i}}{1 + e^{\gamma + \lambda d_i}} \tag{14.11}$$

Note that $\{d_i\}$ can be actual doses or scores assigned to dose. However, Eq. (14.11) represents different models for these two cases.

The hypothesis test problem can be stated as

$$H_0 : \lambda = 0 \text{ vs. } H_a : \lambda = \varepsilon > 0$$

where ε should be to negative for monotonic decreasing response.

An approximate test with continuity correction based on the asymptotically normal deviate is given by

$$z = \frac{(U - \frac{\Delta}{2})}{\sqrt{var(U|H_0 : \lambda = 0)}} = \frac{(U - \frac{\Delta}{2})}{\sqrt{\hat{p}\hat{q} \sum_i n_i (d_i - \bar{d})^2}} \tag{14.12}$$

where $\Delta/2 = (d_i - d_{i-1})/2$ is the continuity correction for equal spaced doses. However, there is no constant Δ exist for unequally spaced doses. Nam pointed out that the familiar Cochran–Armitage test statistic, which obtained from least square theory by formal linear regression analysis for the model $p_i = a + bd_i$, is identical to the square of Eq. (14.12). The advantage of using the Eq. (14.11) is that the sample size formula for the test can be explicitly derived as follows:

$$\Pr(z \geq z_{1-\alpha} | H_a) = 1 - \Phi(u)$$

where

$$u = -E(U - \frac{\Delta}{2}) + z_{1-\alpha} \frac{\sqrt{var(U|H_o)}}{\sqrt{var(U|H_a)}}$$

Thus, we have

$$E(U) - \frac{\Delta}{2} + z_{1-\alpha}\sqrt{var(U|H_o)} + z_{1-\beta}\sqrt{var(U|H_a)}$$

For $\Delta = 0$, i.e., without continuity correction, the sample size is given by

$$n_0^* = \frac{1}{A^2} \left\{ z_{1-\alpha}\sqrt{pq \sum r_i(d_i - \bar{d})^2} + z_{1-\beta}\sqrt{\sum p_i q_i r_i(d_i - \bar{d})^2} \right\}^2 \qquad (14.13)$$

where $A = \sum r_i p_i(d_i - \bar{d})$, $p = \frac{1}{N}\sum n_i p_i$, $q = 1 - p$, and $r_i = n_i/n_0$ is the sample size ratio between the ith group and the control.

On the other hand, sample size with continuity correction is given by

$$n_0 = \frac{n_0^*}{4} \left[1 + \sqrt{1 + 2\frac{\Delta}{An_0^*}} \right]^2 \qquad (14.14)$$

Note that the actual power of the test depends on the specified alternative.

For balance design with equal size in each group, the formula for sample size per group is reduce to

$$n = \frac{n^*}{4} \left[1 + \sqrt{1 + \frac{2}{Dn^*}} \right]^2 \qquad (14.15)$$

where

$$n^* = \frac{1}{D^2} \left\{ z_{1-\alpha}\sqrt{k(k^2 - 1)pq/12} + z_{1-\beta}\sqrt{\sum b_i^2 p_i q_i} \right\}^2 \qquad (14.16)$$

and $b_i = i - 0.5(k - 1)$, and $D = \sum b_i p_i$.

Note that the above formula (Nam, 1987) is based on one-sided test at the α level. For two-sided test, the Type-I error rate is controlled at the 2α level. For equally spaced doses: 1, 2, 3, and 4, the sample sizes required for the five different sets of contracts are given in Table 14.5.

Cochran–Armitage test has been studied by many authors. The one-sided test by Portier and Hoel (1984) was the modification (Neuhauser and Hothorn, 1999) from Armitages' (1955) original two-sided test, which is asymptotically distributed as a standard normal variable under the null hypothesis. Neuhauser and Hothorn (1999) studied the power of Cochran-Armitage test under different true response shape through simulations. Gastwirth(1985) and Podgor et al. (1996) proposed a single maximum efficiency robust test statistic based on prior correlations between

Table 14.5. Sample size from Nam formula

Dose	1	2	3	4	Total n
Response	0.1	0.3	0.5	0.7	28
	0.1	0.4	0.4	0.7	36
	0.1	0.4	0.7	0.5	52
	0.1	0.1	0.1	0.6	44
	0.1	0.6	0.6	0.6	52

Note: The sample size is an approximation due to the normality assumption and small n.

different contrasts, while Neuhauser and Hothorn (1999) proposed a maximum test among two or more contrasts and claim a gain in power.

14.3.3 Time-to-Event Endpoint

Under an exponential survival model, the relationship between hazard (λ), median (T_{median}) and mean (T_{mean}) survival time is very simple:

$$T_{\text{median}} = \frac{\ln 2}{\lambda} = (\ln 2)T_{\text{mean}} \tag{14.17}$$

Let λ_i be the population hazard rate for group i. The contrast test for multiple survival curves can be written as

$$H_0 : L(\mu) = \sum_{i=0}^{k} c_i \lambda_i = 0 \text{ vs. } L(\mu) = \sum_{i=0}^{k} c_i \lambda_i = \varepsilon > 0$$

where contrasts satisfy the condition that $\sum_{i=0}^{k} c_i = 0$.

Similar to other types of endpoints (mean and proportion), the sample size is given by

$$N \geq \left[\frac{z_{1-\alpha}\sigma_0\sqrt{\sum_{i=0}^{k} \frac{c_i^2}{f_i}} + z_{1-\beta}\sqrt{\sum_{i=0}^{k} \frac{c_i^2}{f_i}\sigma_i^2}}{\varepsilon} \right]^2 \tag{14.18}$$

where the variance σ_i^2 can be derived in several different ways. Here we use Lachin and Foulkes's maximum likelihood approach (Lachin and Foulkes, 1986; Chow et al., 2003).

Suppose we design a clinical trial with k groups. Let T_0 and T_s be the accrual time period and the total trial duration, respectively. We then can prove that the variance for uniform patient entry is given by

$$\sigma^2(\lambda_i) = \lambda_i^2 \left[1 + \frac{e^{-\lambda_i T_s}(1 - e^{\lambda_i T_0})}{T_0 \lambda_i} \right]^{-1} \tag{14.19}$$

Let a_{ij} denote the uniform entry time of the jth patient of the ith group, i.e., $a_{ij} \sim \frac{1}{T_0}$, $0 \leq a_{ij} \leq T_0$. Let t_{ij} be the time-to-event starting from the time of the patient's entry for the jth patient in the ith group, $i = 1, \ldots k$, $j = 1, \ldots, n_i$. It is assumed t_{ij} follows an exponential distribution with hazard rate λ_i. The information observed is $(x_{ij}, \delta_{ij}) = \left(\min(t_{ij}, \ T_s - a_{ij}), \ I\left\{t_{ij} \leq T_s - a_{ij}\right\}\right)$. For a fixed i, the joint likelihood for $x_{ij}, \ j = 1, \ldots n_i$ can be written as

$$L(\lambda_i) = \frac{1}{T_0} \lambda_i^{\sum_{j=1}^{n_i} \delta_{ij}} e^{-\lambda_i \sum_{j=1}^{n_i} x_{ij}}$$

Taking the derivative with respect to λ_i and letting it equal to zero, we can obtain the MLE for λ_i which is given by $\hat{\lambda}_i = \frac{\sum_{j=1}^{n_i} \delta_{ij}}{\sum_{j=1}^{n_i} x_{ij}}$. According to the central limit theorem, we have

$$\sqrt{n_i}(\hat{\lambda}_i - \lambda_i) = \sqrt{n_i} \frac{\sum_{j=1}^{n_i}(\delta_{ij} - \lambda_i x_{ij})}{\sum_{j=1}^{n_i} x_{ij}}$$

$$= \frac{1}{\sqrt{n_i} E(x_{ij})} \sum_{j=1}^{n_i} (\delta_{ij} - \lambda_i x_{ij}) + o_p(1) \xrightarrow{d} N(0, \sigma^2(\lambda_i))$$

where

$$\sigma^2(\lambda_i) = \frac{var(\delta_{ij} - \lambda_i x_{ij})}{E^2(x_{ij})}$$

and $\xrightarrow{d}$ denote convergence in distribution. Note that

$$E(\delta_{ij}) = E(\delta_{ij}^2) = 1 - \int_0^{T_0} \frac{1}{T_0} e^{-\lambda_i(T_s-a)} da = 1 + \frac{e^{-\lambda_i T_s}(1 - e^{\lambda_i T_0})}{T_0 \lambda_i}$$

$$E(x_{ij}) = \frac{1}{\lambda_i} E(\delta_{ij}), \quad \text{and} \quad E(x_{ij}^2) = \frac{2E(\delta_{ij} x_{ij})}{\lambda_i}$$

Hence

$$\sigma^2(\lambda_i) = \frac{var(\delta_{ij} - \lambda_i x_{ij})}{E^2(x_{ij})} = \frac{1}{E^2(x_{ij})} \left(E(\delta_{ij}^2) - 2\lambda_i E(\delta_{ij} x_{ij}) + \lambda_i^2 E(x_{ij}^2)\right)$$

$$= \frac{E(\delta_{ij}^2)}{E^2(x_{ij})} = \frac{\lambda_i^2}{E(\delta_{ij})} = \lambda_i^2 \left[1 + \frac{e^{-\lambda_i T_s}(1 - e^{\lambda_i T_0})}{T_0 \lambda_i}\right]^{-1}$$

Example   In a four–arm (the active control, lower dose of test drug, higher dose of test drug and combined therapy) Phase II oncology trial, the objective is to determine if there is treatment effect with time-to-progression as the primary endpoint. Patient enrollment duration is estimated to be $T_0 = 9$ months and the total trial duration $T_s = 16$ months. The estimated median time for the four groups are 14, 20, 22, and 24 months (corresponding hazard rates of 0.0459, 0.0347, 0.0315, and 0.0289/month, respectively). For this Phase II design, we use one-sided $\alpha = 0.05$ and power = 80%. In order to achieve the most efficient design (i.e., minimum sample size), sample sizes from difference contrasts and various designs (balanced or unbalanced) are compared. Table 14.6 are the sample sizes for the balanced design. Table 14.7 provides sample sizes for unbalanced design with specific sample size ratios, i.e., (Control:control, lower dose:Control, higher dose:control, and Combined: control) = (1, 2, 2, 2). This type design are often seen

Table 14.6. Sample sizes for different contrasts (balance design)

Scenario	Contrast				Total n
Average dose effect	−3	1	1	1	666
Linear response trend	−6	1	2	3	603
Median time trend	−6	0	2	4	588
Hazard rate trend	10.65	−0.55	−3.75	−6.35	589

Note: Sample size ratios to the control group: 1, 1, 1, 1.

Table 14.7. Sample sizes for different contrasts (unbalance design)

Scenario	Contrast				Total n
Average dose effect	−3	1	1	1	1036
Linear dose response	−6	1	2	3	924
Median time shape	−6	0	2	4	865
Hazard rate shape	10.65	−0.55	−3.75	−6.35	882

Note: Sample size ratios to the control group: 1, 2 ,2, 2.

in clinical trial where patients are assigned to the test group more than the control group due to the fact that the investigators are usually more interested in the response in the test groups. However, this unbalanced design is usually not an efficient design. An optimal design, i.e., minimum variance design, where the number of patients assign to each group is proportional to the variance of the group, is studied (Table 14.8). It can be seen that from Table 14.8, the optimal design with sample size ratios (1, 0.711, 0.634, 0.574) are generally most powerful and requires fewer patients regardless the shape of the contrasts. In all cases, the contrasts with a trend in median time or the hazard rate works well. The contrasts with linear trend also works well in most cases under assumption of this particular trend of response (hazard rate). Therefore, the minimum variance design seems attractive with total sample sizes 525 subjects, i.e., 180, 128, 114, 103 for the active control, lower dose, higher dose, and combined therapy groups, respectively. In practice, if more patients assigned to the control group is an ethical concern and it is desirable to obtain more information on the test groups, a balanced design should be chosen with a total sample size 588 subjects or 147 subjects per group.

There are many other hypothesis-based dose–response studies. Shirley (1977) proposed a nonparametric William-type test; Chuang and Agresti (1997) reviewed tests for dose–response relationship with ordinal data; Gasprini and Eisele (2000)

Table 14.8. Sample sizes for different contrasts (minimum variance design)

Scenario	Contrast				Total n
Average dose effect	−3	1	1	1	548
Linear dose response	−6	1	2	3	513
Median time shape	−6	0	2	4	525
Hazard rate shape	10.65	−0.55	−3.75	−6.35	516

Note: Sample size ratios (proportional to the variances): 1, 0.711, 0.634, 0.574.

proposed a curve-free method for Phase I trial; Hothorn (2000) compared Cochran-Armitage trend test to multicontrast tests. Liu (1998) studied an order-directed score test for trend in ordered $2 \times K$ tables. Stewart and Ruberg (2000), and Hothorn (2000) proposed multiple contrast tests to increase the robustness of the test. Most of them did not provide close forms for the sample size calculations. However, Whitehead (1993) derived a sample size calculation method for ordered categorical data (Chang, 2004).

14.4 Phase I Oncology Dose Escalation Trial

For non-life-threatening diseases, since the expected toxicity is mild and can be controlled without harm, Phase I trials are usually conducted on healthy or normal volunteers. In life-threatening diseases such as cancer and AIDS, Phase I studies are conducted with limited number of patients due to (1) the aggressiveness and possible harmfulness of cytotoxic treatments, (2) possible systemic treatment effects, and (3) the high interest in the new drug's efficacy in those patients directly.

Drug toxicity is considered as tolerable if the toxicity is manageable and reversible. The standardization of the level of drug toxicity is the common toxicity criteria (CTC) by United States National Cancer Institute (NCI). Any adverse event (AE) related to treatment from the CTC category of Grade 3 and higher is often considered a dose limiting toxicity (DLT). The maximum tolerable dose (MTD) is defined as the maximum dose level with DLT rate occur no more than a predetermined value.

There are usually 5 to 10 predetermined dose levels in a dose escalation study. A commonly used dose sequence is the so-called modified Fibonacci sequence. Patients are treated with lowest dose first and then gradually escalated to higher doses if there is no major safety concern. The rules for dose escalation are predetermined. The commonly employed dose escalation rules are the traditional escalation rules (TER), which also known as the "3 + 3" rule. The "3 + 3" rule is to enter three patients at a new dose level and enter another 3 patients when DLT is observed. The assessment of the six patients will be performed to determine whether the trial should be stopped at that level or to increase the dose. Basically, there are two types of the "3 + 3" rules, namely, TER and strict TER (or STER). TER does not allow dose de-escalation as described in Chapter 4 of this book, but STER does when two of three patients have DLTs (see Figure 14.2). The "3 + 3" STER can be generalized to the A + B TER (see Chapter 4) and STER escalation rules. To introduce the A + B escalation rule, let A,B,C,D, and E be integers. The notation A/B indicates that there are A toxicity incidences out of B subjects and $>$A/B means that there are more than A toxicity incidences out of B subjects. We assume that there are K predefined doses with increasing levels and let p_i be the probability of observing a DLT at dose level i for $1 \leq i \leq K$. In what follows, the general A + B designs without and with dose de-escalation will be described. The closed forms of sample size calculation by Lin and Shih (2001) are briefly reviewed. Sample size estimations by computer simulations are also presented.

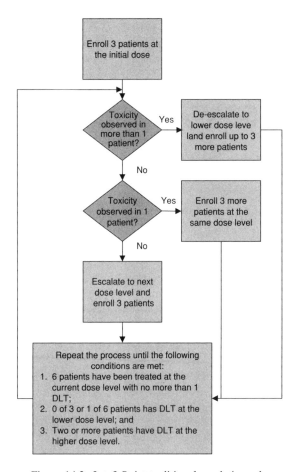

Figure 14.2. $3 + 3$ Strict traditional escalation rule

14.4.1   The A + B Escalation Without Dose De-Escalation

The general A + B designs without dose de-escalation can be described as follows. Suppose that there are A patients at dose level i. If less than C/A patients have DLTs, then the dose is escalated to the next dose level $i + 1$. If more than D/A (where $D \geq C$) patients have DLTs, then the previous dose $i - 1$ will be considered the MTD. If no less than C/A but no more than D/A patients have DLTs, B more patients are treated at this dose level i. If no more than E (where $E \geq D$) of the total of A + B patients have DLTs, then the dose is escalated. If more than E of the total of A + B patients have DLT, then the previous dose $i - 1$ will be considered the MTD. It can be seen that the traditional "3 + 3" design without dose de-escalation is a special case of the general A + B design with $A = B = 3$ and $C = D = E = 1$.

Under the general A + B design without de-escalation, the probability of concluding that MTD has reached at dose i is given by

$$P_i^* = P(\text{MTD} = \text{dose } i) = P\left(\begin{array}{c}\text{escalation at dose } \le i \text{ and} \\ \text{stop escalation at dose } i + 1\end{array}\right)$$

$$= (1 - P_0^{i+1} - Q_0^{i+1})\left(\prod_{j=1}^{i}\left(P_0^j + Q_0^j\right)\right), \quad 1 \le i < K \quad (14.20)$$

where

$$P_0^j = \sum_{k=0}^{C-1}\binom{A}{k}p_j^k(1 - p_j)^{A-k}$$

and

$$Q_0^j = \sum_{k=C}^{D}\sum_{m=0}^{E-k}\binom{A}{k}p_j^k(1 - p_j)^{A-k}\binom{B}{m}p_j^m(1 - p_j)^{B-m}$$

An overshoot is defined as an attempt to escalate to a dose level at the highest level planned, while a undershoot is referred to as an attempt to de-escalate to a dose level at a lower dose than the starting dose level. Thus, the probability of undershoot is given by

$$P_1^* = P(\text{MTD} < \text{dose } 1) = \left(1 - P_0^1 - Q_0^1\right) \quad (14.21)$$

and probability of overshoot is given by

$$P_n^* = P(\text{MTD} \ge \text{dose } K) = \Pi_{j=1}^{K}\left(P_0^j + Q_0^j\right) \quad (14.22)$$

The expected number of patients at dose level j is given by

$$N_j = \sum_{i=0}^{K-1}N_{ji}P_i^* \quad (14.23)$$

where

$$N_{ji} = \begin{cases} \dfrac{AP_0^j + (A + B)Q_0^j}{P_0^j + Q_0^j} & \text{if } j < i + 1 \\[3mm] \dfrac{A\left(1 - P_0^j - P_1^j\right) + (A + B)\left(P_1^j - Q_0^j\right)}{1 - P_0^j - Q_0^j} & \text{if } j = i + 1 \\[3mm] 0 & \text{if } j > i + 1 \end{cases}$$

Note that without consideration of undershoots and overshoots, the expected number of DLTs at dose i can be obtained as $N_i p_i$. As a result, the total expected number DLTs for the trial is given by $\sum_{i=1}^{K}N_i p_i$.

We can use Eq. (14.23) to calculate the expected sample size for given toxicity rate at each dose level. Alternatively, we can also use trial simulation software such as ExpDesign Studio by CTriSoft International to simulate the trial and sample size required (Ctrisoft, 2002). Table 14.9 is an example from ExpDesign Studio. ExpDesign Studio uses an algorithm-based approach instead of using analytical

Table 14.9. Simulation results with 3 + 3 TER

Dose level	1	2	3	4	5	6	7	Total
Dose	10	15	23	34	51	76	114	
DLT rate	0.01	0.014	0.025	0.056	0.177	0.594	0.963	
Expected n	3.1	3.2	3.2	3.4	3.9	2.8	0.2	19.7
Prob. of MTD	.001	.002	.007	.033	.234	.658	.065	

Note: True MTD = 50, mean simulated MTD + 70, mean number of DLTs = 2.9.
Probability of MTD = Percent recommendations of dose as MTD.

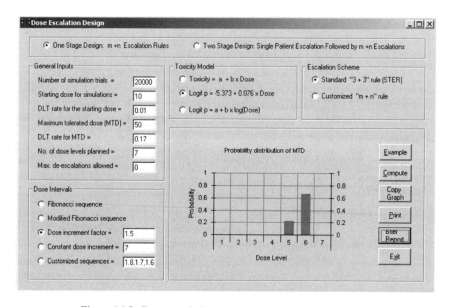

Figure 14.3. Dose-escalation simulations in ExpDesign studio

solution Eq. (14.23), one can do two stage design and Bayesian adaptive and other advanced design with the software.

14.4.2   The A + B Escalation with Dose De-escalation

Basically, the general A + B design with dose de-escalation is similar to the design without dose de-escalation. However, it permits more patients to be treated at a lower dose (i.e., dose de-escalation) when excessive DLT incidences occur at the current dose level. The dose de-escalation occurs when more than D/A (where $D \geq C$) or more than E/(A + B) patients have DLTs at dose level i. In this case, B more patients will be treated at dose level $i - 1$ provided that only A patients have been previously treated at this prior dose. If more than A patients have already been treated previously, then dose $i - 1$ is the MTD. The de-escalation may continue to the next dose level $i - 2$ and so on if necessary.

Similarly, under the general A + B design with dose de-escalation, the probability of concluding that MTD has been reached at dose i is given by

$$P_i^* = P(\text{MTD} = \text{dose } i) = P \left(\begin{array}{c} \text{escalation at dose } \leq i \text{ and} \\ \text{stop escalation at dose } i + 1 \end{array} \right)$$

$$= \sum_{k=i+1}^{K} p_{ik}$$

where

$$p_{ik} = \left(Q_0^i + Q_1^i \right) \left(1 - P_0^k - Q_0^k \right) \left(\prod_{j=1}^{i-1} \left(P_0^j + Q_0^j \right) \right) \prod_{j=i+1}^{k-1} Q_2^j$$

$$Q_1^j = \sum_{k=0}^{C-1} \sum_{m=0}^{E-k} \binom{A}{k} p_j^k (1 - p_j)^{A-k} \binom{B}{m} p_j^m (1 - p_j)^{B-m}$$

and

$$Q_2^j = \sum_{k=0}^{C-1} \sum_{m=E+1-k}^{B} \binom{A}{k} p_j^k (1 - p_j)^{A-k} \binom{B}{m} p_j^m (1 - p_j)^{B-m}$$

Also, the probability of undershoot is given by

$$P_1^* = P(\text{MTD} < \text{dose } 1) = \sum_{k=1}^{K} \left\{ \left(\Pi_{j=1}^{k-1} Q_2^j \right) \left(1 - P_0^k - Q_0^k \right) \right\}$$

and the probability of overshooting is

$$P_K^* = P(\text{MTD} \geq \text{dose } K) = \Pi_{j=1}^{K} \left(P_0^j + Q_0^j \right)$$

The expected number of patients at dose level j is given by

$$N_j = N_{jK} P_K^* + \sum_{i=0}^{K-1} \sum_{k=i+1}^{K} N_{jik} p_{ik}$$

where

$$N_{jn} = \frac{A P_0^j + (A + B) Q_0^j}{P_0^j + Q_0^j}$$

$$N_{jik} = \begin{cases} \dfrac{A P_0^j + (A + B) Q_0^j}{P_0^j + Q_0^j} & \text{if } j < i \\[2ex] A + B & \text{if } i \leq j < k \\[2ex] \dfrac{A \left(1 - P_0^j - P_1^j \right) + (A + B) \left(P_1^j - Q_0^j \right)}{1 - P_0^j - Q_0^j} & \text{if } j = k \\[2ex] 0 & \text{if } j > k \end{cases}$$

Table 14.10. Simulation results with 3+3 STER

Dose level	1	2	3	4	5	6	7	Total
Dose	10	15	23	34	51	76	114	
DLT rate	0.01	0.014	0.025	0.056	0.177	0.594	0.963	
Expected n	3.1	3.2	3.5	4.6	5.5	3	0.2	23
Probability of MTD	0.004	0.013	0.091	0.394	0.481	0.016	0	

Note: True MTD = 50, mean simulated MTD = 41. Mean number of DLTs = 3.3
Prob. of MTD = Percent recommendations of dose as MTD.

and

$$P_1^j = \sum_{i=C}^{D} \binom{A}{k} p_j^k (1 - p_j)^{A-k}$$

Consequently, the total number of expected DLTs is given by $\sum_{i=1}^{K} N_i p_i$,

Table 14.10 is another example as in Table 14.9, but the simulation results are from STER rather than TER. In this example, we can see that the MTD is underestimated and the average sample size is 23 with STER, and three patients more than that with TER. The excepted DLTs also increase with STER in this case. Note that the actual sample size varies from trial to trial. However, simulations will help in choosing the best escalation algorithm or optimal design based on the operating characteristics, such as accuracy and precision of the predicted MTD, expected DLTs and sample size, overshoots, undershoots, and the number of patients treated above MTD.

There are many other dose-escalation designs, see Chapters 4 and 5 of this book and also Crowley (2001).

14.5 Concluding Remarks

We have discussed the sample size calculations for the first three questions in dose–response studies as stated in the beginning of the chapter, i.e., (1) Is there any evidence of the drug effect? (2) What doses exhibit a response different from the control response? (3) What is the nature of the dose-response? The sample size formulations for one and two sample problems (Table 14.1) can be used for the trials that try to answer the first question. Two group design is popular in Phase I and II trials. Single arm design is often used in Phase I and II oncology studies.

Williams' test for minimum effective dose is used to answer the second question in the case of normal response. The test has a strong assumption of monotonic dose response. If the assumption is not realistic, the test is invalid. William' test is not a test for monotonicity. The sample size Eq. (14.7) for Williams' test is very conservative.

Nam's and Cochran-Armitage's methods are equivalent and can be used to answer the third questions when the response is binary. Both methods are regression based methods for testing for a monotonic "trend". However, they are not rigorous tests for monotonicity. Test for true monotonic response is practically difficult without extra assumptions. One possible way to test for monotonic response in a study with $k + 1$ dose levels is to form the following k hypotheses and test them simultaneously:

$$\begin{cases} H_{01}: p_1 \leq p_0 \text{ vs. } H_{a1}: p_1 > p_0 \\ H_{02}: p_2 \leq p_1 \text{ vs. } H_{a2}: p_2 > p_1 \\ \cdots\cdots \\ H_{0k}: p_k \leq p_{k-1} \text{ vs. } H_{ak}: p_k > p_{k-1} \end{cases}$$

However, even when all the null hypotheses are simultaneously rejected, we can only conclude that the monotonicity hold for these prespecified dose levels and we still do not know the response behaviors for doses between the prespecified dose levels.

Contrast tests are very general and can be used to answer all three questions. Two sample tests in Table 14.1 can be reviewed as the special cases of contrast tests where the contrasts $\{c_0, c_1\} = \{-1, 1\}$. The linear trend test (Nam's or Cochran-Armitage's) and contrast test were derived from two different approaches, but the former is a special case of the contrast test. In fact, Nam's test is a contrast test where the contrasts $c_i = d_i - \bar{d}$. In other words, d_i in Nam's test can be dose scores instead of actual dose. The contrast test has been applied to multiple arm (include two arms) trials with three different endpoints (normal, binary, survival) in a very same way in this chapter. The authors have not found sample size formulas for one-sample and multiple (>2) sample survival problems using contrast tests elsewhere in literatures. They are newly proposed.

To use a contrast test, the selection of contrasts should be practically meaningful. If one is interested in a treatment difference among any groups, then any contrasts can be applied. If one is only interested the comparison between Dose level 1 and other dose levels, then one should make the contrast for Dose level 1 have a different sign than that of the contrasts for other dose groups. To test a linear/monotonic "trend", linear/monotonic contrasts should be used, i.e., $(c_0 \leq c_1 \leq \ldots \leq c_k)$ for the corresponding dose $(d_0 \leq d_1 \leq \ldots \leq d_k)$.

Since the power of a contrast test is sensitive to the actual dose response shape, in the case of little knowledge of dose–response nature, multiple contrast tests can be used (Bretz and Hothorn, 2002). Alternatively, we can use a contrast set where each contrast has approximately equal weight (ignoring the sign).

Oncology Phase I dose escalation trial is somewhat unique. The expected sample size is not determined by the error rates (α, β). Instead, it is determined by the escalation algorithm and dose-response (toxicity) relationship and predetermined dose levels. For A + B escalation rules, the sample size has closed form as presented in Section 4. For other designs, sample size can be estimated through computer simulations. Note that the escalation algorithm and dose intervals not only affect the sample size, but also other important operating characteristics such as accuracy and precision in MTD estimation, and the number of DLTS (see also, Chapter 4 of this book). Therefore, selection of an optimal design for an oncology study, just like for other studies, should not be purely based on the (expected) sample size.

References

Armitage, P., 1955. Tests for linear trends in proportions and frequencies. *Biometrics* Sept., 375–386.

Bretz, F., and Hothorn, L.A. 2002. Detecting dose-response using contrasts: Asymptotic power and sample size determination for binary data. *Statistics in Medicine* 21:3325–3335.

Chang, M. 2004. Power and Sample Size Calculations for Dose Response Studies, Dose-Response Trial Design Workshop, November 15, 2004, Philadelphia, PA.

Cochran, W.G. 1954. Some methods for strengthening the common χ^2 tests. *Biometrics* 10:417–451.

Chow, S.C., and Liu, J.P. 2003. *Design and Analysis of Clinical Trials,* 2nd ed. New York: Wiley.

Chow, S.C., Shao, J., and Wang, H. 2003. *Sample Size Calculation in Clinical Research.* New York: Marcel Dekker.

Chuang-Stein, C., and Agresti A. 1997. A review of tests for detecting a monotone dose-response relationship with ordinal response data. *Statistics in Medicine* 16:2599–2618.

Crowley, J. 2001. *Handbook of Statistics in Clinical Oncology,* New York: Marcel Dekker.

CTriSoft Intl. 2002. *Clinical Trial Design with ExpDesign Studio,* www.ctrisoft.net., Lexington, MA, USA: CTriSoft Intl.

Gasprini, M., and Eisele, J. 2000. A curve-free method for Phase I clinical trials. *Biometrics* 56:609–615.

Hothorn, L. A. 2000. Evaluation of animal carcinogenicity studies: Cochran-Armitage trend test vs. multiple contrast tests. *Biometrical Journal* 42:553–567.

Lachin, J.M., and Foukes, M.A. 1986. Evaluation of sample size and power for analysis of survival with allowance for nonuniform patient entry, losses to follow0up, noncompliance, and stratification. *Biometrics* 42:507–519.

Liu, Q. 1998. An order-directed score test for trend in ordered $2 \times K$ Tables. *Biometrics* 54:1147–1154.

Lin, Y., and Shih W. J. 2001. Statistical properties of the traditional algorithm-based designs for Phase I cancer clinical trials. *Biostatistics* 2:203–215.

Nam, J. 1987. A simple approximation for calculating sample sizes for detecting linear tend in proportions. *Biometrics* 43:701–705.

Neuhauser, M., and Hothorn, L. 1999. An exact Cochran-Armitage test for trend when dose-response shapes are a priori unknown. *Computational Statistics and Data Analysis* 30:403–412.

O'Quigley, J., Pepe, M., and Fisher, L. 1990. Continual reassessment method: A practical design for Phase I clinical trial in cancer. *Biometrics* 46:33–48.

O'Quigley, J., and Shen, L. 1996. Continual reassessment method: A likelihood approach. *Biometrics* 52:673–684.

Podgor, M.J., Gastwirth, J.L., and Mehta, C.R. 1996. Efficiency robust tests of independence in contingency tables with ordered classifications. *Statistics in Medicine* 15:2095–2105.

Portier, C., Hoel, D. 1984. Type I error of trend tets in proportions and design of cancer screens. *Communication in Statistics* 13:1–14.

Gastwirth, J.L. 1985. The use of maximum efficiency robust tests in combining contingency tables and survival analysis. *Jouranal of the American Statistical Association* 80:380–384.

Rosenberger, W., and Lachin, J. 2003. *Randomization in Clinical Trials*, New York: Wiley.

Ruberg, S.J. 1995a. Dose response studies: I. Some design considerations. *Journal of Biopharmaceutical Statistics* 5:1–14.

Ruberg, S.J. 1995b. Dose response studies: II. Analysis and interpretation. *Journal of Biopharmaceutical Statistics* 5:1–14.

Shirley, E. 1977. A non-parametric equivalent of William' test for contrasting increasing dose levels of treatment. *Biometrics* 33:386–389.

Stewart, W., and Ruberg, S. J. 2000. Detecting dose response with contrasts. *Statistics in Medicine* 19:913–921.

Whitehead, J 1993. Sample size calculation for ordered categorical data. *Statistics in Medicine* 12:2257–2271.

Whitehead, J. 1997. Bayesian decision procedures with application to dose-finding studies. *International Journal of Pharmaceutical Medicine* 11:201–208.

Williams, D.A. 1971. A test for difference between treatment means when several dose levels are compared with a zero dose control. *Biometrics* 27:103–117.

Williams, D.A. 1972. Comparison of several dose levels with a zero dose control. *Biometrics* 28:519–531.

Index

a priori, 63, 66, 68, 69, 70, 78, 103, 124, 146, 176, 180
A + B design, 52, 53
absorption, 7, 34, 37, 75, 82, 99
absorption, distribution, metabolism, excretion (ADME), 37
accumulation, 11, 42, 43, 100
action, 3, 9, 32–36, 40, 43, 45, 66, 74–82, 106
active control, 90–95, 231, 232
adaptive, 59
adenocarcinomas of gastrointestinal origin, 66
adjacent-categories logit model, 203
adverse (drug) effects, 1, 6, 8
adverse event (AE), 7, 33
agonist, 20
Akaike information criterion (AIC), 157
allocation of sample size, 113
alternative hypothesis, 181, 204, 206, 221, 224–227
analysis of covariance (ANCOVA), 11, 109
angle transformations, 23
antagonist, 20
antibodies, 36
anti-infective drugs, 25
anti-SEA antibodies, 66
anti-tumor activity, 59
area under the curve (AUC), 8, 9
ascending dose studies, 32
association measure, 204–205
asymmetric loss function, 62
asymptotically, 154, 186, 192, 228, 229
average bias, 70
average dose response, 35

balanced design, 181, 225, 231, 232
basal/baseline effect (E0), 127, 150–152
Bayesian approaches, 60
Bayesian C- and D-optimal designs, 60
Bayesian decision theory, 223
Bayesian feasible, 62
Bayesian information criterion (BIC), 157
benefit-risk assessment, 30
beta-agonist, 21
binary dose spacing (BDS), 102
binary outcomes, 184, 186, 188, 190, 192, 194, 196, 198
binding, 20
bioassay, 6
bioavailability, 8, 9, 10, 12, 40, 75, 76
bioequivalence, 8, 9
biologic, 4, 5, 7, 8, 18, 25, 26, 28, 33, 38, 213
biomarkers, 41
bivariate isotonic regression, 55
blood pressure, 1, 10, 11, 20, 33, 36, 41, 44, 80, 92, 139, 140, 145, 200
body surface, 28
body surface area (BSA), 28, 37
Bonferroni method, 193
Bonferroni procedure, 211
Bonferroni–Holm procedure, 211
bootstrap, 154

cancer chemotherapy, 28
cancer phase I clinical, 59, 65, 70
candidate dose-response models, 6, 89
candidate set, 158
carcinogenicity study, 6
carryover effects, 35, 80
categorical data, 11, 95, 198, 200, 201, 210, 216, 233
central limit theory, 186, 192, 231
clearance, 34, 43, 76, 135, 136, 144
clinical development, 4, 13, 14, 30, 89, 92, 94, 101–104, 106, 108

clinical development plan (CDP), 8, 13, 89, 104
clinical endpoint, 89, 91, 92
clinical non-inferiority, 106
clinical similarity, 108–110
clinical trial objectives, 107, 109
clinical trial simulation (CTS), 85, 104, 108, 111
clinically relevant effect, 146
closed testing procedure, 210
closure principle, 174
C_{max}, 8
C_{min}, 9
Cocharan-Armitage Trend test, 209, 219, 221
common toxicity criteria, 63
competitive binding, 21, 23
compliance, 34, 42
concentration controlled clinical trial, 41
confidence interval (CI), 96, 118, 147, 154, 155, 182
continual reassessment method (CRM), 50, 60
continuation-ratio logit model, 203
continuity correction, 228, 229
continuous covariate, 71
contrast, 10, 146
contrast test, 161
covariate utilization, 60
covariates, 63
critical path, 104
crossover design, 35, 93
cross-validation, 159
CTC (*see* common toxicity criteria)
cumulative distribution function, 61
cumulative effect, 80
cumulative odds, 202, 203
cytochlor, 60
cytotoxic agent, 59
cytotoxic drugs, 28
cytotoxic treatments, 233

data models, 108, 111–113, 116–121
decision-theoretic approach, 60
delayed effect, 77–80
design recommendations, 120–124
dichotomous endpoint, 208
disease progress, 73, 75, 83
distribution, 7, 11, 34–37, 43, 50, 61–63, 66–70, 75–80, 100, 103, 114, 115, 145, 155, 159, 161, 162, 175, 176, 180, 185–189, 193–196, 202, 205, 207, 211, 214, 215, 221, 226, 231
D-optimality criterion, 132
dosage regimen, 30
dose allocation, 97, 100, 102
dose escalation, 34, 41–43, 47, 60, 63, 69, 71, 221, 233, 239

dose frequency, 13, 97, 98
dose limiting toxicity (DLT), 49, 59, 67, 70, 233
dose range, 1, 8, 13, 46, 94, 97, 100–115, 119–124, 127, 131, 132, 136, 137, 147, 153, 154, 163, 165, 167
dose regimen, 12, 99
dose response relationship (DRR), 107, 198, 202, 207, 209
dose response (DR), 18
dose selection, 6, 7, 9, 11, 16, 38, 89, 90, 103, 104, 148, 154, 161–163, 166, 167
dose spacing, 97, 102, 104, 113, 114, 120–124
dose spacing pattern, 113
dose titration, 89, 97, 99, 100
dose-dependent and time-dependent changes pharmacokinetics, 41, 43
dose-finding, 30, 32, 34, 36, 38, 40, 42, 44, 46, 48, 49, 50, 52, 54, 55, 56, 155, 162
dose-limiting toxicities, 33, 34, 42, 71
dose-response, 31
dose–toxicity relationship, 49
double-blind, 4, 33, 34, 90, 93, 147, 177
drug label, 12, 13, 14, 16
Dunnett's method, 192

EC_{50}, 77
ED_{50}, 103
ED_{90}, 129
effect, 1, 3, 7, 10, 11, 19–47, 66, 67, 74–86, 90, 96, 100–103, 107, 108, 119, 127–179, 192, 202, 203, 207–215, 220, 221, 224, 227, 231, 232, 238
effectiveness, 15, 32, 73, 93, 94, 146, 195, 220
efficacy, 2–5, 8, 10, 11, 13, 15, 27, 30, 31, 32, 34, 41, 44–46, 59, 77, 79, 90–125, 147, 155, 172, 173, 175, 178, 181, 185, 188, 189, 210, 213, 215, 220, 223, 224, 233
elimination, 43, 75, 76, 80, 82
E_{max} model, 77
equal spaced doses, 228
equally spaced scores, 204
equilibration half-life, 79
escalation algorithm, 238, 239
escalation design, 52, 53
escalation with overdose control (EWOC), 50, 60
estimation of the MTD, 54
EWOC algorithm, 63
ExpDesign Studio, 235
expected sample size, 235, 239
experiment-wise error, 92
exponential model, 151

exposure response, 46, 73, 74
extrapolating dose from animal to
    human, 28

1-factor structure, 194
family-wise error rate (FWE), 159, 174
family-wise experimental error (FWER), 146
feasibility bound, 60
FEV1, 225
Fibonacci sequence, 41, 49
first-order kinetics, 21
first-time in human studies (FIH), 31, 32
fixed dose, 13, 66, 90, 97, 100
formulation, 4, 7, 10, 36, 75, 98, 99, 151, 175,
    189, 227
four-parameter logistic model, 134, 142, 143
Freeman-Tukey transformation, 213
Furosemide, 81

Gaddum, John, 20, 21
gate-keeping procedure, 212
gavage, 26
Glasgow Outcome Scale (GOS), 201
goodness-of-fit, 158
grade III non-hematological toxicity, 49
gross tissue response, 21
group up-and-down design, 54
guinea pig trachea, 21

half-life, 42, 75, 76, 79, 80, 97, 98, 99
hazard rate, 222, 230, 231, 232
hematological grade IV toxicity, 63
heterogeneity, 59
Hill factor, 127, 131
historical control, 93
Hochberg's step-up procedure, 194, 212
Holm's procedure, 194
homogeneous, 221, 224, 225
homoscedasticity, 181
human equivalent dose (HED), 37
hyperbolic E_{max}, 128, 132, 136, 137
hyperparameters, 69

in vitro, 4
in vivo, 4
inclusion and exclusion criteria, 35
independent priors, 69
individual dose response, 73
information criterion, 157
initial parameter values, 138
Institute Review Board, 60
International Conference on Harmonization
    (ICH), 16

investigational drug exemption, 26
investigational new drug (IND), 5, 48, 220
isotonic regression, 54, 158, 181, 209
iterations, 137, 139

Jonckheere–Terpstra statistics, 206, 207

kinetic constants, 23

large sample, 185, 186, 189, 190– 197, 211, 223
law of mass action, 77
least squares, 20
lethal dose in 10% (LD_{10}), 39, 41, 49
life-threatening diseases, 12
Likert scale, 213
linear contrast, 161, 223, 227
linear in log-dose model, 151
linear model, 161
linear regression, 103, 113, 117, 118, 144, 150,
    155, 228
logistic, 61, 69, 94, 103, 117, 118, 134, 142,
    143, 146, 152, 153, 162–168, 218, 219, 228
logistic distribution, 61
logistic models, 203, 214
logistic regression, 103, 118
loss function, 62

malaria, 135, 136, 144
marginal posterior CDF, 62
Marquardt, 137
maximally tolerated dose (MTD), 1, 32–34,
    38–43, 46, 49–55, 59–71, 89, 90, 92, 97, 101,
    102, 107–117, 121, 122, 124, 220, 233–239
maximum effect (E_{max}), 46, 77, 78, 94, 118,
    127–168
maximum effective dose (MaxED), 1
maximum likelihood, 55, 158, 202, 203, 209,
    226, 230
maximum recommended starting dose (MRSD),
    37
maximum safe dose (MaxSD), 172
MCMC sampler, 70
MCP-Mod, 160
mean, 25, 38, 70, 71, 114, 115, 118, 127, 139,
    140, 147, 149, 155, 158, 163, 172, 173, 178,
    181, 192, 196, 200, 205, 206, 209, 210, 218,
    222, 223, 224, 226, 230, 236, 238
mean inhibitory concentration (MIC), 25
mean response model, 206, 209, 218
median, 24, 167, 230, 231, 232
meta-analysis, 104
metabolites, 34, 43
midranks, 205, 206

minimal clinically important difference (MCID), 109
minimal difference, 226
minimally clinically important difference, 95, 102
minimum effect, 20, 172
minimum effective dose (MinED or MED), 2, 95, 146, 153, 172, 181, 212, 220, 221, 226, 238
minimum sample size, 225, 227, 231
minimum variance design, 232
Mithracin, 28
mixed effects E_{max} model, 134
MLE, 231
model selection, 149
model uncertainty, 156, 157, 159
model-based analysis, 100, 104
model-based modeling, 85
modeling, 10
modeling approach, 94, 147, 148, 149, 201, 203, 207, 211, 214
modified Gauss-Newton, 149
modified three-point assay, 18
monotone likelihood ratio, 187
monotonic, 1, 61, 96, 119, 125, 129, 152, 198, 221, 223, 228, 238, 239
monotonic increasing, 61
monotonicity, 56, 147, 173, 174, 175, 177, 203, 204, 226, 228, 238, 239
monotonicity assumption, 173, 174
MSE, 70
MTD uncertainty, 49, 59
multicontrast tests, 233
multinomial distribution, 202, 205, 206
multiple agents, design for, 56
multiple center, 96
multiple comparisons, 94, 210, 211
multiple comparison procedures (MCP), 94, 146
multiple contrast test, 230, 233, 239
multiple dose study, 43
multiple endpoints, 92, 208
multiplicity, 119
multivariate secant method, 137

National Cancer Institute of Canada (NCIC), 63
negative a priori correlation, 68
negative control, 19
new drug application (NDA), 5
new indication, 16
Newton method, 137
no observed adverse effect levels (NOAEL), 37
no observed adverse event level, 7

no observed effect level (NOEL), 27, 38
non-clinical development, 4, 5, 7, 89
non-clinical or preclinical development, 5
non-life-threatening diseases, 92, 233
nonlinear least squares, 149
nonlinear model, 127
NONMEM, 85, 135
non-parametric, 6, 11, 50, 55, 56, 71, 154, 162, 223
non-parametric designs, 50, 55, 56
non-parametric methods, 49–56
nonpeptidomimetic inhibitor of farnesyltransferase (FTase), 62
normal approximation, 185
null hypothesis, 92, 185–189, 202–207, 210, 212, 221, 224–229
numerical integration, 62

oncology, 12, 36, 39, 49, 50, 52, 56, 220, 231, 238, 239
optimal design, 103, 225, 232, 238, 239
oral artesunate, 135
order restricted information criterion (ORIC), 158
ordered groups, design for, 55
ordinal data, 205, 210, 214, 232
ordinal response, 201, 203, 208, 209, 211, 214
outcomes research, 15
overdosing, 59

pA2, 25
Paracelsus, 26
parallel design, 93
parameterization, 76
parametric, 11
partitioning principle, 174
partitioning tests, 184, 186, 188, 190, 192, 194, 196, 198
pathology, 27
patient reported outcome (PRO), 15
patient-specific characteristics, 60
pAx, 24
pharmacodynamics (PD), 8, 48, 73, 74, 75, 84, 92
pharmacoeconomics, 15
pharmacogenetics, 33
pharmacokinetics (PK), 8, 12, 25, 31, 48, 73, 74, 77, 84, 89, 92, 220
pharmacologically active dose (PAD), 37, 38, 40
pharmacology, 4, 6, 12, 20, 22, 27, 30, 32, 38, 40–42, 73, 78, 86, 107
Phase II study, 7, 10, 14, 32, 46, 89, 92, 103, 141, 184

Phase II, 7–11, 14–16, 32, 41, 46, 47, 59, 65, 67, 89–108, 141, 148, 155, 172, 177, 184, 215, 220, 224, 225, 231
phases of drug development, 31
placebo control, 93, 102, 184
PNU, 66
pooled standard deviation, 224
population dose–response, 97
positive control, 19
posterior expected loss, 62
posterior mode, 63
post-marketing, 5
post-translational modification, 62
potency, 3, 6, 19, 20, 23, 24, 25, 107, 109, 111, 112, 114
potential drug, 7
power, 11, 28, 92, 94, 96, 120, 121, 125, 160, 164, 165, 181, 190, 209, 214– 216, 220–231, 239
power model, 151
pre-clinical development, 5
pre-clinical toxicology, 26, 27
pre-determined step-down procedure, 189, 213
primary endpoint, 73, 92, 200, 231
probits, 23
Proc NLIN, 135
Proc NLMIXED, 135
proof-of-activity (PoA), 146
proof-of-concept (PoC), 89, 107, 146, 210
proportion, 10, 22, 33, 59, 60, 61, 65, 67, 70, 71, 77, 222, 223, 227, 230
proportional odds model, 202, 211, 218
protocol, 34, 37, 43, 91, 92, 108, 117, 149

quadratic model, 152
quality of life, 15

radio-immune assays, 25
rat foot edema assay, 18
rate of input, 75
receptor, 18
reference agent, 106, 107, 108, 109, 112, 113, 117
regression coefficients, 115, 206
relative potency (RP), 19, 20, 24, 25, 107, 109, 111, 112, 114
reproductive studies, 6
Research Review Committee, 60
residual sum of squares, 137, 149
responder analysis, 208

response, 1–239
risk minimization, 32

safety, 1–43, 60, 90, 92, 100–107, 114, 133, 147, 155, 177–181, 213, 220, 223, 233
safety evaluation, 26
safety factor, 37, 39, 40
sample size, 10, 11, 33, 50–56, 95–97, 107–113, 121–125, 157, 163, 165, 167, 194, 195, 201, 207, 214–216, 220, 221–235, 238, 239, 240
sample size ratio, 229, 231, 232
sample-determined step-down procedure, 190
SAS, 85
schedule dependence, 81, 82
scores, 178, 204–218, 228, 239
sensitivity, 5, 39, 45, 79, 93, 127, 129
sensitization, 35, 48
sequence of doses, 59
serial dilution, 25
sigmoid, 23
Simes' test, 194
simulation, 53
simulation project objectives, 108, 109, 111, 113, 115, 117, 119
single dose study, 33
size fraction, 224
slope factor, 127, 128, 129, 131, 132, 135, 136, 139, 141, 144, 145
small sample exact tests, 185, 196
specificity, 5
S-Plus, 85
standard deviation, 28, 95, 139, 140, 163, 164, 178, 179, 225
standard or 3+3 design, 53
standardized model, 150
starting dose, 37, 38, 39, 41, 48, 49, 53, 61, 63, 99, 235
starting dose level, 235
starting/initial parameter estimates, 149, 151, 156, 161
starting/initial parameter value, 138, 139
statistical analysis plan, 92, 109
statistical significance, 154
steady state, 43, 76, 80
steepest-descent, 137
step-down procedure, 172, 176, 181, 189–197, 213
STER, 233
stimulus–response, 77
stochastic ordering, 204, 206
stopping rule, 34, 35, 42, 52, 56
subchronic toxicity study, 26

subset pivotality, 192
survival, 11

target dose, 11, 101, 119, 121, 122, 147, 153,
    158, 165, 167, 169, 184
target patient population, 12, 36, 59, 64
target value (TV), 107, 110, 116, 124
TER, 233
test statistic, 180, 186, 192–197, 205–207, 221,
    223, 226, 228, 229
therapeutic index (TI), 3, 108
therapeutic window, 3, 32, 43, 181, 223
thiopental, 79
three-point assay, 18
threshold, 172, 173, 175, 177, 182, 200, 221
time-to-event, 230
time-to-progression, 231
T_{max}, 8
tolerability, 32– 36, 42, 106–123
tolerance, 32, 35
totally positive of order two (MTP_2), 194
toxicity, 2
toxicology, 4, 7, 12, 25–28, 30, 36–43,
    179
traditional or 3+3 design, 50, 52, 233, 234
trend test, 181, 209, 219, 221, 233, 239

tumor progression, 63
turnover, 78, 79, 80, 82
type-I error, 221

umbrella alternative, 214
umbrella-shape, 152
unbiased estimate, 226
unbiased estimator, 223
unbound receptors, 22
union-intersection (UI) method, 175
unit of experimentation, 27
up-and-down design, 50, 51, 52, 54

vague and informative priors, 61
variance, 11, 109, 113–118, 127, 145, 147, 157,
    172, 179, 186, 192, 196, 205, 206, 222, 224,
    230, 232
volume of distribution, 4, 43, 76

warfarin, 80
washout period, 35, 93
Wilcoxon-Mann-Whitney statistics, 211
Williams' test, 220, 221, 227, 238
WinBugs, 85

zero-dose effect, 128

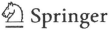

Springer

the language of science

springeronline.com

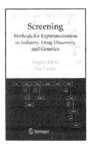

Screening

A. Dean and S. Lewis (Editors)

This book brings together accounts by leading international experts that are essential reading for those working in fields such as industrial quality improvement, engineering research and development, genetic and medical screening, drug discovery, and computer simulation of manufacturing systems or economic models. The aim is to promote cross-fertilization of ideas and methods through detailed explanations, a variety of examples and extensive references.

2005. 384 p. Hardcover ISBN 0-387-28013-8

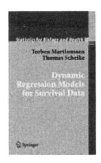

Dynamic Regression Models for Survival Data

T. Martinussen and T. Scheike

This book studies and applies modern flexible regression models for survival data with a special focus on extensions of the Cox model and alternative models with the specific aim of describing time-varying effects of explanatory variables. The book covers the use of residuals and resampling techniques to assess the fit of the models and also points out how the suggested models can be utilised for clustered survival data. The authors demonstrate the practically important aspect of how to do hypothesis testing of time-varying effects making backwards model selection strategies possible for the flexible models considered.

2005. 472 p. (Statistics for Biology and Health) Hardcover ISBN 0-387-20274-9

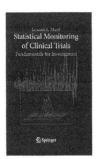

Statistical Monitoring of Clinical Trials

L. Moyé

Statistical Monitoring of Clinical Trials: Fundamentals for Investigators introduces the investigator and statistician to monitoring procedures in clinical research. Clearly presenting the necessary background with limited use of mathematics, this book increases the knowledge, experience, and intuition of investigations in the use of these important procedures now required by the many clinical research efforts.

2005. 280 p. Softcover ISBN 0-387-27781-1

Easy Ways to Order ▶ Call: Toll-Free 1-800-SPRINGER • E-mail: orders-ny@springer.sbm.com • Write: Springer, Dept. S8113, PO Box 2485, Secaucus, NJ 07096-2485 • Visit: Your local scientific bookstore or urge your librarian to order.